Consulting Hematology and Oncology Handbook

Gustavo Rivero • Iberia Romina Sosa
Editors

Consulting Hematology and Oncology Handbook

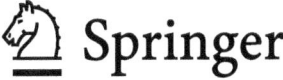 Springer

Editors
Gustavo Rivero
Lombardi Cancer Institute, Georgetown
University School of Medicine
Washington, DC, USA

Iberia Romina Sosa
Department of Hematology/Oncology
Fox Chase Cancer Center
Philadelphia, PA, USA

ISBN 978-3-031-75809-6   ISBN 978-3-031-75810-2   (eBook)
https://doi.org/10.1007/978-3-031-75810-2

This Springer imprint is published by the registered company Springer Nature Switzerland AG
The registered company address is: Gewerbestrasse 11, 6330 Cham, Switzerland

If disposing of this product, please recycle the paper.

Preface

Our medical students, residents, and fellows encounter complex challenges during their rotations on the hematology service. Most of these complexities relate to face-paced molecular discoveries, which have profoundly restructured our patient's therapeutic landscape. Our *Consulting Hematology Handbook* was designed to allow quick disease biology reference, emphasizing personalized molecular therapies when indicated. It is likely that our first edition's work represents unprecedented faculty effort to "bring case complexity into practical knowledge." As a hematology tenured faculty, I enjoyed building our teaching and enduring material portfolio for our Norton Fulbright Award at Baylor College of Medicine, Houston, Texas. To achieve the award, 13 years of experiences and feedback gathered from interactions with learners were incorporated in our handbook. These educational and didactic interactions between our authors and trainees were most recently expanded at Georgetown University School of Medicine in Washington D.C. to illustrate a comprehensive, fast, and up-to-date enduring product. Repeatedly, we were asked by students, residents, and fellows to simplify, albeit maintaining high educational standards, molecular workup for leukemia, lymphomas, and myelomas. Soon after, we realized that their feedback should span challenging benign hematology cases. While we truly appreciate Dr. Sosa's academic contribution to develop benign hematology chapters, we would also like to extend our appreciation to her fellows and medical students at Fox Chase Cancer Center in Philadelphia. Readers will enjoy a handbook that integrates disease complexity into successful consultation and patient outcome. Finally, all the handbook's authors were convinced that success to accrue medical students and residents into hematology fellowship requires not only enthusiastic faculty effort to pursue consults but also effective delivery of high-quality knowledge to learners.

Washington, DC, USA
Philadelphia, PA, USA

Gustavo Rivero
Iberia Romina Sosa

Contents

Part II   Benign Hematology

Contributors

Giuliana Berardi Fox Chase Cancer Center, Philadelphia, PA, USA

Erika Correa Fox Chase Cancer Center, Philadelphia, PA, USA

Department of Hematology, Univerity of Miami, Miami, FL, USA

Diana De Oliveira Baylor College of Medicine, Baylor St Luke's Medical Center, Houston, TX, USA

Garrett Diltz Lombardi Comprehensive Cancer Center, Georgetown University School of Medicine, Washington, DC, USA

Kimberley Doucette Medstar Georgetown University Hospital, Washington, DC, USA

Bittar Gianfranco Baylor College of Medicine, Baylor St Luke's Medical Center, Houston, TX, USA

Colleen Gilstad Lombardi Comprehensive Cancer Center, Georgetown University School of Medicine, Washington, DC, USA

Gregory Hemenway Department of Internal Medicine, Temple University Hospital, Philadelphia, PA, USA

Ishara Lareef Temple University, Philadelphia, PA, USA

Sarah Mudra MedStar Georgetown University Hospital, Washington, DC, USA

Division of Hematology and Oncology, Georgetown University School of Medicine, Washington, DC, USA

Lombardi Cancer Institute, Georgetown University School of Medicine, Washington, DC, USA

Grace Park Division of Pharmacy, The University of Texas MD Anderson Cancer Center, Houston, TX, USA

Gustavo Rivero Lombardi Cancer Institute, Georgetown University School of Medicine, Washington, DC, USA

Paul Sackstein Georgetown University School of Medicine, Washington, DC, USA

Georgetown University School of Medicine, MedStar Georgetown University Hospital, Washington, USA

Iberia Romina Sosa Department of Hematology/Oncology, Fox Chase Cancer Center, Philadelphia, PA, USA

Sravanti Teegarapavu Dan L Duncan Comprehensive Cancer Center at Baylor College of Medicine, Houston, TX, USA

Baylor College of Medicine, Houston, TX, USA

Olivia Wilkins Medstar Georgetown University Hospital, Washington, DC, USA

Alexis K. Williams Baylor College of Medicine, School of Medicine, Houston, TX, USA

Department of Medicine, New York University, New York, NY, USA

Lacey Williams MedStar Georgetown University Hospital, Washington, DC, USA

Division of Hematology and Oncology, Georgetown University School of Medicine, Washington, DC, USA

Lombardi Cancer Institute, Georgetown University School of Medicine, Washington, DC, USA

Rachel Zemel Medstar Georgetown University Hospital, Washington, DC, USA

Linda Zhang Graduate Program in Translational Biology and Molecular Medicine, Baylor College of Medicine, Houston, TX, USA

Part I
Malignant Hematology

Chapter 1
What Should We Quickly Know About Hemopoietic Malignancies?

Gustavo Rivero

Acute Leukemia

Acute Myelogenous Leukemia

Definitions

Acute myelogenous leukemia (AML) is a cytogenetic and molecular heterogeneous disease characterized by expansion of undifferentiated myeloid progenitor. Studies suggest that 21,450 adults were diagnosed with AML in 2019 [1]. Age represents a strong risk factor for disease acquisition with an age-adjusted incidence of 20.1 per 100,000 person-years vs 2.0 per 100,000 person-years in patients older versus younger than 65 years, respectively [2]. AML presents as de novo disease or secondary when previous myeloid disorders, such as myelodysplastic syndrome (MDS), myeloproliferative neoplasm (MPN), or previous chemotherapy exposure, has induced stem cell/progenitor injury that initiates myeloid transformation.

Classification

The world health organization (WHO) 2016 classification for AML designates subgroups based on recurrent cytogenetic and molecular defects. Recent modifications include incorporation of *BCR ABL1* as unusual de novo AML and designation of APL with *PML-RARA* to capitalize that *PML-RARA* fusion could be cryptic or initiated by cytogenetic abnormalities different from t(15;17)(q24.1; q21.2) [3].

G. Rivero (✉)
Lombardi Cancer Institute, Georgetown University School of Medicine, Washington, DC, USA
e-mail: garivero@bcm.edu

© The Author(s), under exclusive license to Springer Nature Switzerland AG 2024
G. Rivero, I. R. Sosa (eds.), *Consulting Hematology and Oncology Handbook*, https://doi.org/10.1007/978-3-031-75810-2_1

3

Table 1.1 summarizes entities included in AML and related neoplasms classification. Additionally, the WHO incorporates myeloid specific mutations with known prognostic value for outcome, such as *CEBPA* biallelic, *NPM1,* and in the case of *RUNX1* only for those cases without myelodysplastic syndrome (MDS)-related

Table 1.1 WHO 2016 classification of acute myelogenous leukemia (AML)

Acute myelogenous leukemia and related neoplasms
AML with recurrent cytogenetic abnormalities
AML with t(8;21)(q22;q22.1);*RUNX1-RUNX1T1*
AML with inv(16)(p13.1q22) or t(16;16)(p13.1;q22); CBFB-MYH11
AML with *PML-RARA*
AML with t(9;11)(p21.3;q23.3); *MLLT3-KMT2A*
AML with t(6;9)(p23;q34.1); *DEK-NUP214*
AML with inv(3)(q21.3q26.2) or t(3;3)(q21.3;q26.2); *GATA2, MECOM*
AML (megakaryoblastic) with t(1;22) (p13.3;q13.3);*RBM12-MKL1*
Provisional entity: AML with *BCR-ABL1*
AML with mutated *NPM1*
AML with biallelic mutations of *CEBPA*
Provisional entity: AML with mutated *RUNX1*
AML with myelodysplasia-related changes
Therapy-related myeloid neoplasms
AML, NOS
AML with minimal differentiation
AML without maturation
Acute myelomonocytic leukemia
Acute monoblastic/monocytic leukemia
Pure erythroid leukemia
Acute megakaryocytic leukemia
Acute basophilic leukemia
Acute panmyelosis with myelofibrosis
Myeloid sarcoma
Myeloid proliferation related to Down syndrome
Transient abnormal myelopoiesis (TAM)
Myeloid leukemia associated with Down syndrome

cytogenetic abnormalities. MDS and therapy-related myeloid neoplasms were maintained within the classification. However, a distinction for therapy-related MDS or AML was recommended for prognostic and therapeutic consideration [3].

Etiology

Leukemogenesis is a process that requires sequential steps leading to highly proliferative malignant hemopoietic disease. In general, inherited predisposition, aging associated risk, and drug-induced genotoxic effect are the most prominent factors contributing individually or in combination to leukemia initiation in susceptible patients.

Germline Predisposition

Germline sequencing has uncovered large number of mutations associated with hemopoietic malignancies (Table 1.2). These mutations could correlate with clinical and laboratory manifestations such as high incidence of thrombocytopenia among family members with *RUNX1* germline mutation. Early onset of gray hair in 20 s and cytopenias may signal *TERT/TERC* mutation predisposition. In patients who harbor *P53* and *FANCA* genes defects, concurrent or previous history of solid tumors is frequently observed.

Aging Associated Risk

In patients without MDS or AML, myeloid mutations at low allele frequency (usually less than 2%) may develop years before diagnosis (Fig. 1.1). These mutations are classically found in epigenetic regulators including DNA methyltransferase 3A

Table 1.2 Genes mutated in patients with germline predisposition for hematologic malignancies

Gene	Incidence among families with predisposing genetic defects	Phenotype	References
DDX41	2–6%	MDS and AML	[4]
CEBPA	10%	AML	[5]
GATA2	7–15%	MonoMac syndrome[a], MDS and AML	[6]
RUNX1	12%	AML, ALL	[7]
FANCA	1%	Bone marrow failure, MDS, AML	[7]
TERT	5%	Bone marrow failure, MDS	[7]
P53	1%	MDS, AML	[7]

[a]MonoMac syndrome = mycobacterial infections, monocytopenia, B lymphopenia and pulmonary alveolar proteinosis (MonoMac syndrome) or primary lymphoedema, cutaneous warts

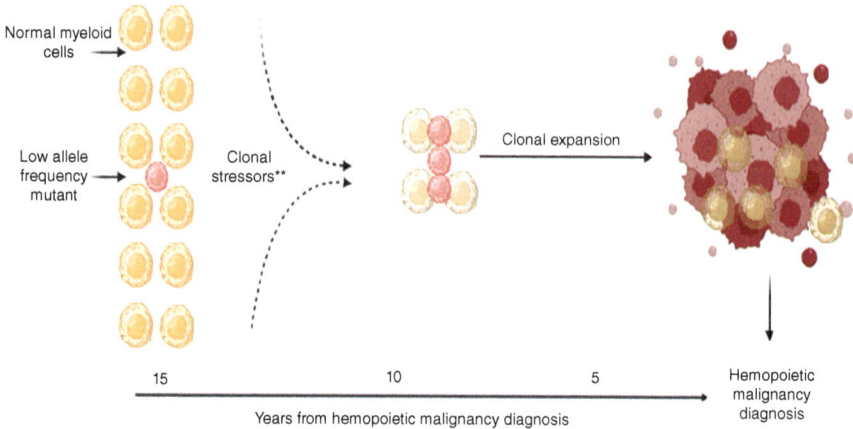

** Smocking, aging, alcohol, advanced glycosilation

Fig. 1.1 Clonal expansion and dominance of myeloid clones under leukemia stressor factors

(*DNMT3A*), Ten–Eleven Translocation 2 (*TET2*), and additional sex combs like 1 (*ASXL1*) genes. This entity is collectively termed clonal hematopoiesis of undetermined prognosis (CHIP) [8]. A strong correlation with aging suggested that somatic hemopoietic stem cell/progenitor mutation acquisition likely results from accumulation of unrepaired DNA followed by repeated DNA replicative rounds and subsequent clonal expansion under selection. Development of clonality is not entirely characterized; however, it possible that complex mechanisms interplay between cell intrinsic (i.e., germline predisposition, aging) and cell extrinsic factors such as smoking; autoimmunity, among others, contributes to clonal dominance (Fig. 1.1) [9]. Progression from aplastic anemia to MDS represents an illustration of cytokine-induced hemopoietic stress initiated by autologous T cells within marrow microenvironment. In this condition, stem cell/progenitor attrition, cytogenetic abnormalities, and mutation acquisition frequently develop during clonal evolution toward MDS/ AML. *DNMT3A, ASXL1,* and *TET2* (DAT mutations) impair cellular differentiation posing permissible state toward hemopoietic transformation [10]. DAT and spliceosome (*SF3B1, SRS2F2* and *U2AF1*) mutations are known elderly leukemia founder defects.

Drug-Induced Genotoxic Effect

Chemotherapy drugs are not selective to cancer cells, but also damage rapidly dividing cells, especially hemopoietic cells. In fact, the world health organization acknowledges therapy-related AML as a late event after exposure to cytotoxic therapy or radiation [3]. After genomic injury by cytotoxic agents, mutant clones exhibit quiescent trajectory, whereas others demonstrate a clonal expansion (i.e., *P53* and *PPM1D*) [10]. Myeloid-related hemopoietic malignancies occurs 5–10 years after alkylating agents or radiation and frequently present as therapy-related myelodysplastic syndromes. After DNA topoisomerase II inhibitor therapy, AML commonly presents after 1–5 years of exposure [11]. In anthracycline-induced therapy-myeloid neoplasm (t-MN), chromosomic abnormalities involving chromosome 5 and/or 7, complex karyotypes, and *TP53* mutations are frequently observed. In contrast, translocations involving KMT2A at 11q23.3 and RUNX1 at 21q22.1 prevalent in t-MN are initiated by topoisomerase inhibitors [12]. The disease is conventionally associated with poor response to standard chemotherapy and dismal outcome.

Clinical Context

Chapter 4 describes in detail clinical manifestations of AML. In general, de novo AML may present as a highly proliferative disease and severe hyperleukocytosis. Expression of adhesion molecules can induce leukemia aggregation and organ ischemia by limiting blood vessels flow. On the other hand less proliferative secondary leukemias in the elderly presents with life-threatening cytopenias.

Laboratory Investigation

Peripheral blood smear examination is important to identify Acute Promyelocytic Leukemia (APL). Heavily granulated promyelocytes with Auer Rods support APL diagnosis. Hypersegmented neutrophils, pseudo-Pelger-Huet anomaly and hypogranular large platelets suggest that MDS likely initiated AML in elderly patients. A bone marrow aspirate, flow cytometry, and biopsy are needed for diagnosis. Chromosome metaphase karyotyping, in situ fluorescent hybridization (FISH), and next-generation sequencing (NGS) for myeloid-specific mutations would allow AML risk stratification.

Acute Lymphoblastic Leukemia

Definitions

Acute lymphoblastic leukemia (ALL) compromises a complex genetic and molecular subtype of leukemia in adults. The disease is broadly classified in B- and T-cell phenotype and accounts for 0.4% of all leukemia diagnosed in the United States [13]. B-cell ALL represents the larger proportion of patients. This entity can be associated with aggressive behavior, especially if initiated by Philadelphia chromosome or a Philadelphia-like gene signature [14]. T-ALL accounts for approximately 25% of ALL cases [15], and it is characterized by the presence of activating mutations in *NOTCH1* in 50% of patients. The disease presents in a bimodal distribution with initial peak observed at age five and a second peak around age 50. While cure rates are more than 90% in pediatric patients, only 20–40% of adults survive at 5 years [16].

Classification

The WHO 2016 classification of ALL subcategorizes the disease in B and T phenotypes based on lineage specification. During the recent 2016 revision, two additional B-cell subgroups were incorporated to account for "Ph-like" B-ALL associated with tyrosine kinases or cytokine receptors translocations and those with intrachromosomal amplification of chromosome 21 [3]. Both entities exhibit inferior response to conventional chemotherapy and are associated with poor prognosis [17]. Table 1.3 summarizes proposed WHO 2016 ALL classification.

Table 1.3 Acute lymphoblastic leukemia classification

B-lymphoblastic leukemia/lymphoma, NOS
B-lymphoblastic leukemia/lymphoma with recurrent genetic Abnormalities
B-lymphoblastic leukemia/lymphoma with t(9;22) (q34.1;q11.2);BCR-ABL1
B-lymphoblastic leukemia/lymphoma with t(v;11q23.3);KMT2A Rearranged
B-lymphoblastic leukemia/lymphoma with t(12;21)(p13.2;q22.1); ETV6-RUNX1
B-lymphoblastic leukemia/lymphoma with hyperdiploidy
B-lymphoblastic leukemia/lymphoma with hypodiploidy
B-lymphoblastic leukemia/lymphoma with t(5;14)(q31.1;q32.3) IL3-IGH
B-lymphoblastic leukemia/lymphoma with t(1;19) (q23;p13.3);TCF3-PBX1
Provisional entity: B-lymphoblastic leukemia/lymphoma, BCR-ABL1–like
Provisional entity: B-lymphoblastic leukemia/lymphoma with iAMP21
T-lymphoblastic leukemia/lymphoma
Provisional entity: Early T-cell precursor lymphoblastic leukemia
Provisional entity: Natural killer (NK) cell lymphoblastic Leukemia/lymphoma

Etiology

Acute lymphoblastic leukemia can initiate from germline predisposition syndromes and/or submicroscopic genomic alterations important for leukemogenesis [18]. Additional, genetic studies using high-throughput sequencing have uncovered molecular landscapes in major subgroups of B-ALL, a frequent ALL observed in pediatric, adolescent, and adults. In this section, we summarize recent advances in ALL germline predisposition and chromosomic abnormalities that are important in disease pathogenesis.

Germline Predisposition

Down syndrome, ataxia telangiectasia, and Nijmegen breakage syndrome (SBS) are known ALL predisposing syndromes. However, genomic wide association studies (GWAS) have revealed common loci in gene transcription factors involved in ALL predisposition [19]. Germline susceptibly clusters seem to aggregate patients by ethnic background suggesting that ancestry is an important factor for ALL subtype and disease behavior. Notably, *GATA3* is associated with specific ALL subgroups such as Ph-like ALL among patients of Hispanic ancestry [20]. In African American, germline predisposition involving *TP63, PTPRJ,* and *ETV6-RUNX1* ALL is frequently observed [21]. Table 1.4 summarizes commonly genetic abnormalities, mutational frequencies, and associated phenotypes in patients with ALL predisposition.

Table 1.4 Genetic abnormalities and genes mutated in patients with germline predisposition for acute lymphoblastic leukemia

Genetic abnormalities	Incidence among families with predisposing genetic defects	Phenotype	References
+21		Down syndrome AML (150 fold increased risk in first 5 years of life), MDS, and ALL	[19]
ATM	0.14%	Ataxia telangiectasia (T-cell rather B-cell ALL)	[22]
NBN	0.08	Nijmegen breakage syndrome (T-cell phenotype)	
NF1	0.12%	Neurofibromatosis 1	[22]
PAX5		B-cell ALL	[19]
TP53	2%	Li-Fraumeni syndrome (low hypodiploid ALL, AML)	[19]
IKZF1	1%	B-cell ALL	[19]
ETV6	1%	B-cell ALL, MDS, AML, mixed lineage phenotype acute leukemia	[19]
SH2B3	Case reports	B- and T-cell ALL, especially in Ph-like B-cell ALL	[23]

Chromosomic Abnormalities

Recurrent cytogenetic abnormalities are unequally distributed among pediatric and adults diagnosed with B-cell ALL patients. Higher proportion of hyperdiploid karyotype is observed in pediatric cases (Fig. 1.2), as opposed to poor risk *P53* hypodiploid disease normally seen in adults [24]. Less favorable cytogenetic and genomic subgroups such as t (9; 22) (q34; q11) initiating *BCR-ABL1*, t (4; 11) (q21; q23), and (24) Philadelphia-like, ("Ph-like") B-cell ALL are frequent in adults rather than pediatric patients suggesting that aging drives aggressive genomic and phenotype (Fig. 1.2). The success achieved in treating Philadelphia B-cell ALL with tyrosine kinase inhibitors (TKIs) prompted genome sequencing investigation across ALL to identify similar potential targets. In ALL patients lacking *BCR-ABL1* fusion, gene expression (GE) reproduced a similar BCR-ABL prolife that clinically retained poor prognosis. Median age ranges from 5.3 to 40 years. While most of "Ph-like" cases are associated with *IKZF1* deletion [25], *CRKF2* overexpression, *JAK* mutations with and without JAK2 fusions, and *EPOR and ABL* class rearrangements are observed (Fig. 1.3) [26–28].

Clinical Context

ALL patients present with leukocytosis and peripheral blood lymphoblasts with high nucleocytoplasmic ratio. Cytoplasm is frequently basophilic with hypogranulation and few vacuoles. Anemia and thrombocytopenia are commonly associated with initial presentation. Additionally, tumor lysis syndrome (TLS), which signals highly proliferative disease and disseminated intravascular coagulation (DIC), can be observed.

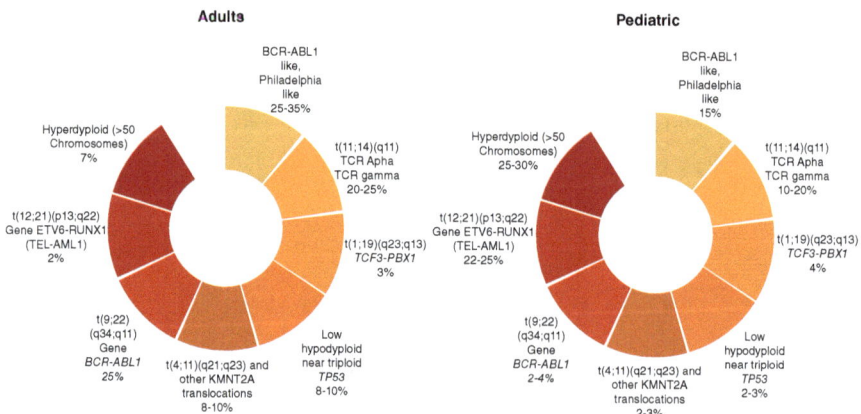

Fig. 1.2 Chromosomic and genomic abnormalities in B-cell ALL distributed by age at disease onset "Created with BioRender.com"

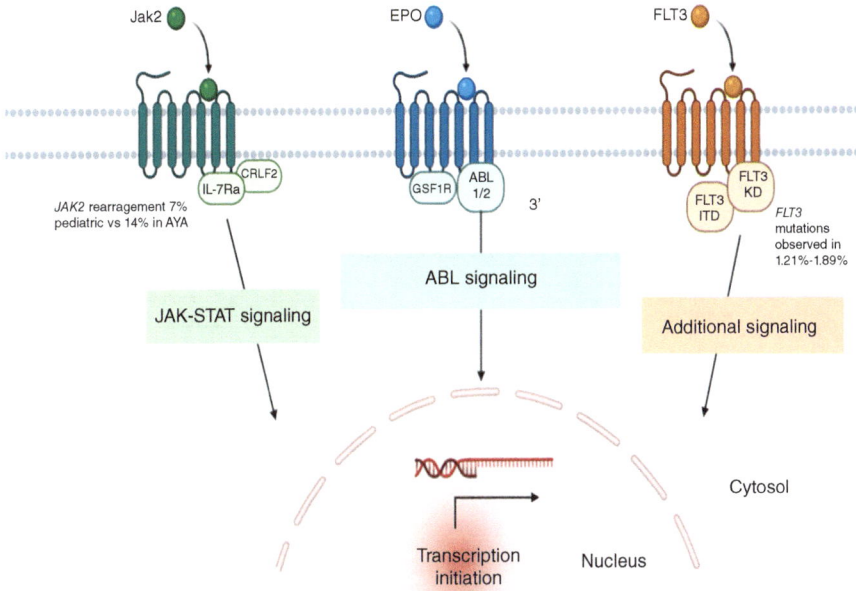

Fig. 1.3 Philadelphia like B-cell ALL (Ph-like) common genomic abnormalities. A combination of mutations, especially *JAK* type, fusion genes, deletions result in upregulation of cytokine receptors such as CRLF2, EPOR and IL-7. "Created with BioRender.com"

Laboratory Investigation

Flow cytometry is needed to determine whether B- or T-lineage ALL phenotype is present. Immunophenotype is also used to identify potential targets including CD20, CD19, and CD22. Bone marrow karyotypic analysis, ALL FISH, and next-generation sequencing are needed for risk stratification. Reverse transcription polymerase chain reaction (RT-PCR) for *BCR-ABL* can assist with diagnosis and monitoring of Philadelphia-positive B-cell ALL.

What Are the Basic Principles for Initial Evaluation of Myeloproliferative Neoplasms?

According to the WHO, myeloproliferative neoplasms (MPNs) are classified like myeloid entities initiated by clonal expansion (i.e., *BCR-ABL, JAK2,* among others) that result in specific disease phenotype [3]. A general approach to evaluate an undiagnosed MPN is summarized in Fig. 1.4.

A close examination of peripheral smear is helpful to characterize MPN type. In chronic myelogenous leukemia (CML), increased number of myelocytes,

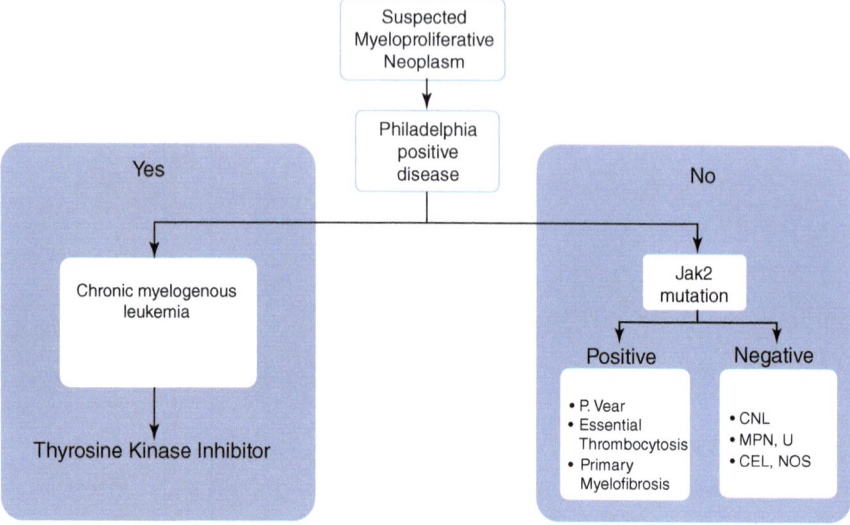

Fig. 1.4 Algorithm to establish MPN diagnosis. *P. Vera* polycythemia vera, *CNL* chronic neutro-philic leukemia; *MPN, U* myeloproliferative neoplasm, unclassifiable; *CEL, NOS* chronic eosino-philic leukemia, not otherwise specified

promyelocytes, and basophils suggest the presence of *BCR-ABL* fusion gene. Similar myeloid proliferation can be observed in proliferative stage of *JAK2-617F* myelofibrosis. Thrombocytosis may otherwise signal essential thrombocytosis (ET) and even atypical presentation for CML. In this section, we will review useful information that could assist with initial consultation of patients diagnosed with CML.

Chronic Myeloid Leukemia

Definitions

Chronic myelogenous leukemia (CML) is a clonal myeloproliferative disorder characterized by bone marrow expansion of immature myeloid cells and compromises 15% of leukemias in adults [29]. The key feature of CML is the presence of the translocation t (9; 22), which initiates *BCR-ABL* fusion. *BCR-ABL* fusion leads to constitutive active tyrosine kinase activity. CML is an infrequent disease with an annual age-adjusted incidence of 1 case per 100,000 in Europe, contrasting with 1.6 per 100,000 based on previous publication from the Surveillance Epidemiology and End Results Program (SEER). Differences in incidence could be attributed to diverse ethnic populations and under or overreporting leading to inclusion of Philadelphia negative myeloproliferative disorders [30]. Recently, the European Treatment and Outcome Study (EUTOS) of CML reported that median age among 2342 patients was 55 years, with 53% of CML cases being male [31]. Patients older than 70 years represent >20% of cases and children/adolescents <5% [32]. Age and comorbidities are important risk factors for therapy selection, especially since higher number of comorbid conditions are seen in older patients.

Clinical Context

Leukocytosis with or without basophilia is a frequent presenting feature of CML. Patients can develop varying degree of splenomegaly. The disease natural outcome includes three phases: (1) chronic phase (CP), (2) accelerated phase (AP), and (3) terminal blast phase (BP). According to EUTOS population-based registry, AP and BP CML accounts for 4% and 2% of diagnosis [33]. Table 1.5 illustrates proposed criteria for definition of accelerated and blast phase CML.

Risk Stratification

Risk scores are important tools for physicians to predict response and long-term survival in patients receiving tyrosine kinase inhibitors (TKI). The Sokal score, albeit originally designed to predict survival in patients receiving chemotherapy and/or interferon, is frequently used along the EUTOS long-term survival score

Table 1.5 Definition for chronic myelogenous leukemia accelerated and blast phase by MDACC, ELN and WHO

MDACC[a]	European LeukemiaNet	WHO[b]
Accelerated phase		
Peripheral (P) blast 15–29%	P or marrow (M) blast 15–29%	P or M blast 10–19%
P blast plus promyelocytes >30%	P blast plus promyelocytes >30%	
P basophils >20%	P basophils >20%	P basophils >20%
Platelets <100 × 10⁹/L (without relation to therapy)	Platelets <100 × 10⁹/L (without relation to therapy)	Platelets <100 × 10⁹/L (without relation to therapy) or > 1000 × 10⁹ (unresponsive to therapy
Splenomegaly (unresponsive to therapy)		Splenomegaly (unresponsive to therapy)
Cytogenetic evolution on therapy	Cytogenetic evolution on therapy	Additional chromosomic abnormalities/ Ph[c]+ major route, complex karyotype, or 3q26.2 abnormality at diagnosis
Blast phase		
P or M blast >30%		P or M blast>20%
EM[d] blast proliferation		EM blast proliferation

[a]*MDACC* MD Anderson Cancer Center
[b]*WHO* World Health Organization
[c]*Ph* Philadelphia chromosome
[d]*EM* Extramedullary

Table 1.6 CML-risk stratification

Risk score	Calculation	Risk category	
Sokal	Exp 0.0116x (age-42.4) + 0.0345 × (spleen-7.51) + 0.188 × [(platelet count ÷ 700)^2 − 0.563] ÷ 0.0887 × (blasts-2.10)	Low	<0.8
		Intermediate	0.8–1.2
		High	>1.2
EUTOS long-term survival (ELTS) score	0.0025 × *age/10)^3 + 0.0615 × spleen size cm below costal margin + 0.1052 × blasts in PB^a ÷ 0.4104 × (platelet count/1000)$^{-0.5}$	Low	<1.5680
		Intermediate	>1.5680 but <2.2185
		High	>2.2185

^{a}*PB* peripheral blood

(ELTS) subsequently developed to evaluate survival in patients receiving TKIs. Age at diagnosis, spleen size, platelet, and blast counts are considered for Sokal and ELTS scores estimation. Table 1.6 summarizes risk score systems commonly used in newly diagnosed CML patients.

The superiority of ELTS system predicting failure-free, overall survival has been demonstrated in multiple studies [34]. Risk stratification tools are also used to select chronic phase CML patients for risk-adapted TKI therapy. Cases identified as intermediate risk by the ELTS score may benefit more from initial second-generation-TKI therapy in achieving better failure- and progression-free survivals [34]. In patients considered low risk, the preferred regimens include Imatinib, Bosutinib, Dasatinib, or Nilotinib. However, in high-risk patients, the National Comprehensive Cancer Network (NCCN) normally recommends Bosutinib, Dasatinib, or Nilotinib.

Risk of TKIs Toxicity

Most of TKI's side effects are mild and resolved without complications. However, severe side effects can be observed. Diabetes, hypertension, and dyslipidemia increase proportionally with age diagnosis. The Charlson Comorbidity Index (CCI) clearly predicted strong association between number of comorbid conditions and CML outcome demonstrating an 8-years survival of 48% and 91% for patients with score >5 and 2, respectively [35]. Careful history and documentation of coronary-artery disease (CAD) is important for TKI therapy selection. The risk of arterio-occlusive events was significantly higher in hypertensive patients treated with Ponatinib [36]. Previous studies have demonstrated increased risk of pleural effusion with Dasatinib [37] and renal dysfunction mostly associated with Imatinib and Bosutinib [38].

Laboratory Investigation

Complete blood count (CBC) and differential, chemistry profile, bone marrow aspirate/biopsy for morphologic examination, metaphases cytogenetic, quantitative RT-PCR (qPCR), and hepatitis B panel are needed for investigation of patients presenting with leukocytosis and suspected CML.

Useful Tools

Sokal and ELTS Scores Can Be Accessed Via the Below Link

https://www.leukemia-net.org/content/leukemias/cml/euro__and_sokal_score/
   index_eng.html
https://www.leukemia-net.org/content/leukemias/cml/elts_score/index_eng.html

References

1. Siegel RL, Miller KD, Fuchs HE, Jemal A. Cancer statistics, 2022. CA Cancer J Clin. 2022;72(1):7–33.
2. Shallis RM, Wang R, Davidoff A, Ma X, Zeidan AM. Epidemiology of acute myeloid leukemia: recent progress and enduring challenges. Blood Rev. 2019;36:70–87.
3. Arber DA, Orazi A, Hasserjian R, Thiele J, Borowitz MJ, Le Beau MM, et al. The 2016 revision to the world health organization classification of myeloid neoplasms and acute leukemia. Blood. 2016;127(20):2391–405.
4. Sebert M, Passet M, Raimbault A, Rahme R, Raffoux E, Sicre de Fontbrune F, et al. Germline DDX41 mutations define a significant entity within adult MDS/AML patients. Blood. 2019;134(17):1441–4.
5. Pabst T, Eyholzer M, Haefliger S, Schardt J, Mueller BU. Somatic CEBPA mutations are a frequent second event in families with germline CEBPA mutations and familial acute myeloid leukemia. J Clin Oncol. 2008;26(31):5088–93.
6. Wlodarski MW, Hirabayashi S, Pastor V, Stary J, Hasle H, Masetti R, et al. Prevalence, clinical characteristics, and prognosis of GATA2-related myelodysplastic syndromes in children and adolescents. Blood. 2016;127(11):1387–97. quiz 1518
7. Rio-Machin A, Vulliamy T, Hug N, Walne A, Tawana K, Cardoso S, et al. The complex genetic landscape of familial MDS and AML reveals pathogenic germline variants. *Nature*. Communications. 2020;11(1):1044-020-14829-5.
8. Jaiswal S, Ebert BL. Clonal hematopoiesis in human aging and disease, vol. 366. Science (New York, NY); 2019. p. 6465. https://doi.org/10.1126/science.aan4673.
9. King KY, Huang Y, Nakada D, Goodell MA. Environmental influences on clonal hematopoiesis. Exp Hematol. 2020;83:66–73.
10. McNerney ME, Le Beau MM. The harmful consequences of increased fitness in hematopoietic stem cells. Cell Stem Cell. 2018;23(5):634–5.
11. Zhou Y, Tang G, Medeiros LJ, McDonnell TJ, Keating MJ, Wierda WG, et al. Therapy-related myeloid neoplasms following fludarabine, cyclophosphamide, and rituximab (FCR) treatment in patients with chronic lymphocytic leukemia/small lymphocytic lymphoma. Mod Pathol. 2012;25(2):237–45.
12. Liu YC, Illar GM, Al Amri R, Canady BC, Rea B, Yatsenko SA, et al. Therapy-related myeloid neoplasms with different latencies: a detailed clinicopathologic analysis. Mod Pathol. 2022;35:625–31.
13. Aldoss I, Forman SJ, Pullarkat V. Acute lymphoblastic leukemia in the older adult. J Oncol Pract. 2019;15(2):67–75.
14. Advani A. Acute lymphoblastic leukemia (ALL). Best Pract Res Clin Haematol. 2017;30(3):173–4.
15. Hunger SP, Mullighan CG. Acute lymphoblastic leukemia in children. N Engl J Med. 2015;373(16):1541–52.

16. Paul S, Kantarjian H, Jabbour EJ. Adult acute lymphoblastic leukemia. Mayo Clin Proc. 2016;91(11):1645–66.
17. Gavralidis A, Brunner AM. Novel therapies in the treatment of adult acute lymphoblastic leukemia. Curr Hematol Malig Rep. 2020;15(4):294–304.
18. Holmfeldt L, Wei L, Diaz-Flores E, Walsh M, Zhang J, Ding L, et al. The genomic landscape of hypodiploid acute lymphoblastic leukemia. Nat Genet. 2013;45(3):242–52.
19. Klco JM, Mullighan CG. Advances in germline predisposition to acute leukaemias and myeloid neoplasms. Nat Rev Cancer. 2021;21(2):122–37.
20. Perez-Andreu V, Roberts KG, Harvey RC, Yang W, Cheng C, Pei D, et al. Inherited GATA3 variants are associated with ph-like childhood acute lymphoblastic leukemia and risk of relapse. Nat Genet. 2013;45(12):1494–8.
21. Ellinghaus E, Stanulla M, Richter G, Ellinghaus D, te Kronnie G, Cario G, et al. Identification of germline susceptibility loci in ETV6-RUNX1-rearranged childhood acute lymphoblastic leukemia. Leukemia. 2012;26(5):902–9.
22. Schutte P, Moricke A, Zimmermann M, Bleckmann K, Reismuller B, Attarbaschi A, et al. Preexisting conditions in pediatric ALL patients: Spectrum, frequency and clinical impact. Eur J Med Genet. 2016;59(3):143–51.
23. Perez-Garcia A, Ambesi-Impiombato A, Hadler M, Rigo I, LeDuc CA, Kelly K, et al. Genetic loss of SH2B3 in acute lymphoblastic leukemia. Blood. 2013;122(14):2425–32.
24. DeAngelo DJ, Jabbour E, Advani A. Recent advances in managing acute lymphoblastic leukemia. Am Soc Clin Oncol Educ Book. American Society of Clinical Oncology Annual Meeting. 2020;40:330–42.
25. Roberts KG, Pei D, Campana D, Payne-Turner D, Li Y, Cheng C, et al. Outcomes of children with BCR-ABL1-like acute lymphoblastic leukemia treated with risk-directed therapy based on the levels of minimal residual disease. J Clin Oncol. 2014;32(27):3012–20.
26. Yadav V, Ganesan P, Veeramani R, Kumar VD. Philadelphia-like acute lymphoblastic leukemia: a systematic review. Clin Lymphoma Myeloma Leuk. 2021;21(1):e57–65.
27. Iacobucci I, Mullighan CG. Genetic basis of acute lymphoblastic leukemia. J Clin Oncol Off J Am Soc Clin Oncol. 2017;35(9):975–83.
28. Zhang Y, Zhang Y, Wang F, Wang M, Liu H, Chen X, et al. The mutational spectrum of FLT3 gene in acute lymphoblastic leukemia is different from acute myeloid leukemia. Cancer Gene Ther. 2020;27(1–2):81–8.
29. How J, Venkataraman V, Hobbs GS. Blast and accelerated phase CML: room for improvement. Hematology Am Soc Hematol Educ Program. 2021;2021(1):122–8.
30. Hoglund M, Sandin F, Hellstrom K, Bjoreman M, Bjorkholm M, Brune M, et al. Tyrosine kinase inhibitor usage, treatment outcome, and prognostic scores in CML: report from the population-based swedish CML registry. Blood. 2013;122(7):1284–92.
31. Hoffmann VS, Baccarani M, Hasford J, Castagnetti F, Di Raimondo F, Casado LF, et al. Treatment and outcome of 2904 CML patients from the EUTOS population-based registry. Leukemia. 2017;31(3):593–601.
32. Hochhaus A, Baccarani M, Silver RT, Schiffer C, Apperley JF, Cervantes F, et al. European LeukemiaNet 2020 recommendations for treating chronic myeloid leukemia. Leukemia. 2020;34(4):966–84.
33. Hoffmann VS, Baccarani M, Hasford J, Lindoerfer D, Burgstaller S, Sertic D, et al. The EUTOS population-based registry: incidence and clinical characteristics of 2904 CML patients in 20 European countries. Leukemia. 2015;29(6):1336–43.
34. Zhang XS, Gale RP, Huang XJ, Jiang Q. Is the Sokal or EUTOS long-term survival (ELTS) score a better predictor of responses and outcomes in persons with chronic myeloid leukemia receiving tyrosine-kinase inhibitors? Leukemia. 2022;36(2):482–91.
35. Saussele S, Krauss MP, Hehlmann R, Lauseker M, Proetel U, Kalmanti L, et al. Impact of comorbidities on overall survival in patients with chronic myeloid leukemia: results of the randomized CML study IV. Blood. 2015;126(1):42–9.

36. Cortes JE, Kim DW, Pinilla-Ibarz J, le Coutre PD, Paquette R, Chuah C, et al. Ponatinib efficacy and safety in Philadelphia chromosome-positive leukemia: final 5-year results of the phase 2 PACE trial. Blood. 2018;132(4):393–404.
37. Cortes J. How to manage CML patients with comorbidities. Hematology Am Soc Hematol Educ Program. 2020;2020(1):237–42.
38. Cortes JE, Gambacorti-Passerini C, Kim DW, Kantarjian HM, Lipton JH, Lahoti A, et al. Effects of bosutinib treatment on renal function in patients with Philadelphia chromosome-positive leukemias. Clin Lymphoma Myeloma Leuk. 2017;17(10):684–695.e6.

Chapter 2
Acute Myeloid Leukemia Risk Stratification

Linda Zhang

Acute Myelogenous Leukemia Risk Stratification

Case Demonstration

A 33-year-old male presented with fatigability and easy bruising. His WBC was 120 K/uL and his CBC differential showed peripheral blood blasts, which were observed during microscope examination (Fig. 2.1). Flow cytometry demonstrated CD34, CD33, and CD117 positive myeloblasts. Karyotype was normal. His next-generation sequencing for myeloid-specific mutations showed *KRAS* c.35G>C and *U2AF1* p.R156H mutations with allele frequencies of 26% and 22.5%, respectively. He received anthracycline plus cytarabine intravenously as induction followed by high-dose cytarabine per 2 cycles. Patient was HLA typed and received allogeneic matched sibling donor transplantation as consolidation.

Definitions

Acute myelogenous leukemia (AML) is an oligoclonal disease characterized by rapid accumulation of undifferentiated myeloid progenitors in bone marrow. Without therapy, the disease rapidly progresses resulting in life-threatening cytopenias and severe infections and bleeding. Administration of intravenous chemotherapy induces remission and reestablishes normal hematopoiesis. However, without adequate consolidation, relapse would frequently occur. A comprehensive evaluation for relapse risk includes careful consideration of clinical, cytogenetic, and

L. Zhang (✉)
Graduate Program in Translational Biology and Molecular Medicine, Baylor College of Medicine, Houston, TX, USA
e-mail: linda.zhang@bcm.edu

© The Author(s), under exclusive license to Springer Nature Switzerland AG 2024
G. Rivero, I. R. Sosa (eds.), *Consulting Hematology and Oncology Handbook*,
https://doi.org/10.1007/978-3-031-75810-2_2

Fig. 2.1 Peripheral blood blasts observed in AML patient. Cells revealed prominent nuclei with scant cytoplasm lacking granules

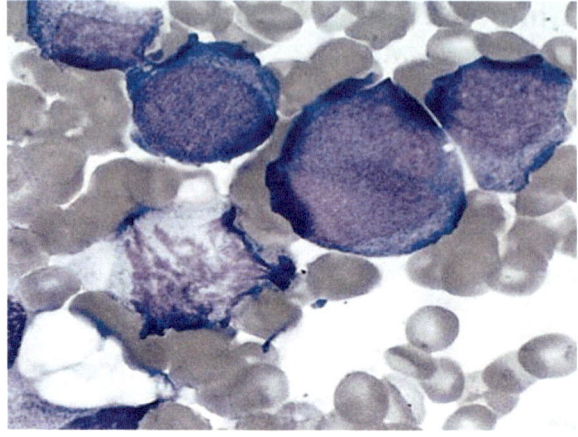

Table 2.1 Favorable and unfavorable clinical factors that should be considered while risk stratifying acute myelogenous leukemia [1–3]

Favorable	Unfavorable
• Age < 50 • Karnofsky score > 60% • MDR[a] 1-negative phenotype • No antecedent hematologic disorder or prior chemo/ radiotherapy	• Age > 60 • Karnofsky score < 60% • MR 1-positive phenotype • Therapy-related AML, prior myelodysplastic syndrome, myeloproliferative, or other hematologic disorder

[a]*MRD* measurable residual disease

genomic AML features. This would allow careful selection of patients for allogenic stem cell transplantation and risk adaptive targeted intervention that could improve leukemia outcome. In this chapter, we will discuss important clinical AML features that assist with recognition of AML patients with high risk for relapse.

Clinical Context

AML can present as *novo* or secondary to "preexisting" conditions such as myelo-dysplastic syndrome (MDS), myeloproliferative neoplasms (MPN), and previous exposure to chemotherapy agents (i.e., anthracycline and topoisomerase inhibitors). The latter is classically described as secondary AML. Secondary AML are typically associated with inferior outcome even after allogeneic bone marrow transplantation (Table 2.1). Risk of relapse is better determined based on chromosomal abnormalities detected by metaphase karyotyping and myeloid-specific mutations obtained by next-generation sequencing.

Important clinical and laboratory features that are associated with inferior outcome include (a) age > 60 years, (b) hyperleukocytosis (WBC > 100 K/uL), (c) evidence of extramedullary leukemia [i.e., adenopathy confirmed to be myeloid sarcoma by tissue biopsy, CNS involvement], and (d) hepatosplenomegaly.

Laboratory Investigation

Patients admitted with suspected AML should obtain the following:

(a) Complete blood count and differential.
(b) Peripheral blood smear for morphologic examination.
(c) Peripheral blood flow cytometry.
(d) Bone marrow aspirate and biopsy.
(e) Metaphase karyotyping.
(f) Fluorescent in situ hybridization (FISH). This technique would be important to uncover "cryptic" metaphase karyotyping abnormalities such as inversion 16. Additionally, in older patients, particularly those between age 60 to 65 years, it may assist in quickly identifying high-risk karyotypic abnormalities individually or in combination [i.e., monosomy 7, deletion 7p, monosomy 5, inversion 3, deletion 17p, KMT2A (mixed lineage leukemia) to consider more effective induction therapy.
(g) Next-generation sequencing analysis for myeloid-specific mutations.

Useful Tools

European LeukemiaNet (ELN) Risk Stratification of Adult AML

An AML patient's response to treatment and overall survival may be predicted based on certain molecular and cytogenetic features of their disease. In 2022, the European LeukemiaNet (ELN) panel categorized these features into three risk categories: favorable, intermediate, and adverse (Table 2.2). These risk categories inform therapeutic decision, more of which is discussed in Chap. 4 (Management of Adult AML).

It is also important to note that while numerous studies have found *DNMT3A*, *IDH1*, *IDH2*, and several other genes to be commonly mutated in adult leukemias, the ELN panel did not estimate there was enough evidence accumulated yet to warrant their assignment to a prognostic group. However, several modifications were incorporated in the newest 2022 risk stratification including the following: (1) *FLT3 ITD* mutation independently of allelic ratio is no longer considered adverse risk, but should retain intermediate prognosis; (2) new myelodysplasia-related genes including *ASXL1 BCOR, EZH2, RUNX1, SF3B1, SRSF2, STAG2, U2AF1*, and *ZRSR2 are* prognostically allocated to adverse ELN2022 subgroup; (3) association of adverse cytogenetic in a *NPM1*-mutated AML should be considered unfavorable risk; (4) bZIP in-frame-mutated *CEBPA* retains favorable prognosis independently of

Table 2.2 European Leukemia Network 2022 risk stratification of acute myelogenous leukemia [4]

Risk category	Molecular markers	
Favorable	• t(8;21)(q22;q22.1) • *RUNX1-RUNX1T1* • inv16(p13.1q22) or t(16;16)p(13.1;q22) • *CBFB-MYH11* • Mutated *NPM1*[a] without co-occurring *FLT3-ITD*[b] • bZIP in-frame-mutated *CEBPA*[c]	
Intermediate	• Mutated *NPM1 and FLT3-ITD* • Wild-type *NPM1* with *FLT3-ITD*[low] (without adverse-risk genetic lesions) • t(9;11) (p21.3;q23.3)/MLLT3::KM2TA • Cytogenetic and/or molecular abnormalities not classified as favorable or adverse	
Adverse	• t(6;9)(p23;134.1) • *DEK-NUP214*[d] • t(v;11q23.3) • *KMT2A* rearranged • t(9;22)(q34.1;q11.2) • *BCR-ABL1* • t(8;16) (p11.2;p13.3)/ KAT6A::*CREBBP* • inv.(3)(q21.3q26.2) or t(3.3)(q21.3;q26.2) • *GATA2, MECOM(EVI1)*	• -5 or del(5q) • -7 • -17/abn(17p) • Complex karyotypes • Mutated *ASXL1*[e], *BCOR, EZH2, RUNX1*[f], *SF3B1, SRSF2, STAG2, U2AF1*, and or *ZRSR2* • Mutated p53

[a]*NPM1* Nucleophosmin
[b]*FLT3-ITD* FMS-related tyrosine kinase-Internal tandem duplication
[c]*CEBPA* CCAAT/enhancer-binding protein alpha
[d]*DEK-NUP214* DEK proto-oncogene (DEK) and nucleoporin 214 (NUP214)
[e]*ASXL1* Putative Polycomb group protein ASXL1
[f]*RUNX1* Runt-related transcription factor 1

biallelic or monoallelic genomic insult; (5) newest high-risk chromosomal aberrations including t(8;16); and (6) karyotypes exhibiting hyperdiploidy with multiple trisomies are not considered complex karyotype or adverse risk.

AML Relapse Risk

Relapse is defined by the re-emergence of leukemic cells in the bone marrow, peripheral blood, or extramedullary site several months to several years after achieving complete molecular remission. About 40–50% of fit patients have relapsed disease after hematopoietic stem cell transplantation [5], and nearly all elderly patients have relapse or refractory disease after non-intensive therapy [6].

Patients suspected of relapse should be evaluated with a bone marrow aspiration followed by pathologic review, immunophenotyping, cytochemistry, and cytogenetics to assess the clonal evolution of disease. These results will help determine prognostic stratification, summarized in Table 2.3. A study done by Chavellier et al. in

Table 2.3 Prognostic stratification of patients with relapsed AML [7]

Prognostic factor	Favorable (0 adverse factors)	Intermediate (1 adverse factor)	High risk (2–3 adverse factors)	p-Value
Number of patients	36	54	43	
Relapse <12 months	0	36 (67%)	43 (100%)	
FLT3-ITD+	0	11 (20%)	26 (60%)	
High-risk cytogenetics	0	7 (13%)	19 (44%)	
Allograft post-GO[a]	14 (39%)	17 (31%)	14 (33%)	0.75
OR[b] after GO	26 (72%)	41 (76%)	18 (42%)	0.001
Two-year EFS[c]	45 ± 9%	31 ± 7%	12 ± 5%	0.001
Two-year OS[d]	58 ± 8%	38 ± 7%	12 ± 6%	$<10^{-4}$

[a]*GO* Gemtuzumab (anti-CD33 monoclonal antibody)
[b]*OR* overall response
[c]*EFS* event free survival
[d]*OS* overall survival

2011 identified three independent adverse prognostic factors: time to relapse (<12 months), FLT3-ITD+ molecular status, and poor cytogenetics.

References

1. Olesen LH, Aggerholm A, Andersen BL, Nyvold CG, Guldberg P, Norgaard JM, et al. Molecular typing of adult acute myeloid leukaemia: significance of translocations, tandem duplications, methylation, and selective gene expression profiling. Br J Haematol. 2005;131(4):457–67. https://doi.org/10.1111/j.1365-2141.2005.05791.x.
2. Estey EH. Therapeutic options for acute myelogenous leukemia. Cancer. 2001;92(5):1059–73. https://doi.org/10.1002/1097-0142(20010901)92:5<1059::aid-cncr1421>3.0.co;2-k
3. Sekeres MA, Peterson B, Dodge RK, Mayer RJ, Moore JO, Lee EJ, et al. Differences in prognostic factors and outcomes in African Americans and whites with acute myeloid leukemia. Blood. 2004;103(11):4036–42. https://doi.org/10.1182/blood-2003-09-3118.
4. Dohner H, Estey E, Grimwade D, Amadori S, Appelbaum FR, Buchner T, et al. Diagnosis and management of AML in adults: 2017 ELN recommendations from an international expert panel. Blood. 2017;129(4):424–47. https://doi.org/10.1182/blood-2016-08-733196.
5. Thol F, Ganser A. Treatment of relapsed acute myeloid leukemia. Curr Treat Options in Oncol. 2020;21(8):66. https://doi.org/10.1007/s11864-020-00765-5.
6. Dombret H, Seymour JF, Butrym A, Wierzbowska A, Selleslag D, Jang JH, et al. International phase 3 study of azacitidine vs conventional care regimens in older patients with newly diagnosed AML with >30% blasts. Blood. 2015;126(3):291–9. https://doi.org/10.1182/blood-2015-01-621664.
7. Chevallier P, Labopin M, Turlure P, Prebet T, Pigneux A, Hunault M, et al. A new leukemia prognostic scoring system for refractory/relapsed adult acute myelogeneous leukaemia patients: a GOELAMS study. Leukemia. 2011;25(6):939–44. https://doi.org/10.1038/leu.2011.25.

Chapter 3
How to Diagnose Acute Myelogenous Leukemia

Linda Zhang and Gustavo Rivero

Diagnosis of acute leukemias is determined by a combination of clinical, morphologic, and immunophenotypic features along with cytogenetics and molecular genetic studies. The use of genetic data has allowed for risk and prognostic stratification and has helped guide therapeutic decision-making as discussed in the previous section. When faced with a patient with suspected leukemia, diagnostic workup should include the following (summarized in Fig. 3.1).

Clinical Manifestations

- Cytopenias (anemias, neutropenia, thrombocytopenia).
- Severe fatigue, shortness of breath, pallor.
- Fever and/or chills.
- Frequent infections.
- Hemorrhagic findings (ecchymosis, gingival bleeding, menorrhagia).
- Unintentional weight loss.
- Organomegaly (adenopathy, hepatomegaly, splenomegaly).

L. Zhang (✉)
Graduate Program in Translational Biology and Molecular Medicine, Baylor College of Medicine, Houston, TX, USA
e-mail: linda.zhang@bcm.edu

G. Rivero
Lombardi Cancer Institute, Georgetown University School of Medicine, Washington, DC, USA
e-mail: garivero@bcm.edu

G. Rivero, I. R. Sosa (eds.), *Consulting Hematology and Oncology Handbook*,
https://doi.org/10.1007/978-3-031-75810-2_3

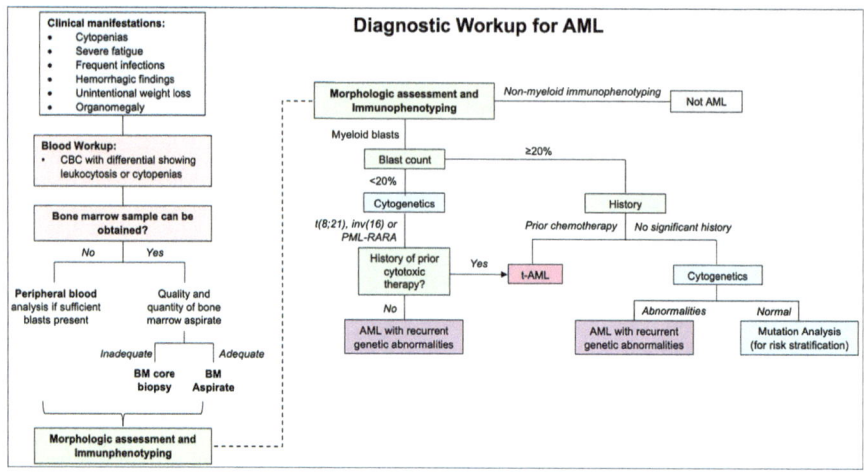

Fig. 3.1 Workflow for the diagnostic workup of a patient suspected to have AML

Table 3.1 Cell surface and cytoplasmatic markers for immunophenotypic diagnosis of AML [1]

Lineage	Marker
Precursors	CD34, CD117, CD33, CD13, HLA-DR
Granulocytes	CD65, cytoplasmic MPO
Monocytes	CD14, CD36, CD64
Megakaryocytic	CD41 (glycoprotein IIb/IIIa), CD61 (glycoprotein IIIa)
Erythroid	CD235a (glycophorin A), CD36

Tests to Establish a Diagnosis

- CBC with differential.
- Bone marrow aspirate.
- Bone marrow trephine biopsy if initial aspiration inadequate (dry tap).
- Immunophenotyping (Table 3.1) and/or cytochemistry to determine cell of origin.

Genetic Analyses

- **Cytogenetic studies** with karyotypic analysis +/− fluorescence in situ hybridization (FISH) or reverse-transcriptase polymerase chain reaction (RT-PCR).
- **Mutation analysis** including *NPM1, CEBPA, RUNX1, FLT3, TP53,* and *ASXL1.*
- **Germ-line investigation:** This should be considered in patients with strong family history of hemopoietic malignancies and/or bone marrow failure occurring at early diagnosis age. Importantly, older AML patients may still harbor germline predisposition syndromes (i.e., DDX41) [2].

Morphology

- From a 500-cell differential count, a blast percentage of ≥20% in the bone marrow or peripheral blood is required for the diagnosis.
- The presence of certain genetic abnormalities including t (8; 21), t (15; 17), inv. (16), or t(16;16) is considered diagnostic of AML *without* regard to blast count [3].

Additional Tests or Procedures at Diagnosis

- Demographics and detailed medical history including analysis of comorbidities.
- Performance status (ECOG/WHO Score/Karnofsky).
- Electrolytes, uric acid, liver, and renal function tests.
- Coagulation profile, including PT, aPTT, and fibrinogen.
- Hepatitis A, B, C; HIV-1 testing.
- Biobanking (pretreatment leukemic bone marrow and blood).

Differential Diagnoses to Consider

- Other malignancies.
  - Some ALLs can co-express myeloid markers; CML in blast crisis.
  - Non-hematopoietic tumors (small cell carcinoma of the lung).
- Clinical presentation predominated by *cytopenias* can be caused by the following:
  - Aplastic anemia.
  - Myelofibrosis.
  - Myelodysplastic syndrome.
  - Medications.
  - Nutritional deficiencies (Vit B12, folate, copper).
  - Bone marrow suppression (alcohol, infection).
  - Felty syndrome.

References

1. Arber DA, Orazi A, Hasserjian R, Thiele J, Borowitz MJ, Le Beau MM, et al. The 2016 revision to the world health organization classification of myeloid neoplasms and acute leukemia. Blood. 2016;127(20):2391–405.

2. Rio-Machin A, Vulliamy T, Hug N, Walne A, Tawana K, Cardoso S, et al. The complex genetic landscape of familial MDS and AML reveals pathogenic germline variants. Nat Commun. 2020;11(1):1044-020-14829-5.
3. Mrozek K, Bloomfield CD. Clinical significance of the most common chromosome translocations in adult acute myeloid leukemia. J Natl Cancer Inst Monogr. 2008;39:52–7.

Chapter 4
Preparing Your Patient for Chemotherapy

Linda Zhang and Gustavo Rivero

Leukostasis

Case Demonstration

A 43-year-old male presented with fatigability and easy bruising. His WBC was 158 K/µL. MPO, CD34, CD33, and CD117 positive myeloblasts were detected by flow cytometry. His bone marrow was 90% hypercellular with more than 80% blasts. His next-generation sequencing (NGS) showed *FLT3 ITD* at allele frequency of 0.86%. Soon after his admission, he complained of right arm and leg weakness. His Brain Magnetic Resonance Imaging (MRI) showed left insular cortex and left parietal subcortical white matter acute and subacute infarcts (Fig. 4.1).

Definitions

Leukostasis

The complication is a life-threatening condition associated with highly proliferative myeloid blast overexpressing adhesion molecules such as CD11, CD49, and L-selecting [1].

L. Zhang
Graduate Program in Translational Biology and Molecular Medicine, Baylor College of Medicine, Houston, TX, USA
e-mail: Linda.zhang@bcm.edu

G. Rivero (✉)
Lombardi Cancer Institute, Georgetown University School of Medicine, Washington, DC, USA
e-mail: garivero@bcm.edu

© The Author(s), under exclusive license to Springer Nature Switzerland AG 2024
G. Rivero, I. R. Sosa (eds.), *Consulting Hematology and Oncology Handbook*, https://doi.org/10.1007/978-3-031-75810-2_4

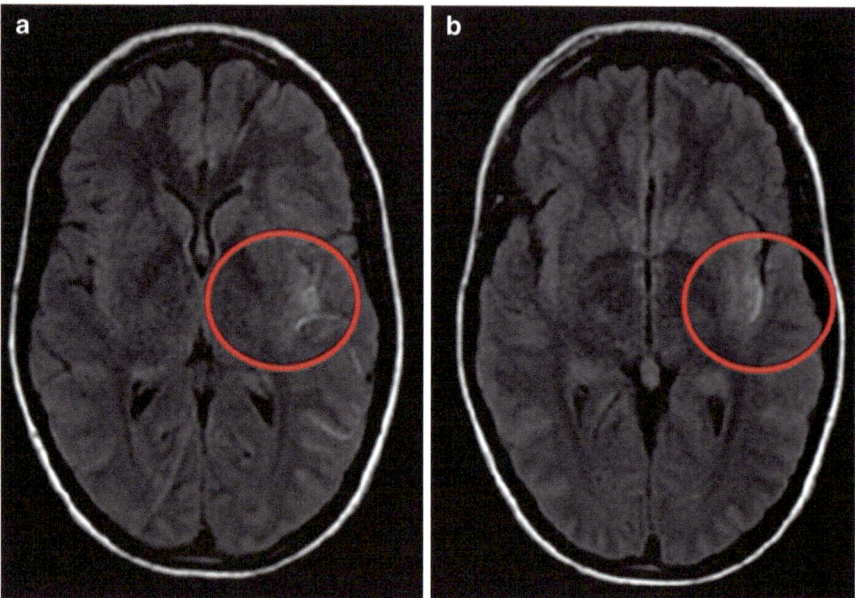

Fig. 4.1 Brain Magnetic Resonance Imaging (MRI). Panel **a** and **b** demonstrate left insular cortex and left parietal subcortical white matter acute and subacute infarcts

Clinical Context

It is commonly observed among AML patients with hyperleukocytosis, which is defined as an elevated white blood cell (WBC) count of more than 100,000/μL. 5–13% of AML cases present with the complication [2]. Pathophysiologically, high viscosity, disruption of vessel wall, and lack of AML blast deformity ability contribute to restricted blood flood. The condition results in high early mortality attributable to organ failure, tumor lysis, and disseminated intravascular coagulation (DIC) [2–4]. Organs frequently involved include central nervous system (CNS0, lungs, cardiovascular system, and gastrointestinal tract. Monocytic and myelo-monocytic AML (M4/M5 French-American-British [FAB] classification) and myeloid specific mutations such as *FLT3 ITD*, *NRAS*, *DNMT3A*, *TET2*, and *NPM1* are additional risk factors for the complication [5].

Laboratory Investigation

(a) Complete blood count and differential.
(b) Coagulation profile including PT, PTT, fibrinogen.

(c) Comprehensive metabolic profile (CMP).
(d) Peripheral blood flow cytometry.

Other Investigation

(a) Electrocardiogram.
(b) Echocardiogram.
(c) Chest X-ray.
(d) Head computerized tomography (CT) scan in the event of neurologic symptoms and/or deficit.

Management

Several interventions can be implemented including the following:

(a) *Leukapheresis*: It is an emergency procedure intended to rapidly reduce peripheral blood white cell count and prevent organ failure attributable to leukostasis. *Careful investigation of acute promyelocytic leukemia (APL) to avoid leukapheresis should be always done*. APL is frequently associated with DIC, which can result in severe hemorrhagic complication during insertion of catheter for the procedure. Teamwork is needed with blood bank personnel and surgical team to ensure Quinton catheter access prior leukapheresis. The intervention has not demonstrated superiority over other interventions including continuous intravenous (IV) infusion of cytarabine [4, 6].
(b) *Pharmacologic Cytoreduction*

   1. Hydroxycarbamide (hydroxyurea) is an orally available antiproliferative drug that impairs DNA synthesis and decreases adhesion molecule expression in AML cells frequently used prior initiation of chemotherapy. Usually, 1000 mg orally every 12 h is a standard initial dose; however, dose can be increased to 2000 mg every 8 h if needed for WBC control [7].
   2. Cytarabine infusion: In our center, this is the preferred intervention leading to rapid peripheral blood blast reduction. An initial dose of 100–200 mg/m^2 intravenously in continuous infusion is recommended. As cytoreduction proceeds, it is important to monitor uric acid and renal function given extremely high risk for tumor lysis syndrome. Figure 4.2 depicts recommended algorithm for initial management of AML patients with evidence of hyperleukocytosis.

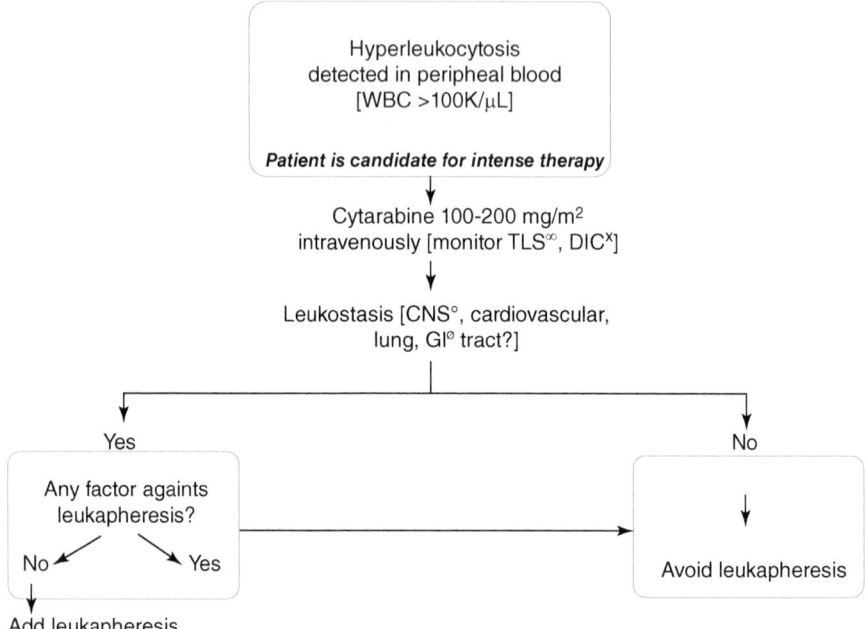

Fig. 4.2 Initial management of AML patients presenting with hyperleukocytosis. ∞*TLS* tumor lysis syndrome; ×*DIC* disseminated intravascular coagulation; °*CNS* central nervous system; ⁰*GI* gastrointestinal tract [8]

Case Demonstration (Continued)

Cytarabine infusion at 100 mg/m2 initiated. 24 h later, patient regained muscle strength in his arm and leg. He reported increasing nose and gum bleeding. His CBC showed a WBC of 23,000/μL, hemoglobin 9 g/dL, and platelets of 23,000/μL. His PT, INR, PTT, and fibrinogen were 23 s, 2.1, 67 s, and 134 mg/dL, respectively. A PTT mixing study showed a normalized PTT of 32 s. Patient was diagnosed with DIC.

Disseminated Intravascular Coagulation

Definition

Leukemia induced hyperfibrinolytic disseminated intravascular coagulation (DIC) is a life-threating complication associated with activation of coagulation system. DIC can result in bleeding and thrombosis [9]. Extensive and uncontrolled coagulation activation leads to severe hemostatic factor depletion and hemorrhagic manifestation. Particularly, APL is strongly associated with the complication.

Clinical Context

Clinical manifestations are heterogeneous and include severe/life-threatening bleeding and thrombosis, which is frequently observed during induction therapy. The incidence in non-APL cases, including acute lymphoblastic leukemia, varies between 8.5–25% [9]. In non-APL cases, the presence of Nucleophosmin 1 (*NMP1*) [10], and FMS-like tyrosine kinase 3 internal tandem duplication (*FLT3-ITD*) [11] are predictors for DIC. M5 FAB myelomonocytic leukemias harbor high proportion of *NPM1* mutations and are associated with significant DIC risk [10]. A significant number of AML cases with hyperleukocytosis develop thrombohemorrhagic complications and typically present with concomitant DIC and TLS. Thrombocytopenia and coagulation parameter modifications may signal overt DIC. In this context, high level of suspicious should be maintained to establish the diagnosis, especially if AML patients are receiving chemotherapy. The International Society of Thrombosis and Hemostasis (ISTH) scoring system (Table 4.1) is a helpful tool to facilitate recognition of the complication [12, 13].

Laboratory Investigation

(a) Coagulation profile including PT, PTT, fibrinogen, and soluble fibrin monomers/fibrin degradation products.
(b) Peripheral blood smear for investigation of red cell fragmentation.
(c) CBC differential.

Table 4.1 ISTH coring system for diagnosis of disseminated intravascular coagulation [12, 13]

Risk assessment: Does the patient have an underlying disorder known to be associated with overt DIC
If yes, proceed; if not, do not use this algorithm
Order global coagulation tests (platelet count, PT, fibrinogen, soluble fibrin monomers, or fibrin degradation products
Score Global Coagulation Test Results
Platelet count (>100 × 10^9/L, 0; <100 × 10^9/L, 1; <50, 2)
Elevated fibrin-related marker (i.e., soluble fibrin monomers/fibrin degradation products) (no increase = 0; moderate increase = 2; strong increase = 3)
Prolonged PT (<3 s, 0; >3 s but <6 s, 1, >6 s, 2)
Fibrinogen level (>1.0 g/L = 0; <1.0 g/L = 1)
Calculate Score
If ≥5, compatible with overt DIC

Management

Supportive Care

In patients with DIC and active bleeding:

(a) Platelets should be maintained $>50 \times 10^9/L$.
(b) Consider fresh frozen plasma (FFP) (15–30 mL × kg).
(c) Fibrinogen should be replaced with 2 units of cryoprecipitate in patients with persistent bleeding and fibrinogen below 150mg/dL [14].

In patients with DIC at risk of bleeding necessitating surgery or invasive procedures:

(a) Consider two doses of platelets if platelet count is less than $30 \times 10^9/L$ in APL and less than $20 \times 10^9/L$ in non-APL cases [14].

Caveats

In patients with active DIC and fibrinolysis, fibrinogen and platelets lifespan is significantly reduced requiring frequent monitoring. AML patients who develop neutropenic sepsis and hypotension can present with more severe coagulation factor deficiency, lower platelet and fibrinogen levels given impaired synthetic liver function.

Case Demonstration (Continued)

Patient's coagulopathy is resolved after completion of intravenous cytarabine for 7 days and idarubicin for 3 days [7 + 3 regimen]. On induction day 14, patient developed 103F temperature associated with tachycardia and blood pressure of 80/50 mmHg. Vancomycin plus cefepime intravenously were initiated.

Neutropenic Fever

Definition

Neutropenia refers to a decline in the absolute neutrophil count (ANC) below physiologic acceptable range of less than 1500 U/L. Neutrophils are frontline innate immunity protective mechanism. During administration of cytotoxic chemotherapy, direct bone marrow cytotoxicity results in progressive decline of absolute neutrophil count. Additionally, chemotherapy induced disruption of intestinal, lung, and skin barrier integrity facilitating bloodstream and tissue microbial invasion [15].

Neutropenia is defined as an absolute neutrophil count (ANC) of 0.5 K/μL or an ANC, which is expected to decline to 0.5 K/μL during the next 48 h.

Profound neutropenia is classically referred as an ANC <0.1 K/μL.

Functional neutropenia is conventionally defined as a qualitative neutrophil defect (i.e., impaired phagocytosis leading to defective bacterial eradication) developed from preexisting hemopoietic malignancies such as myelodysplastic syndrome [15].

Clinical Context

Risk and severity of infections in patients receiving chemotherapy are variable, but for better understanding, we should consider factors associated with the host, disease, and type of chemotherapy. Host-dependent factors include age and comorbid conditions such as diabetes, renal failure, and autoimmune disorders, especially if patient have received previous immunosuppressive therapy. As discussed in the previous chapters, AML can develop as de novo or secondary to preexisting hemopoietic conditions, such as MDS, MPN, or prior chemotherapy exposure (therapy-related AML). Risk for infection in AML and MDS increases with severity and duration of neutropenia. Particularly, MDS induces differentiation defects resulting in impaired neutrophil function. Studies have demonstrated that dysplastic neutrophils exhibit lower antimicrobial efficiency when compared to health donors [16]. Lastly, the type of chemotherapy, including commonly used regimens like 7 + 3, fludarabine+ cytarabine+ Idarubicin+ granulocyte colony stimulating factor (FLAG) and cladribine+ cytarabine+ granulocyte colony stimulating factor (CLAG), could induce profound and prolonged myeloid aplasia leading to higher infection risk. Fludarabine, high-dose steroids, cyclophosphamide, and bortezomib may impair T-cell function providing unique propensity for viral infection [17]. Recently approved regimens including hypomethylating agents (HMA) plus BCL-2 inhibitors are associated with a lower but still meaningful risk for infections. Treatment of neutropenic fever will not be our primary objective in this chapter. For a more detailed guidelines for the management of neutropenic host after chemotherapy, please refer to Chap. 8 for details. Here, we will emphasize the importance of careful clinical evaluation and timing after chemotherapy exposure to better address post AML therapy infections.

Important Timelines After Chemotherapy Exposure

AML patients receiving induction chemotherapy can develop severe infections, which are directly correlated with magnitude of absolute neutrophil count (ANC) decline. Additional host-dependent factors such as the mucositis enhance oral and gastrointestinal microbial translocation and bloodstream infections. In particular, hemolytic alpha streptococcus bacteremia may be observed among AML patients exposed to chemotherapy agents associated with oral and gastrointestinal mucosa ulceration. Figure 4.3 shows important timelines when evaluating febrile AML patient after induction therapy.

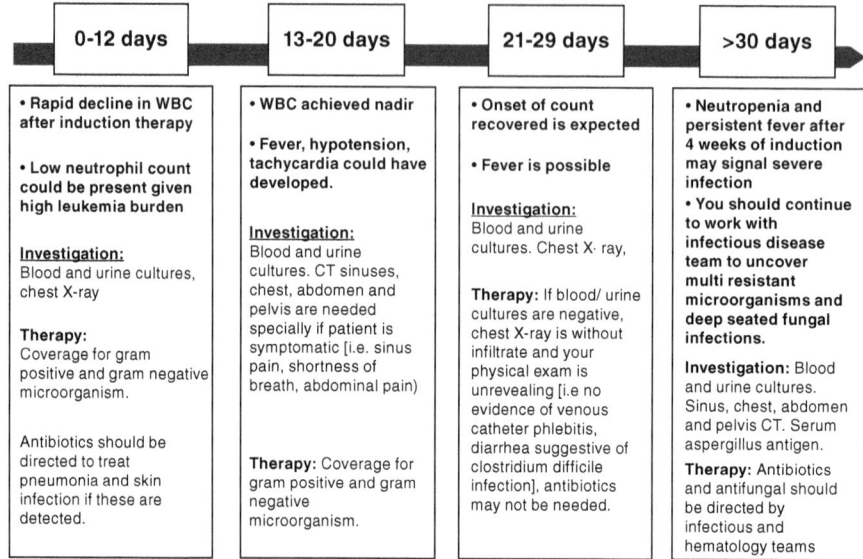

Fig. 4.3 Timeline for infections in febrile acute myelogenous leukemia patients receiving induction chemotherapy

Laboratory Investigation

(a) CBC differential.
(b) Comprehensive metabolic panel.
(c) Blood and urine cultures.
(d) If fungal infection is considered, especially "aspergillosis" [i.e., *A. fumigatus*, *A. flavus*, *A. niger*, and *A. terreus*], galactomannan antigen could assist in diagnosis.
(e) PCR for *Aspergillus* DNA for patients with suspected fungal infection.

Other Diagnostic Tools

(a) Sinus, chest, abdomen, and pelvis CT scan. Sinus and chest CT would be important, especially if diagnosis of sinus or lung fungal infection is considered. Imaging combined with serologic or bronchoalveolar lavage (BAL) cultures yields better diagnostic results [18].

Caveats

In AML patients undergoing induction or re-induction for relapsed disease, it would be important to obtain a careful history of previous infections. It is possible that colonization with resistant microorganism exits prior chemotherapy exposure. In these cases, antibiotic therapy should be directed to address the possibility that methicillin-resistant staphylococcus (MRSA) or vancomycin-resistant enterococci (VRE) are culprit. For AML patients being investigated for fungal infection who has received piperacillin-tazobactam, false-positive galactomannan antigen is possible given the presence of galactomannan in the antibiotic [19].

Tumor Lysis Syndrome

Case Demonstration

A 67-year-old patient was admitted with white blood cell count (WBC) of 120,000 u/l. His peripheral smear showed myeloblasts. Flow cytometry revealed CD34-negative CD117 CD33-positive blast consistent with acute myelogenous leukemia (AML). His lactate dehydrogenase was 3000 U/L. Her creatinine, uric acid, potassium, and phosphorous were 1.8 mg/dL, 9.5 m/dL, 5.6 mmol/L, and 4.9 mmol/dL, respectively. Azacitidine plus BCL-2 inhibitor were initiated. Intravenous (IV) fluid plus allopurinol orally at 200 mg were administered. On day 2, her creatinine was 2.2 mg/dL and uric acid 9 mg/dL.

Definition

Tumor lysis syndrome (TLS) is a life-threatening condition resulting from rapid spontaneous and/or drug-induced tumor cell death. Acute tubular necrosis associated with overwhelming accumulation of uric acid is central to renal dysfunction [1] TLS is a unique complication that requires prompt recognition and therapy. Management should be directed to prevention and restoration of organ functions once complication has initiated.

Clinical Context

- High hemopoietic tumor burden and/or leukocytosis.
- Higher risk for patients with myelomonocytic leukemia and white blood cell count [WBC] > 50 K/uL.

Clinical Manifestations

- Rapid weight gain.
- Electrolyte abnormalities and arrhythmias.
- Oliguria or anuria.
- Shortness of breath as results of volume overload and/or metabolic acidosis.
- Acute renal failure.

Laboratory Investigation

- Lactate dehydrogenase, uric acid, creatinine, phosphate.

Risk Stratification

The risk for severe TLS complications should be promptly considered in high-risk patients. Uric acid, WBC, evidence of bulky adenopathy, and LDH (Table 4.2) can guide initial management (Fig. 4.4 and Table 4.3).

Table 4.2 Risk stratification for tumor lysis syndrome [20]

Low risk	High risk
• Serum uric acid <8 mg/dL	• Serum uric acid >8 mg/dL
• White blood cell count <25 K/uL	• White blood cell count >100 K/uL
• Lack of bulky adenopathies	• Bulky adenopathies [stage 3/4 lymphoma]
• Absence of bulky myeloid sarcoma	• Large myeloid sarcoma
• Lactate dehydrogenase <2 upper limit of normal	• Lactate dehydrogenase >2 upper limit of normal

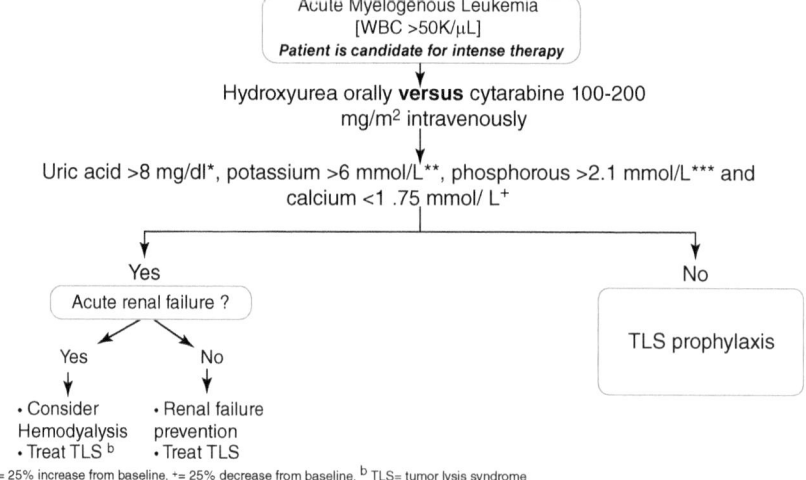

****= 25% increase from baseline, += 25% decrease from baseline, b TLS= tumor lysis syndrome

Fig. 4.4 Pharmacologic and supportive management of TLS based on clinical and laboratory findings

Table 4.3 Management of tumor lysis syndrome [20]

Low risk	High risk	
Most of patients treated as outpatients Allopurinol	**2 factors?**	
	Yes	No
	IV fluids Allopurinol Rasburicase Correct electrolytes Close monitoring of kidney function Hemodialysis if rapid renal function deterioration	IV fluids Allopurinol Monitor electrolytes

Management

Caveats

Chronic lymphocytic leukemia (CLL) patients treated with venetoclax or fludarabine are at high risk for tumor lysis syndrome. Risk for TLS is at the highest during 1–3 cycle of therapy and significantly decrease thereafter.

Specific Considerations

- Intravenous fluid (preferred saline 0.9%) at 75–150 cc per hour.
- Consider allopurinol at 300 mg orally daily. Renal adjustment is needed for this medication.
- Patients who are at high risk of renal failure and under specific circumstances rasburicase are indicated.
- In elderly patients diagnosed with AML and lymphoma with impaired ejection fraction, fluids should be cautiously administered and weight should be recorded and monitor during admission.

References

1. Stucki A, Rivier AS, Gikic M, Monai N, Schapira M, Spertini O. Endothelial cell activation by myeloblasts: molecular mechanisms of leukostasis and leukemic cell dissemination. Blood. 2001;97(7):2121–9.
2. Bruserud O, Liseth K, Stamnesfet S, Cacic DL, Melve G, Kristoffersen E, et al. Hyperleukocytosis and leukocytapheresis in acute leukaemias: experience from a single centre and review of the literature of leukocytapheresis in acute myeloid leukaemia. Transfus Med. 2013;23(6):397–406.
3. Nan X, Qin Q, Gentille C, Ensor J, Leveque C, Pingali SR, et al. Leukapheresis reduces 4-week mortality in acute myeloid leukemia patients with hyperleukocytosis—a retrospective study from a tertiary center. Leuk Lymphoma. 2017;58(9):1–11.

4. Stahl M, Shallis RM, Wei W, Montesinos P, Lengline E, Neukirchen J, et al. Management of hyperleukocytosis and impact of leukapheresis among patients with acute myeloid leukemia (AML) on short- and long-term clinical outcomes: a large, retrospective, multicenter, international study. Leukemia. 2020;34(12):3149–60.
5. Tien FM, Hou HA, Tsai CH, Tang JL, Chen CY, Kuo YY, et al. Hyperleukocytosis is associated with distinct genetic alterations and is an independent poor-risk factor in de novo acute myeloid leukemia patients. Eur J Haematol. 2018;101(1):86–94.
6. Coffe C, Pouthier F, Barisien C, Slimane M, Sheytanova A. Therapeutic leukapheresis and thrombapheresis in medical emergencies. Transfus Apher Sci. 2020;59(6):102997.
7. Mamez AC, Raffoux E, Chevret S, Lemiale V, Boissel N, Canet E, et al. Pre-treatment with oral hydroxyurea prior to intensive chemotherapy improves early survival of patients with high hyperleukocytosis in acute myeloid leukemia. Leuk Lymphoma. 2016;57(10):2281–8.
8. Rollig C, Ehninger G. How I treat hyperleukocytosis in acute myeloid leukemia. Blood. 2015;125(21):3246–52.
9. Guo Z, Chen X, Tan Y, Xu Z, Xu L. Coagulopathy in cytogenetically and molecularly distinct acute leukemias at diagnosis: comprehensive study. Blood Cells Mol Dis. 2020;81:102393.
10. Cheng Z, Hu K, Tian L, Dai Y, Pang Y, Cui W, et al. Clinical and biological implications of mutational spectrum in acute myeloid leukemia of FAB subtypes M4 and M5. Cancer Gene Ther. 2018;25(3–4):77–83.
11. Marasca R, Maffei R, Zucchini P, Castelli I, Saviola A, Martinelli S, et al. Gene expression profiling of acute promyelocytic leukaemia identifies two subtypes mainly associated with flt3 mutational status. Leukemia. 2006;20(1):103–14.
12. Thachil J, Falanga A, Levi M, Di Nisio M, Scientific and Standardization Committee of the International Society on Thrombosis and Hemostasis. Management of cancer-associated disseminated intravascular coagulation: guidance from the SSC of the ISTH. J Thromb Haemost. 2015;13(4):671–5.
13. Kunwar S, Alam M, Ezekwueme F, Yasir M, Lawrence JA, Shah S, et al. Diagnostic scores and treatment options for acute disseminated intravascular coagulation in children. Cureus. 2021;13(9):e17682.
14. Wada H, Matsumoto T, Department of Hematology and Oncology, Mie University School of Medicine, Mie, Japan, Aota T, Yamashita Y, Suzuki K, Katayama N. Management of cancer-associated disseminated intravascular coagulation: guidance from the SSC of the ISTH: comment. J Thromb Haemost. 2016;14(6):1314–5.
15. Freifeld AG, Bow EJ, Sepkowitz KA, Boeckh MJ, Ito JI, Mullen CA, et al. Clinical practice guideline for the use of antimicrobial agents in neutropenic patients with cancer: 2010 update by the infectious diseases society of America. Clin Infect Dis. 2011;52(4):e56–93.
16. Fianchi L, Leone G, Posteraro B, Sanguinetti M, Guidi F, Valentini CG, et al. Impaired bactericidal and fungicidal activities of neutrophils in patients with myelodysplastic syndrome. Leuk Res. 2012;36(3):331–3.
17. Sharpley FA, De-Silva D, Mahmood S, Sachchithanantham S, Ramsay I, Garcia Mingo A, et al. Cytomegalovirus reactivation after bortezomib treatment for multiple myeloma and light chain amyloidosis. Eur J Haematol. 2020;104(3):230–5.
18. Gavalda J, Len O, San Juan R, Aguado JM, Fortun J, Lumbreras C, et al. Risk factors for invasive aspergillosis in solid-organ transplant recipients: a case-control study. Clin Infect Dis. 2005;41(1):52–9.
19. Walsh TJ, Shoham S, Petraitiene R, Sein T, Schaufele R, Kelaher A, et al. Detection of galactomannan antigenemia in patients receiving piperacillin-tazobactam and correlations between in vitro, in vivo, and clinical properties of the drug-antigen interaction. J Clin Microbiol. 2004;42(10):4744–8.
20. Mato AR, Riccio BE, Qin LDF, et al. A predictive model for the detection of tumor lysis syndrome during AML induction therapy. Leuk Lymphoma. 2006;47(5):877–83.

Chapter 5
Acute Chemotherapy Administration and Complications

Linda Zhang and Gustavo Rivero

Management of Adult AML

In patients without hyperproliferative disease and/or organ compromise, it would be adequate to initiate chemotherapy once *NPM1* and *FLT3* sequencing data is available, which could take 72 h.

Initial efforts should be made to stabilize the patient's conditions and control complications. Initiation of chemotherapy should be started after assessment of the patient's medical fitness, which is determined by performance status combined with the severity of their medical comorbidities. The following are **performance status** measures (Table 5.1) that are considered acceptable for intensive induction chemotherapy:

- Eastern Cooperative Oncology Group (ECOG) PS: 0 to 1.
- Karnofsky PS ≥ 80.

The severity of **medical comorbidities** can be assessed using the hematopoietic cell transplantation-specific comorbidity index (IICT-CI) (Table 5.2). HCT-CI <3 is considered acceptable for further intensive treatment.

L. Zhang (✉)
Graduate Program in Translational Biology and Molecular Medicine, Baylor College of Medicine, Houston, TX, USA
e-mail: Linda.zhang@bcm.edu

G. Rivero
Lombardi Cancer Institute, Georgetown University School of Medicine, Washington, DC, USA
e-mail: garivero@bcm.edu

© The Author(s), under exclusive license to Springer Nature
Switzerland AG 2024
G. Rivero, I. R. Sosa (eds.), *Consulting Hematology and Oncology Handbook*,
https://doi.org/10.1007/978-3-031-75810-2_5

Table 5.1 Acceptable performance status measures (ECOG and Karnofsky) to determine patient's medical fitness

ECOG		Karnofsky	
Score	Definition	Score	Definition
0	Fully active, no performance restrictions	100	Normal, no complaints or evidence of disease
1	Strenuous physical activity restricted, ambulatory and able to carry light work	90	Able to carry normal activity, minor signs, or symptoms
2	Capable of self-care but unable to do any work activities; up and about >50% of waking hours	80	Normal activity with effort, some signs, or symptoms
3	Capable of only limited self-care; confined to bed or chair >50% waking hours	70	Cares for self, unable to carry normal activity or do active work
4	Completely disabled; cannot carry out any self-care; totally confined to bed or chair	60	Requires occasional assistance but able to care for most needs
5	Dead	50	Requires considerable assistance and frequent medical care
		40	Disabled, requires special care
		30	Severely disabled, hospitalization indicated, death not imminent
		20	Hospitalization necessary, very sick, active supportive treatment necessary
		10	Moribund, fatal processes, progressing rapidly
		0	Dead

Acute Promyelocytic Leukemia

APL is a clinically distinct variant of AML characterized most commonly by the balanced translocation of t(15;17)(q22;q12-21) which leads to the fusion of the promyelocytic leukemia (*PML*) gene with the retinoic acid receptor alpha (*RARA*) gene [1]. This fusion leads to the arrest of granulocyte differentiation and the abnormal accumulation of promyelocytes in the bone marrow. Patients with APL typically present as medical emergencies, often with significant hemorrhage due to severe coagulopathies and disseminated intravascular thromboses. Therefore, patients suspected of APL should be immediately initiated on *all-trans* retinoic acid (ATRA) therapy to prevent hemorrhagic complications and mortality. The use of ATRA combination therapy with arsenic trioxide (ATO) and other chemotherapies has allowed APL to be a curable disease among hematologic malignancies.

Case Demonstration

A 38-year-old female presents with weakness and frequent nosebleeds. Her white count is 120 K, and promyelocytes were observed in the peripheral blood smear (Fig. 5.1). Flow cytometry demonstrated CD34$^-$, HLA-DR$^-$, CD33$^+$, CD117$^+$

Table 5.2 Hematopoietic stem cell transplantation-specific comorbidity index (HCT-CI) for evaluation of patient's medical fitness [1]

Hematopoietic stem cell transplantation-specific comorbidity index (HCT-CI)		
	Definition	Score
Pulmonary disease		
Mild	Dyspnea with moderate activity and/or FEV1 81–90%	0
Moderate	Dyspnea on slight activity and/or FEV1 66–80%	2
Severe	Dyspnea at rest or requires O2, and/or FEV1 $\leq$ 65%	3
Cardiac disease		
General	CAD, CHF, MI, or EF $\leq$ 50%	1
Arrhythmia	Afib or flutter, sick sinus syndrome, ventricular arrhythmias	1
Heart valve disease	Except mitral valve prolapse	3
Hepatic disease		
Mild	Chronic hepatitis, Bilirubin > 1–1.5× ULN, AST/ALT > 1–2.5× ULN	1
Moderate–Severe	Cirrhosis or fibrosis; Bilirubin >1.5× ULN or AST/ALT > 2.5× ULN	3
Renal disease		
Mild	Creatinine 1.2–2 mg/dL	0
Moderate–Severe	Creatinine >2 mg/dL, renal dialysis, or renal transplant	2
Other malignancies		
Prior solid tumor	Treated at any point in the patient's past history, excluding nonmelanoma skin cancer	3
Other comorbidities		
Diabetes	Requiring treatment with insulin or oral hypoglycemics but not diet alone	1
Cerebrovascular disease	Transient ischemic attack or cerebrovascular accident	1
Rheumatologic	SLE, RA, polymyositis, mixed CTD, or polymyalgia rheumatica	2
Peptic ulcer	Requiring treatment	2
Psychiatric disturbance	Depression or anxiety requiring psychiatric consult or treatment	1
Infection	Requiring continuation of antimicrobial after day 0	1
Inflammatory bowel disease	Crohn's disease or ulcerative colitis	1
Obesity	BMI >35 kg/m^2	1

myeloblasts. Her fibrinogen was 130, platelets were 23 K. FISH was positive for PML/RARA and next-generation sequencing revealed a FLT3-ITD mutation. Patient was initiated on high-risk induction therapy with ATRA + ATO + IDA.

Fig. 5.1 Acute
promyelocytic leukemia.
Red arrow demonstrate
promyelocyte exhibiting
significant granulation

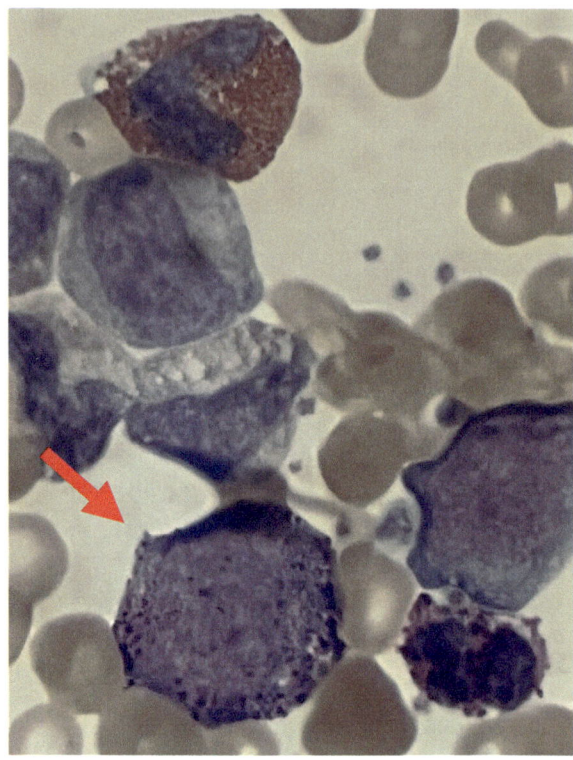

Table 5.3 Risk stratification
for patients with APL

Risk stratification	WBC
Low	<10,000/μL
High	>10,000/μL

APL Risk Stratification

Prognostic factors were identified by the Italian Group for Adult Hematologic Diseases (GINEMA) and Spanish PETHEMA group who determined risk stratification based on WBC and platelet counts. However, National Comprehensive Cancer Network (NCCN) recommend stratification based on WBC only (Table 5.3) [2].

Treatment of APL

Choice of therapy regimen for APL is based on the patient's risk stratification. A key component of APL therapy includes the use of ATRA, which leads to the differentiation of leukemic promyelocytes into mature granulocytes. However, during ATRA remission-induction, patients may develop hyperleukocytosis and severe side effects. Therefore, ATRA must be used in combination with arsenic trioxide

(ATO) or other cytoreductive therapies such as hydroxyurea to prevent hyperleuko-cytosis and the incidence of relapse [3].

Upon suspicion of APL, patients should be immediately started on ATRA therapy at 45 mg/m^2/day in two divided doses. Avoid any invasive procedures and leukapheresis before and during induction therapy due to high risk of hemorrhagic complications. Additionally, supportive measures should be taken to correct any coagulopathies, and the following parameters should be achieved via transfusions if necessary:

- Platelets > 30 × 10^9/L.
- Fibrinogen > 100 mg/dL.
- INR < 1.5–2.0.

  - Monitor PTT, aPTT, thrombin time, fibrinogen, and fibrinogen degradation products daily until resolution of coagulopathies.

Low-Risk Induction

Clinical trials comparing ATRA+ATO to ATRA+chemotherapy (idarubicin) showed that ATRA-ATO resulted in fewer deaths during induction therapy, significantly less toxicity, and fewer short- and long-term relapses [4–6] in patients with low- and intermediate-risk APL.

- **ATRA Dosing**: Daily divided oral dose of 45 mg/m^2 dose until complete remission.
- **ATO Dosing**: Therapeutic advantage has been achieved using two different dosing schedules based on the Italian-German and NCRI clinical trials. While the total amount of ATO administered is almost identical, the main differences are in scheduling and duration of treatment.

  - *Italian-German Trial*: 0.15 mg/kg daily until complete remission [6].
  - *NCRI Trial*: 0.3 mg/kg on days 1–5; 0.25 mg/kg twice weekly for 7 weeks [5].

High-Risk Induction

In patients with high-risk APL (>10,000 WBC), there is less consensus on the optimal treatment regimen. There are currently two potential treatment options for high-risk patients:

- ATRA + ATO + [cytoreduction therapy with **idarubicin** (IDA) *or* **gemtuzumab ozogamicin** (GO)].
- ATRA + anthracycline-containing chemotherapy.

  - ATRA + Daunorubicin + Cytarabine.
  - ATRA + Idarubicin.

GO is an anti-CD33 monoclonal antibody conjugated to calicheamicin, a class of antitumor antibiotics derived from bacteria. Studies have shown that inclusion of GO was well tolerated and resulted in a 3-year overall survival rate of 86% in patients with high-risk APL [7]. However, many centers currently do not have GO readily available. In these settings, IDA can be used instead for patients with normal left ventricular ejection [8]. In the United States and Europe, the FDA and EMA have restricted the use of ATO to non-high-risk patients only making ATO-containing regimens problematic in these regions [9]. Clinical trials combining ATRA with anthracycline-containing chemotherapies have shown 90–95% CR rates and 85–90% rates of long-term survival [10, 11], offering a favorable alternative to ATO-containing regimens.

Neither treatment options have shown superiority in clinical trials. Due to the heterogeneity of studies of ATRA + ATO + different schedules of chemotherapies, there are currently no officially recommended treatment regimens for high-risk APL patients from European LeukemiaNet guidelines. However, the NCCN guidelines recommend age-adjusted idarubicin at 6–12 mg/m^2 on days 2, 4, 6, and 8 plus arsenic trioxide at 0.15 mg/kg on days 9–36. Alternatively, in patients with impaired ejection fraction, gemtuzumab ozogamicin could be administered at 9 mg/m^2 or 6 mg/m^2, per 1 dose depending whether arsenic trioxide is given at 0.15 mg/kg/day or 0.3 mg/kg/day, respectively.

Caveats

APL patients on ATRA and/or ATO therapy may develop *differentiation syndrome (DS)*, which occurs in ~20% of patients approximately 1–2 weeks after induction of therapy but can also occur later (Table 5.4) [12]. DS is caused by the large burden of rapidly maturing granulocytes leading to a systemic inflammatory response due to the release of cytokines.

All patients should be closely monitored for *clinical manifestations of DS* [13], which include:

- Dyspnea.
- Unexplained fever.
- Hypotension.
- Peripheral edema.
- Weight gain.
- Pleuro-pericardial effusion.
- Acute renal failure.
- Musculoskeletal pain.
- Hyperbilirubinemia.

Table 5.4 Acute differentiation syndrome in APL patients receiving ATRA plus ATO

Caveat	Management
Significant leukocytosis at presentation (WBC > 10×10^9/L)	Cytoreductive therapy should be initiated immediately even if molecular testing still pending • ATRA + chemotherapy (idarubicin or daunorubicin +/− cytarabine) • For patients being treated with ATRA + ATO, cytoreduction can be achieved with idarubicin (12 mg/m^2) or GO (6–9 mg/m^2) Avoid leukapheresis Can give prophylactic steroids to reduce risk of DS
Significant increase in WBC *after* treatment induction with ATRA and/or ATO	Treat with one of the following: • **Hydroxyurea** (2 g/d) • 1–2 doses of **IDA** (12 mg/m^2) or • **GO** (6–9 mg/m^2) in cases of extreme hyperleukocytosis
Management of ATO therapy	Carefully monitor electrolytes: • K > 4 mEq/L • Mg > 1.8 mg/dL Monitor QT/QTc by ECG at least twice weekly • Withhold ATO and replete electrolytes if QT or QTc interval is prolonged >500 ms until interval returns to ~460 ms
Fluid overload	Monitor weight daily and input/outputs Diuretics to keep fluid balance even
CNS prophylaxis for extramedullary disease	Only for patients with hyperleukocytosis • Delay CNS prophylaxis until achieving CR due to high risk of hemorrhagic complications associated with lumbar puncture

Additional diagnostic evaluations may also show the following abnormalities [14]:

- *CBC and blood chemistries*: Elevated WBC, anemia, thrombocytopenia, coagulopathy, elevated creatinine.
- *Chest radiographs*: Pleural effusions, increased cardiothoracic ratio, septal lines and peribronchial cuffing, increased vascular pedicle width.

Management of DS

Prophylactic steroids should be promptly initiated if DS is suspected.

- If ≥1 clinical feature, immediately start dexamethasone 10 mg IV every 12 h in conjunction with ongoing diagnostic evaluation [15].
- Dosing schedule can be increased to every 6 h if response to initial treatment is inadequate.
- Continue dexamethasone for 3 days until symptoms subside before tapering.
- Monitor for recurrence of DS during steroid taper.
- Hold ATRA + ATO only in cases of severe DS until symptoms resolved.

Minimal Residual Disease (MRD) Monitoring after Induction

At the end of induction therapy, molecular assessment of a new marrow sample should be performed. Real-time quantitative polymerase chain reaction (RQ-PCR) is the standard method for molecular monitoring in APL.

Consolidation

Due to advances in treatment regimens, complete remission is currently attainable in all APL patients with genetically confirmed PML/RARA fusions.

- *For patients treated with ATRA + ATO (low-risk ALP)*: ATO 0.15 mg/kg/day for 4 weeks every 8 weeks for a total of 4 cycles and ATRA 45 mg/m^2 for 2 weeks every 4 weeks for a total of 7 cycles.
- *For patients treated with ATRA + chemotherapy (high-risk AP)*: 4 weeks consolidation therapy with ATRA at 45 mg/m^2 plus ATO (0.15 mg/kg/day, for 4 week per 1 cycle, followed by ATRA at 45 mg/m^2 for 7 days every 2 weeks for 3 cycles plus ATO at 0.15 /kg/day for 5 weeks per 1 cycle.

- Or

- ATO 0.15 mg/kg/day, 5 days for 5 weeks every 7 weeks for a total of 2 cycles, and then ATRA 45 mg/m^2 for 7 days plus 2 courses of anthracycline-based chemotherapy should be given for consolidation.

A new marrow sample should be assessed by RQ-PCR for molecular remission upon completion of consolidation therapy.

Management After Consolidation

Prolonged MRD monitoring can be avoided in non-high-risk patients who achieve complete remission, MRD$^-$ status regardless of treatment regimen. These patients should receive CBC assessment every 3 months and do not require maintenance therapy.

High-risk patients should receive CBC + RQ-PCR of peripheral blood every 3 months for 2–3 years. In patients with molecular persistence of disease even after consolidation therapy, hematopoietic stem cell transplantation should be considered.

Management of Non-APL Acute Myeloid Leukemia

Case Demonstration

A 47-year-old patient presents with recurrent headaches and weight loss over the past month, multiple bruises, and fatigue. His WBC count was 118 K/uL at presentation, and he was subsequently admitted for further evaluation of suspected AML. Bone marrow analysis revealed hypercellular marrow with 80% blasts and flow cytometry demonstrated CD13, CD33, CD117 positivity. Molecular studies revealed *DNMT3A* R882H and *FLT3-ITD* mutations, and cytogenetics were significant for t(8;21)(q22;q22.1).

Hyperleukocytosis in Newly Diagnosed AML

For our patient with hyperleukocytosis (defined as WBC $\geq 100 \times 10^9$/L), the main initial goal is to rapidly reduce his WBC due to the high mortality rate related to leukostasis, hyperviscosity, organ failure, DIC, and tumor lysis syndrome [16]. In highly specialized centers, three strategies could be considered:

Leukapheresis

Exchange transfusions are used to mechanically separate leukocytes from blood to achieve rapid cytoreductions in hyperleukocytosis-presenting AML patients with symptoms of leukostasis. If apheresis equipment is unavailable at the treatment center, careful phlebotomies with concurrent blood/plasma replacements may be used.

- Carefully monitor O_2 saturation, blood pressure, and heart rate during intervention. Transfer to ICU if necessary for continuous monitoring.
- RBC transfusions should only be given at the end of leukapheresis to avoid further increase in blood viscosity.
- Leukapheresis can be performed daily until symptoms of leukostasis disappear or WBC $< 100 \times 10^9$/L.

Caveats

In patients necessitating access, carefully evaluate the possibility of DIC development. This procedure should always be avoided in patients with APL. PT, PTT, fibrinogen, and platelet count should be available before catheter insertion. Quick coagulopathy correction could be achieved with fresh frozen plasma, cryoprecipitate infusions.

- May aggravate preexisting thrombocytopenia. One study found a reduction in almost 50% of platelets after two cycles of leukapheresis [17].

- Leukapheresis may also only result in a transient reduction in WBC, as the blasts originating in the bone marrow are not eliminated using this procedure. There is risk for rebound hyperleukocytosis that must be monitored [18].
- Hypocalcemia may occur due to calcium chelation from citrate anticoagulation in the apheresis equipment. Monitor patient for signs of hypocalcemia-induced paresthesia.

Hydroxyurea (HU)

Studies have shown that pretreatment with oral hydroxyurea prior to intensive induction therapy can improve early survival of AML patients presenting with hyperleukocytosis [19].

- Oral 50–60 mg/kg per day until the WBC count is 20×10^9/L [20].

Cytarabine Infusion

Standard- or high-dose cytarabine can be initiated after diagnosis of hyperleukocytosis-AML is made [21, 22].

Caveats

Due to the high burden of leukocyte cell death by HU and cytarabine, efforts should be made to prevent tumor lysis syndrome.

- Increase IV hydration, treat with allopurinol or rasburicase to decrease serum uric acid, and control of urine pH.
- Cytoreduction using HU is slower compared to leukapheresis.

While leukapheresis has been the preferred method in some centers, recent systematic reviews questioned the clinical benefit of this procedure regarding early mortality [18]. Additionally, another studied showed a lack of evidence for the superiority of leukapheresis, HU/low-dose cytarabine compared to standard-dose induction therapy [23]. Due to the lack of randomized trials and the critical timeliness of decision-making upon diagnosis, the management of hyperleukocytosis AML continues to remain a challenge.

A recent study published in 2021 achieved rapid, profound, and sustained cytoreduction using a single high-dose treatment with cyclophosphamide (HDC, 60 mg/kg IV) [24]. A major caveat to this study, however, is that 30–67% of patients received adjunct therapies such as HU or leukapheresis in conjunction with HDC for cytoreduction. However, this is not considered current standard therapy for initial management of AML.

Pretreatment Evaluation

Additional evaluation and procedures must be performed on the patient in preparation for chemotherapy.

- **In-depth history and physical exam** (especially history of prior hematologic disorders or cytotoxic therapies).
- *Laboratory Studies*.
  - *Baseline blood chemistries* pertinent to tumor lysis syndrome monitoring: uric acid, LDH, phosphate, calcium, potassium, renal functions.
  - CBC with differential, coagulation studies, viral serologies, liver function tests, urinalysis for renal function.
  - *HLA typing* for future consideration of transfusions and hematopoietic stem cell transplantation.
  - Germline mutation screening when indicated, especially if matched sibling donors are considered for allogeneic transplantation.
- **Other**.
  - 2D or 3D echocardiogram for cardiac evaluation
  - Neurologic evaluation (lumbar puncture in patients with high-risk features, avoid in APL patients).
  - Fertility counseling for patients with child-bearing potential.
  - Establish venous access via PICC line.

"7 + 3" Induction Therapy for Medically Fit Patients

This regimen consists of 7 days of continuous cytarabine (Ara-C) along with shorter infusions of anthracycline on days 1–3. These treatments require adequate cardiac, hepatic, and renal functions which should be assessed in the pretreatment evaluation.

- **Cytarabine (Ara-C)**: 100–200 mg/m^2 daily as continuous infusion for 7 days.
- **Anthracycline Chemotherapy**.
  - Idarubicin: 12 mg/m^2 on days 1–3 **or**
  - Daunorubicin: 60–90 mg/m^2 on days 1–3.

Acute Chemotherapy Complications

Patients will typically be admitted during induction therapy due to high risk of developing cytopenias, infections, infusion reactions, and more.

- *"Cytarabine Syndrome"*: Patients may develop fever, rash, rigors, diaphoresis, myalgias, arthralgias, conjunctivitis, and, occasionally, hypotension, which may develop within 6–12 h of infusion [25].

  - Acetaminophen and/or glucocorticoids before and after each day's drug infusion may help with both treatment and prevention of symptoms [26, 27].

- *Anthracycline-Related Infusion Reactions*: Erythema at the infusion site, flushing, dyspnea, facial edema, headache, chills, tightness of the chest or throat [28].

  - Occurs more often with liposomal anthracyclines [29].
  - Pretreatment with diphenhydramine and/or glucocorticoids can prevent symptoms [30].

- *Profound Cytopenias*: Monitor with CBC w/ differential and coagulation studies.

  - Be wary of signs of neutropenic fever and infection.
  - Transfuse with leukocyte-depleted, irradiated blood products if necessary (maintain Hg between 8–9 g/dL).

- *Tumor Lysis Syndrome (TLS)*: Massive tumor cell lysis leads to the release of life-threatening levels of potassium, phosphate, and nucleic acids into circulation.

  - Laboratory criteria V (Cairo-Bishop Definition) [31]:

    - Uric acid ≥ 8 mg/dL.
    - Potassium ≥ 6 mEq/L.
    - Phosphorus: ≥ 4.5 mg/dL.
    - Calcium ≤ 7 mg/dL.

  - Clinical signs include cardiac arrhythmias and seizures.
  - *Laboratory studies for monitoring*: Serum concentrations of uric acid, phosphate, potassium, creatinine calcium, and LDH; urine I/Os.
  - For more on TLS, please refer to Chap. 4.

- *Disseminated intravascular coagulation (DIC)*: DIC is a medical emergency caused by the abnormal activation of coagulation and fibrinolysis leading to massive bleeding. Coagulation studies should be monitored closely during induction therapy as DIC can be triggered by chemotherapy. Abnormal findings indicative of acute DIC include:

Parameter	Acute DIC findings
• Thrombin time	• Prolonged
• Prothrombin time (PT)	• Prolonged
• Activated partial thromboplastin time (aPTT)	• Prolonged
• Fibrinogen	• Reduced
• Factors V and VIII	• Reduced
• Fibrin degradation products	• Elevated
• D-dimers	• Elevated

  - For more on DIC, please refer to Chap. 4.

Additional Therapies to Backbone 7 + 3

Depending on the patient's mutation status, an additional monoclonal antibody or targeted therapy may be added to the 7 + 3 regimen to improve the chances for achieving CR.

- *FLT3* + patients: Patients with FLT3-ITD or FLT3-TKD mutations will benefit from the addition of **midostaurin (Rydapt)**, a multitargeted kinase inhibitor. A phase 3, multi-institutional, international clinical trial (RATIFY) showed the addition of midostaurin led to superior outcomes in young patients compared to those who received 7 + 3 therapy only [32].

  - 50 mg orally BID on days 8–21 of induction therapy.
  - Four 28-day cycles of consolidation therapy with high-dose cytarabine (3000 mg/m^2 over a period of 3 h q12 h on days 1, 3, 5). Midostaurin administered 40 mg BID on days 8–21.
  - Hold midostaurin if corrected QT interval is >500 ms.
  - Be careful co-administering with other strong CYP34A inhibitors.

- *CD33+ patients*: Patients with CD33+ disease, especially in favorable core binding factor [t(8;21) and inv(16) AML], shown by flow cytometry can receive IV **gemtuzumab ozogamicin (Mylotarg** or **GO)**. A phase 3 clinical trial (ALFA-0701) found that GO significantly improved event-free survival (EFS), but did not affect rates of CR. Although the OS trended higher in the GO arm, the difference did not reach statistical significance (27.5 months in GO group vs. 21.8 months in the control group) [33].

  - 3 mg/m^2 on days 1, 4, and 7 during 7 + 3 induction.
  - 3 mg/m2 on day 1 of consolidation therapy (two rounds).
  - Acquire baseline liver function tests and monitor for hepatotoxicity, veno-occlusive disease, infusion-related reactions, and infection.

Liposomal Daunorubicin Plus Cytarabine

CPX-351 dual drug liposomal cytarabine plus daunorubicin demonstrated CR rate of about 29–32% in patients harboring *P53* abnormalities. It is currently recommended for patients younger and older than 60 years who are candidate for intense treatment strategies.

Treatment Options for Medically Unfit Patients

Older patients with multiple comorbidities cannot receive high-intensity induction therapy. Although treatment alternatives for these patients remain a challenge, current options include:

- Supportive care.
- Clinical trials.
- Low-intensity chemotherapy.

  - Hypomethylating agents (HMA).
  - Low-dose cytarabine (LDAC).
  - Targeted therapies (IDH1/2 and FLT3 inhibitors).

Case Demonstration

A 72-year-old patient presents with a 30-lb unintentional weight loss, fever, fatigue, and petechiae. His WBC count was 3.4 K/uL and he was admitted for further evaluation. His bone marrow aspiration showed 80% myelomonocytic blasts and flow cytometry demonstrated positivity for CD15, CD34, and MPO. Further cytogenetic analysis revealed −7 deletion and mutational analysis showed *NRAS* G12D and *STAG2* R216* mutations.

Low-Intensity Therapy Options

The patient described in the case demonstration would not be a candidate for intense 7 + 3 induction therapy. However, low-intensity interventions with hypomethylating agents, especially if combined with BCL-2 inhibitor, have demonstrated improvement in complete remission rate and overall survival.

Hypomethylating Agents (Monotherapy)

A phase 3 clinical trial (AZA-AML-001) published in 2015 showed the hypomethylating agent (HMA), **azacitidine**, had superior median OS compared to three strategies of conventional therapies including LDAC, supportive care, or 7 + 3 [34].

- Azacitidine 75 mg/m^2 subcutaneously daily for seven consecutive days/28 day cycles.
- Treat for at least 6 cycles.
- Treatment may be delayed as needed until blood counts recover.

Similarly, **decitabine** was also found to significantly improve median OS and EFS compared to LDAC or supportive care in the phase 3 DACO-016 clinical trial [35]. Additionally, in contrast to standard therapy, the presence of high-risk karyotypes and *TP53* mutations did not affect sensitivity to HMAs [36].

- $20 \ mg/m^2$ IV over 1 h, daily × 5 consecutive days, repeated every 4 weeks

Caveats

A population-based study later found that the median OS of elderly AML patients treated with azacitidine or decitabine was 7.1 and 8.2 months, respectively [37], suggesting that these therapies are insufficient for achieving long-term remission.

BCL-2 Inhibitor Combination Therapies

The combination of the BCL2 inhibitor, Venetoclax, was shown to work synergistically with LDAC *or* azacitidine to significantly increase median OS, CR, and EFS in the VIALE-C and VIALE-A clinical trials [38, 39] when compared to LDAC or HMA monotherapy.

- **VIALE-C**: Venetoclax (600 mg QD PO × 28 days) + LDAC ($20 \ mg/m^2$ subcutaneously daily on days 1–10).
- **VIALE-A**: Venetoclax (400 mg QD PO × 28 days) + Azacitidine ($75 \ mg/m^2$ subcutaneously or IV on days 1–7).
  - To mitigate TLS, dose of Venetoclax was 100 mg on day 1, 200 mg on day 2, and 400 mg on days 3–28.

Caveats

Significant thrombocytopenia and febrile neutropenia occurred in patients treated with Venetoclax.

- Venetoclax dose adjustments are necessary when combined with strong CYP3A4 inhibitors (antifungals, fluoroquinolones).
- Retrospective analysis suggests that once patients become unresponsive to Ven/Aza, the prognosis is very poor.

Targeted Therapies

- *IDH1 and 2 inhibitors*: Older patients (≥ 75 years) with *IDH1*- or *IDH2*-mutated newly diagnosed and relapsed or refractory AML can receive targeted therapy with **Ivosidenib** [40] and **enasidenib** [41], respectively, based on phase I/II clinical trials.

- **Ivosidenib**: 500 mg PO QD.

  21.6% of patients achieved CR and duration of response was 6.5 months. Median duration of response was 8.2 months [40].

- **Enasidenib**: 100 mg PO QD.

  Overall response rate was 40% with a median response duration of 5.8 months. Median OS was 9.3 months, which increased to 19.7 months for the 19% of patients who achieved CR [41].

Caveats: IDH differentiation syndrome, as described earlier in this chapter, has been reported in 10–20% of patients treated with IDH inhibitors [42].

Can treat with systemic corticosteroids until improvement.
Leukocytosis can be treated with hydroxyurea [41] (Table 5.5).

Table 5.5 Summary of treatment recommendations for patients with AML

Medically fit • ECOG < 2 • Karnofsky ≥ 80 • HCT-CI < 3	*Medically unfit* • ECOG ≥ 2 • Karnofsky < 80 • HCT-CI > 3	
Induction therapy (Also known as "7 + 3") 7 days continuous cytarabine +3 days anthracycline +/− additional targeted agents depending on cytogenetics ($FLT3^{mut+}$)	**Unfit, but not frail** Either ECOG ≥3 OR CCI ≥3, but not both	**Unfit and frail** ECOG ≥3 *and* CCI ≥3
Bone marrow biopsy day 14–21 to assess initial response to therapy	Focus on stabilizing comorbidities to move towards medical fitness/ induction therapy	Focus on symptom relief and improving quality of life through supportive care Hydroxyurea to avoid symptomatic leukostasis Consider clinical trial
Complete remission in 60–80% younger adults and 40–60% older patients	If medical fitness cannot be achieved, use hypo-methylating agents (HMA), only if no severe liver of kidney disease, and no prior HMA therapy – HMA + Bcl2 inhibitor – HMA + targeted therapy (such as IDH inhibitors)	
Post-remission therapy – Consolidation therapy – Autologous hematopoietic stem cell transplantation (HSCT) – Allogeneic HSCT from matched-related or unrelated donor Choice of therapy dependent on ELN risk group of patient's AML		
Favorable-risk: 2–4 cycles of HIDAC Intermediate-risk: Allogeneic HSCT – 2–4 cycles of IDAC Adverse-Risk: Allogeneic HSCT	*If patient ineligible for HMA therapy, consider*: – IDH inhibitors (ivosidenib for *IDH1* and enasidenib for *IDH2*) – Low-dose cytarabine (LoDAC), better for low-intermediate risk AML – LoDAC combination therapy – Gemtuzumab (anti-CD33 monoclonal antibody) – Clofarabine – Gilteritinib (mutant FLT3 inhibitor) Medically unit, frail patients with certain molecular features may be offered targeted agents listed above	

Table 5.6 Salvage regimens for patients not responding to a first induction cycle or with relapsed disease who are medically fit to undergo intensive therapy

Treatment regimen	Dosing
HIDAC (with or without anthracycline)	HIDAC: 2000–3000 mg/m^2
FLAG-IDA	• Fludarabine 30 mg/m^2 IV, days 2-6 • Cytarabine 1500–2000 mg/m^2 IV over 3 h, starting 4 h after fludarabine infusions, days 2–6 • Idarubicin 10 mg/m^2 IV, days 2–4 • G-CSF 5 ug/kg, SC, days 1–5
MEC	• Mitoxantrone 8 mg/m^2, days 1–5 • Etoposide 100 mg/m^2, days 1–5 • Cytarabine 1000 mg/m^2, days 1–5
Allogeneic HCT	Consider transplantation for patients in: • Primary refractory disease • Second complete remission • Major cytoreduction but still active disease following salvage therapy

Relapsed/Refractory Disease

The main goal for AML patients with relapsed/refractory who are candidate for allogeneic stem cell transplantation is quick cytoreduction. Table 5.6 summarizes approved standard of therapy regimens. Next-generation sequencing could inform the presence of actionable mutations and allow the incorporation of targeted therapy.

References

1. Sorror ML, Maris MB, Storb R, Baron F, Sandmaier BM, Maloney DG, et al. Hematopoietic cell transplantation (HCT)-specific comorbidity index: a new tool for risk assessment before allogeneic HCT. Blood. 2005;106(8):2912 9. https://doi.org/10.1182/blood-2005-05-2004.
2. Grimwade D, Lo Coco F. Acute promyelocytic leukemia: a model for the role of molecular diagnosis and residual disease monitoring in directing treatment approach in acute myeloid leukemia. Leukemia. 2002;16(10):1959–73. https://doi.org/10.1038/sj.leu.2402721.
3. Sanz MA, Lo Coco F, Martin G, Avvisati G, Rayon C, Barbui T, et al. Definition of relapse risk and role of nonanthracycline drugs for consolidation in patients with acute promyelocytic leukemia: a joint study of the PETHEMA and GIMEMA cooperative groups. Blood. 2000;96(4):1247–53.
4. Wang ZY, Chen Z. Differentiation and apoptosis induction therapy in acute promyelocytic leukaemia. Lancet Oncol. 2000;1:101–6. https://doi.org/10.1016/s1470-2045(00)00017-6.
5. Platzbecker U, Avvisati G, Cicconi L, Thiede C, Paoloni F, Vignetti M, et al. Improved outcomes with retinoic acid and arsenic trioxide compared with retinoic acid and chemotherapy in non-high-risk acute promyelocytic leukemia: final results of the randomized Italian-German APL0406 trial. J Clin Oncol. 2017;35(6):605–12. https://doi.org/10.1200/JCO.2016.67.1982.
6. Burnett AK, Russell NH, Hills RK, Bowen D, Kell J, Knapper S, et al. Arsenic trioxide and all-trans retinoic acid treatment for acute promyelocytic leukaemia in all risk groups (AML17): results of a randomised, controlled, phase 3 trial. Lancet Oncol. 2015;16(13):1295–305. https://doi.org/10.1016/S1470-2045(15)00193-X.

7. Lo-Coco F, Avvisati G, Vignetti M, Thiede C, Orlando SM, Iacobelli S, et al. Retinoic acid and arsenic trioxide for acute promyelocytic leukemia. N Engl J Med. 2013;369(2):111–21. https://doi.org/10.1056/NEJMoa1300874.
8. Lancet JE, Moseley AB, Coutre SE, DeAngelo DJ, Othus M, Tallman MS, et al. A phase 2 study of ATRA, arsenic trioxide, and gemtuzumab ozogamicin in patients with high-risk APL (SWOG 0535). Blood Adv. 2020;4(8):1683–9. https://doi.org/10.1182/bloodadvances.2019001278.
9. Abaza Y, Kantarjian H, Garcia-Manero G, Estey E, Borthakur G, Jabbour E, et al. Long-term outcome of acute promyelocytic leukemia treated with all-trans-retinoic acid, arsenic trioxide, and gemtuzumab. Blood. 2017;129(10):1275–83. https://doi.org/10.1182/blood-2016-09-736686.
10. Sanz MA, Fenaux P, Tallman MS, Estey EH, Lowenberg B, Naoe T, et al. Management of acute promyelocytic leukemia: updated recommendations from an expert panel of the European LeukemiaNet. Blood. 2019;133(15):1630–43. https://doi.org/10.1182/blood-2019-01-894980.
11. Sanz MA, Montesinos P, Rayon C, Holowiecka A, de la Serna J, Milone G, et al. Risk-adapted treatment of acute promyelocytic leukemia based on all-trans retinoic acid and anthracycline with addition of cytarabine in consolidation therapy for high-risk patients: further improvements in treatment outcome. Blood. 2010;115(25):5137–46. https://doi.org/10.1182/blood-2010-01-266007.
12. Kanamaru A, Takemoto Y, Tanimoto M, Murakami H, Asou N, Kobayashi T, et al. All-trans retinoic acid for the treatment of newly diagnosed acute promyelocytic leukemia. Japan Adult Leukemia Study Group. Blood. 1995;85(5):1202–6.
13. Montesinos P, Bergua JM, Vellenga E, Rayon C, Parody R, de la Serna J, et al. Differentiation syndrome in patients with acute promyelocytic leukemia treated with all-trans retinoic acid and anthracycline chemotherapy: characteristics, outcome, and prognostic factors. Blood. 2009;113(4):775–83. https://doi.org/10.1182/blood-2008-07-168617.
14. Lo-Coco F, Avvisati G, Vignetti M, Breccia M, Gallo E, Rambaldi A, et al. Front-line treatment of acute promyelocytic leukemia with AIDA induction followed by risk-adapted consolidation for adults younger than 61 years: results of the AIDA-2000 trial of the GIMEMA Group. Blood. 2010;116(17):3171–9. https://doi.org/10.1182/blood-2010-03-276196.
15. Sanz MA, Montesinos P. How we prevent and treat differentiation syndrome in patients with acute promyelocytic leukemia. Blood. 2014;123(18):2777–82. https://doi.org/10.1182/blood-2013-10-512640.
16. Rollig C, Ehninger G. How I treat hyperleukocytosis in acute myeloid leukemia. Blood. 2015;125(21):3246–52. https://doi.org/10.1182/blood-2014-10-551507.
17. Villgran V, Agha M, Raptis A, Hou JZ, Farah R, Lim SH, et al. Leukapheresis in patients newly diagnosed with acute myeloid leukemia. Transfus Apher Sci. 2016;55(2):216–20. https://doi.org/10.1016/j.transci.2016.07.001.
18. Oberoi S, Lehrnbecher T, Phillips B, Hitzler J, Ethier MC, Beyene J, et al. Leukapheresis and low-dose chemotherapy do not reduce early mortality in acute myeloid leukemia hyperleukocytosis: a systematic review and meta-analysis. Leuk Res. 2014;38(4):460–8. https://doi.org/10.1016/j.leukres.2014.01.004.
19. Mamez AC, Raffoux E, Chevret S, Lemiale V, Boissel N, Canet E, et al. Pre-treatment with oral hydroxyurea prior to intensive chemotherapy improves early survival of patients with high hyperleukocytosis in acute myeloid leukemia. Leuk Lymphoma. 2016;57(10):2281–8. https://doi.org/10.3109/10428194.2016.1142083.
20. Dohner H, Estey EH, Amadori S, Appelbaum FR, Buchner T, Burnett AK, et al. Diagnosis and management of acute myeloid leukemia in adults: recommendations from an international expert panel, on behalf of the European LeukemiaNet. Blood. 2010;115(3):453–74. https://doi.org/10.1182/blood-2009-07-235358.
21. Dohner H, Estey E, Grimwade D, Amadori S, Appelbaum FR, Buchner T, et al. Diagnosis and management of AML in adults: 2017 ELN recommendations from an international expert panel. Blood. 2017;129(4):424–47. https://doi.org/10.1182/blood-2016-08-733196.

22. Ferrara F, Schiffer CA. Acute myeloid leukaemia in adults. Lancet. 2013;381(9865):484–95. https://doi.org/10.1016/S0140-6736(12)61727-9.
23. Pastore F, Pastore A, Wittmann G, Hiddemann W, Spiekermann K. The role of therapeutic leukapheresis in hyperleukocytotic AML. PLoS One. 2014;9(4):e95062. https://doi.org/10.1371/journal.pone.0095062.
24. Zhao J, Bewersdorf JP, Jaszczur S, Kowalski A, Perreault S, Schiffer M, et al. High dose cyclophosphamide for cytoreduction in patients with acute myeloid leukemia with hyperleukocytosis or leukostasis. Leuk Lymphoma. 2021;62(5):1195–202. https://doi.org/10.1080/1042819 4.2020.1856835.
25. Williams SF, Larson RA. Hypersensitivity reaction to high-dose cytarabine. Br J Haematol. 1989;73(2):274–5. https://doi.org/10.1111/j.1365-2141.1989.tb00267.x.
26. Castleberry RP, Crist WM, Holbrook T, Malluh A, Gaddy D. The cytosine arabinoside (Ara-C) syndrome. Med Pediatr Oncol. 1981;9(3):257–64. https://doi.org/10.1002/mpo.2950090309.
27. Ek T, Jarfelt M, Mellander L, Abrahamsson J. Proinflammatory cytokines mediate the systemic inflammatory response associated with high-dose cytarabine treatment in children. Med Pediatr Oncol. 2001;37(5):459–64. https://doi.org/10.1002/mpo.1230.
28. Castells MC, Tennant NM, Sloane DE, Hsu FI, Barrett NA, Hong DI, et al. Hypersensitivity reactions to chemotherapy: outcomes and safety of rapid desensitization in 413 cases. J Allergy Clin Immunol. 2008;122(3):574–80. https://doi.org/10.1016/j.jaci.2008.02.044.
29. Alberts DS, Garcia DJ. Safety aspects of pegylated liposomal doxorubicin in patients with cancer. Drugs. 1997;54(Suppl 4):30–5. https://doi.org/10.2165/00003495-199700544-00007.
30. Rahman A, Treat J, Roh JK, Potkul LA, Alvord WG, Forst D, et al. A phase I clinical trial and pharmacokinetic evaluation of liposome-encapsulated doxorubicin. J Clin Oncol. 1990;8(6):1093–100. https://doi.org/10.1200/JCO.1990.8.6.1093.
31. Coiffier B, Altman A, Pui CH, Younes A, Cairo MS. Guidelines for the management of pediatric and adult tumor lysis syndrome: an evidence-based review. J Clin Oncol. 2008;26(16):2767–78. https://doi.org/10.1200/JCO.2007.15.0177.
32. Stone RM, Mandrekar SJ, Sanford BL, Laumann K, Geyer S, Bloomfield CD, et al. Midostaurin plus chemotherapy for acute myeloid leukemia with a FLT3 mutation. N Engl J Med. 2017;377(5):454–64. https://doi.org/10.1056/NEJMoa1614359.
33. Lambert J, Pautas C, Terre C, Raffoux E, Turlure P, Caillot D, et al. Gemtuzumab ozogamicin for de novo acute myeloid leukemia: final efficacy and safety updates from the open-label, phase III ALFA-0701 trial. Haematologica. 2019;104(1):113–9. https://doi.org/10.3324/haematol.2018.188888.
34. Dombret H, Seymour JF, Butrym A, Wierzbowska A, Selleslag D, Jang JH, et al. International phase 3 study of azacitidine vs conventional care regimens in older patients with newly diagnosed AML with >30% blasts. Blood. 2015;126(3):291–9. https://doi.org/10.1182/blood-2015-01-621664.
35. Kantarjian HM, Thomas XG, Dmoszynska A, Wierzbowska A, Mazur G, Mayer J, et al. Multicenter, randomized, open-label, phase III trial of decitabine versus patient choice, with physician advice, of either supportive care or low-dose cytarabine for the treatment of older patients with newly diagnosed acute myeloid leukemia. J Clin Oncol. 2012;30(21):2670–7. https://doi.org/10.1200/JCO.2011.38.9429.
36. Middeke JM, Teipel R, Rollig C, Stasik S, Zebisch A, Sill H, et al. Decitabine treatment in 311 patients with acute myeloid leukemia: outcome and impact of TP53 mutations—a registry based analysis. Leuk Lymphoma. 2021;62(6):1432–40. https://doi.org/10.1080/10428194.202 0.1864354.
37. Zeidan AM, Wang R, Wang X, Shallis RM, Podoltsev NA, Bewersdorf JP, et al. Clinical outcomes of older patients with AML receiving hypomethylating agents: a large population-based study in the United States. Blood Adv. 2020;4(10):2192–201. https://doi.org/10.1182/bloodadvances.2020001779.
38. Wei AH, Strickland SA Jr, Hou JZ, Fiedler W, Lin TL, Walter RB, et al. Venetoclax combined with low-dose cytarabine for previously untreated patients with acute myeloid leukemia:

results from a phase Ib/II study. J Clin Oncol. 2019;37(15):1277–84. https://doi.org/10.1200/JCO.18.01600.

39. DiNardo CD, Jonas BA, Pullarkat V, Thirman MJ, Garcia JS, Wei AH, et al. Azacitidine and venetoclax in previously untreated acute myeloid leukemia. N Engl J Med. 2020;383(7):617–29. https://doi.org/10.1056/NEJMoa2012971.

40. DiNardo CD, Stein EM, de Botton S, Roboz GJ, Altman JK, Mims AS, et al. Durable remissions with Ivosidenib in IDH1-mutated relapsed or refractory AML. N Engl J Med. 2018;378(25):2386–98. https://doi.org/10.1056/NEJMoa1716984.

41. Stein EM, DiNardo CD, Pollyea DA, Fathi AT, Roboz GJ, Altman JK, et al. Enasidenib in mutant IDH2 relapsed or refractory acute myeloid leukemia. Blood. 2017;130(6):722–31. https://doi.org/10.1182/blood-2017-04-779405.

42. Norsworthy KJ, Mulkey F, Scott EC, Ward AF, Przepiorka D, Charlab R, et al. Differentiation syndrome with Ivosidenib and enasidenib treatment in patients with relapsed or refractory IDH-mutated AML: a U.S. Food and Drug Administration Systematic Analysis. Clin Cancer Res. 2020;26(16):4280–8. https://doi.org/10.1158/1078-0432.CCR-20-0834.

Chapter 6
Acute Differentiation Syndrome

Sarah Mudra and Lacey Williams

Case 1

A 35-year-old obese Hispanic male presents with WBC of 11 K/UL, Hb 7 g/dL, and platelet 23 K/UL. Bone marrow biopsy showed promyelocytes. PML-RARA FISH was positive. NGS showed *FLT3ITD* mutation. Patient was initiated on ATRA. Thirty-six hours later, his nurse informs you that his weight increased by 1.5 kg. Creatinine increased from 1.4 to 1.8 mg/dL.

Acute APL Differentiation Syndrome (DS)

Definition

All-trans retinoic acid (ATRA), a vitamin A derivative, is used to treat acute promy-elocytic leukemia (APL). ATRA reverses coagulopathy and reduces life-threatening bleeding; however, differentiation syndrome (DS) is a serious and potentially life-threatening complication of this therapy.

S. Mudra (✉) · L. Williams
MedStar Georgetown University Hospital, Washington, DC, USA

Division of Hematology and Oncology, Georgetown University School of Medicine, Washington, DC, USA

Lombardi Cancer Institute, Georgetown University School of Medicine, Washington, DC, USA
e-mail: Sarah.e.mudra@medstar.net; Lacey.s.williams@medstar.net

© The Author(s), under exclusive license to Springer Nature Switzerland AG 2024
G. Rivero, I. R. Sosa (eds.), *Consulting Hematology and Oncology Handbook*,
https://doi.org/10.1007/978-3-031-75810-2_6

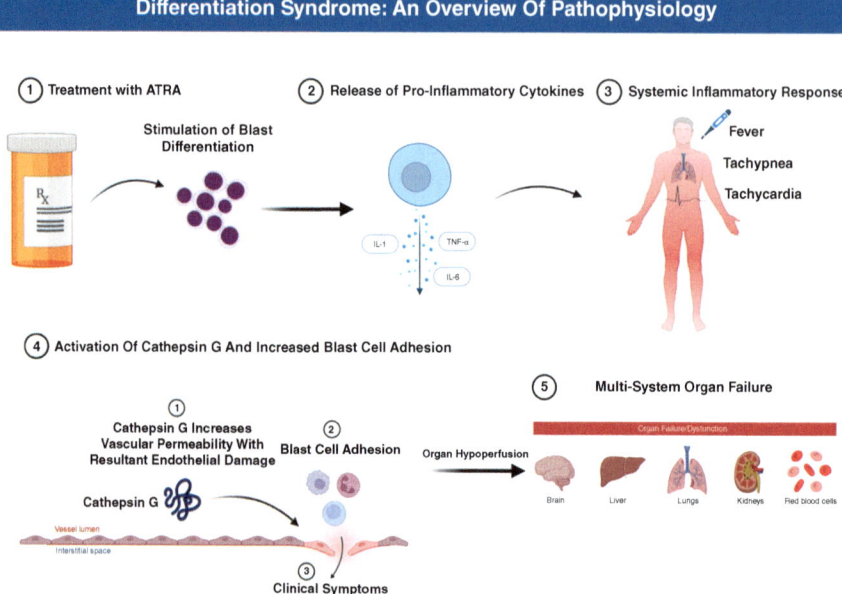

Fig. 6.1 Pathophysiology of differentiation syndrome. Treatment with ATRA induces terminal blast cell differentiation. In the process, massive release of pro-inflammatory cytokines coupled with increased vascular permeability results in SIRS. Leukostasis and adhesion of blasts can rapidly progress to shock and multiorgan failure

Pathogenesis

ATRA treatment induces terminal differentiation of blasts and releases pro-inflammatory cytokines including IL-1, IL- β, IL-6, IL-8, and TNF-α [1]. This widespread release of inflammatory mediators results in systemic inflammatory response syndrome (SIRS). In particular, the release of cathepsin G from azurophilic granules causes endothelial damage and increases vascular permeability [2]. Adhesion of blast cells to endothelial tissue causes leukostasis and leads to ischemia. Without prompt treatment, DS can result in shock, end-organ ischemia and multiorgan failure (Fig. 6.1).

Incidence and Timing of Onset

Approximately 15–25% of those receiving initial therapy with ATRA develop DS [3].

Clinical Manifestations

Hallmarks of differentiation syndrome include the following [3]:

- Fever (>38 °C).
- Weight gain (>5 kg).
- Hypotension.
- Hypoxemia.
- Dyspnea.
- Pulmonary infiltrates.
- Pleural or pericardial effusion.
- Acute kidney injury.

Grading of DS

The above features are used to grade disease severity [4]:

- ≥4 features: Severe.
- 3 features: Moderate.
- 1–2 features: Indeterminate.

Rarely, DS can result in diffuse alveolar hemorrhage. Neutrophil invasion into the dermis can also cause acute febrile neutrophilic dermatosis.

Laboratory and Radiologic Investigation

As weight gain and edema may be initial manifestations of DS, daily weights and fluid balance should be monitored. A net even fluid balance should be maintained.
    Initial diagnostic investigation should include the following:

- CBC with differential: WBC >100 k confers a high index of suspicion for DS.
- CMP.
- PT/PTT/INR, fibrinogen.
- Oxygen saturation, via pulse oximetry or ABG.
- Infectious workup with blood cultures, urine cultures, respiratory viral panel.
- Chest radiography.

Case 1 Continued

Following 3 days of therapy, the patient complained of shortness of breath. Chest x-ray reveals diffuse pulmonary edema. CBC reveals a WBC of 90,000.

Pulmonary Manifestations of Acute DS

- Dyspnea.
- Hypoxia.
- Respiratory distress.
- Pulmonary edema.
- Diffuse pulmonary infiltrates.
- Pleural effusions.

Patients often present with dyspnea and hypoxia requiring supplemental oxygen. In severe cases, respiratory failure may result, necessitating intubation and mechanical ventilation.

Imaging with chest X-ray reveals diffuse pulmonary infiltrates with or without pleural effusions. Chest computed tomography (CT) may be pursued to further characterize the pattern of pulmonary infiltrates and extent of pleural effusions. Widespread ground glass opacities with bilateral pleural effusions may be evident (Fig. 6.2).

Cardiovascular Manifestations of Acute DS

- Cardiomegaly.
- Heart failure.
- Pericardial effusion.
- Arrythmias: QT prolongation, polymorphic ventricular tachycardia, torsade de pointes, ventricular fibrillation.

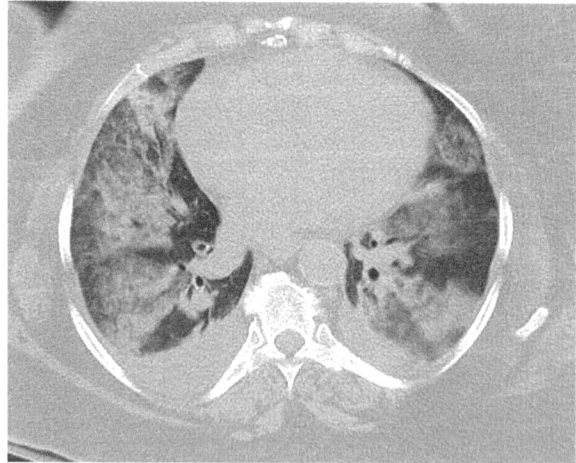

Fig. 6.2 Chest CT demonstrating diffuse ground glass opacities and bilateral pleural effusions [5]

Acute DS may cause pericardial effusions (Fig. 6.3); in one large case series, pericardial effusions were seen in 11–23% of those with moderate to severe DS [6]. Fluid retention also increases stretch of cardiac myocytes, generating brain natriuretic peptide (BNP) which may result in acute heart failure. Certainly, those with underlying cardiac dysfunction are at increased risk. Myopericarditis has also been rarely reported in the literature [7–11]. Arrythmias, particularly polymorphic ventricular tachycardia, torsade de pointes, and progression to ventricular fibrillation, are typically a consequence of arsenic trioxide and QT prolongation rather than DS itself. Nevertheless, serum electrolytes should be maintained with $K > 4$ and $Mg > 1.8$.

Management

Management of DS involves prompt corticosteroid initiation and aggressive supportive care including intubation, mechanical ventilation, renal replacement therapy, and correction of underlying coagulopathy (Fig. 6.4).

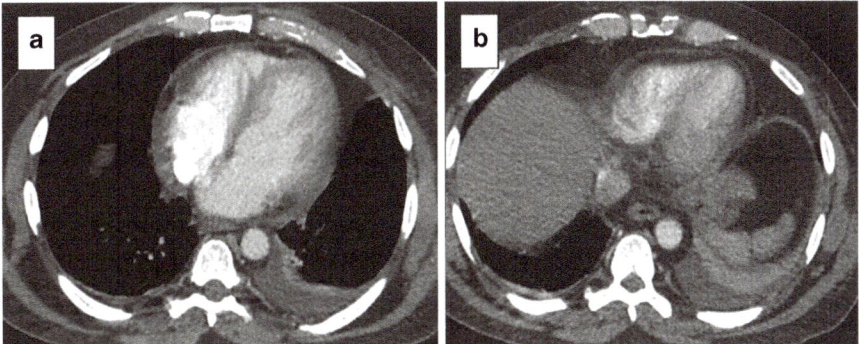

Fig. 6.3 Trace pericardial effusion (**a**, **b**) in a patient with differentiation syndrome as visualized on CT chest [12]

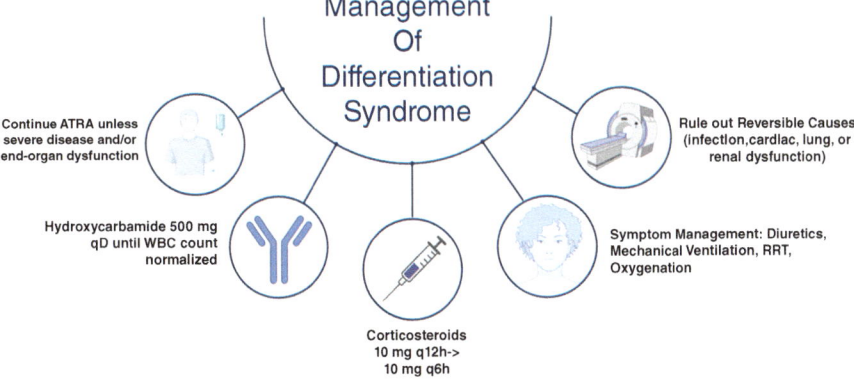

Fig. 6.4 Differentiation syndrome management

Steroids

At the first sign of respiratory compromise (i.e., dyspnea, hypoxia, pulmonary edema, pleural or pericardial effusions), steroids should be initiated.

Corticosteroid dosing:

- Dexamethasone 10 mg q12 h.
- If no improvement within 24 h, increase to dexamethasone 10 mg q6 h.

NCCN guidelines propose 10 mg q12 h for 3–5 days followed by a gradual taper over 2 weeks [13, 14]. Others have suggested dexamethasone should be tapered when clinical improvement is evident or with count recovery [3].

Interruption in ATRA or ATO Therapy

Ceasing therapy with ATRA or ATO is not required in acute DS management. However, ATRA or ATO should be stopped in the following cases: (1) severe grade DS, (2) end-organ dysfunction (i.e., respiratory or renal failure), (3) ICU-level care, and (4) lack of improvement with steroid administration [3].

Cytoreductive Strategies

If DS remains recalcitrant to both steroid administration and interruption in ATRA or ATO therapy, then cytoreductive agents including hydroxyurea, anthracyclines, or gemtuzumab ozogamicin may be administered until WBC normalizes. In particular, ATRA or ATO is inadequate for the treatment of high-risk APL. In such cases, cytoreduction during induction has improved outcomes.

Hydroxyurea

Hydroxyurea at 2–3 g/day may be preferred in those with cardiac dysfunction over idarubicin. However, a 50% dose reduction is necessary for those with renal impairment (CrCl <60 mL/min).

Chemotherapy

The anthracycline idarubicin at a dose of 12 mg/m^2 may also be used for cytoreduction.

Gemtuzumab Ozogamicin

Gemtuzumab ozogamicin (GO) is an anti-CD33 monoclonal antibody conjugated to an anthracycline. In high-risk patients, studies have added GO at doses of 6 or 9 mg/m^2 on day 1. Caution should be exercised in those with hepatic dysfunction.

DS Prophylaxis

Patients with WBC >10,000 are at high risk of developing DS.

In these cases, prophylaxis with corticosteroids is indicated. Regimens include prednisone 0.5 mg/kg on day 1 through or dexamethasone 10 mg q12 h. Corticosteroids are then tapered over several days if DS does not develop.

However, the PETHEMA group observed that a WBC >5000 was associated with an increased risk of severe DS. Thus, some trials have administered steroid prophylaxis to those with WBC >5000 (i.e., LPA96 trial) [6].

Caveats

For patients with severe disease and coagulopathy, bronchoscopy with bronchoalveolar lavage may be considered to evaluate for diffuse alveolar hemorrhage. Pulmonary embolism should be ruled out with contrasted chest CT.

Predictors of DS

An analysis of two large trials identified prognostic factors for the development of moderate and severe DS [6].

- Moderate DS: WBC > 10,000.
- Severe DS: WBC > 5000 and creatinine >1.4.

Case 2

68 years borderline ESRD presented with pancytopenia. WBC was 1.4 K/UL, HB 9 g/dL and platelets 17 K/uL. Bone marrow showed CD34 and HLADR negative; CD33 and CD117+ positive AML. +8 was detected in metaphase karyotyping. NGS revealed *IDH1* + mut. Given significant comorbid condition, primary treating team opted for single-agent IDH inhibitor. After 72 h of therapy, the patient developed fever, WBC of 16 K/uL, and mild hypoxemia with SpO2 of 89%. O2 at 2 L was administered intranasally. Fig. 6.5 shows chest X ray.

Fig. 6.5 Chest radiograph
demonstrating diffuse
pulmonary edema [15]

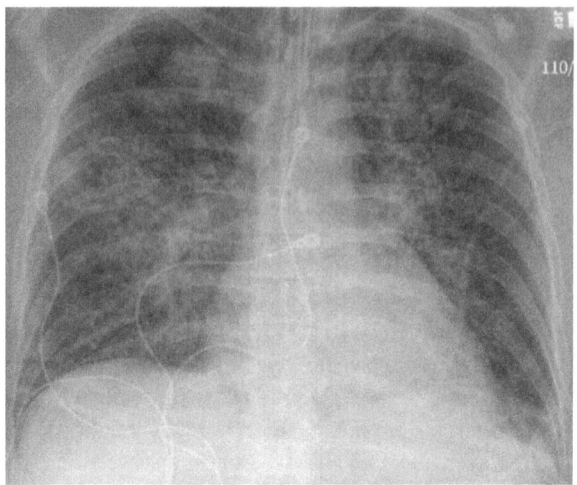

Table 6.1 Incidence of IDH
and FLT3 inhibitor-associated
differentiation syndrome

IDH inhibitors	Incidence
Ivosidenib (IDH1i)	19–25% [20]
Enasidenib (IDH2i)	14% [21]
FLT3 inhibitors	
Gilteritinib	3% [22, 23]
Midostaurin	Not reported
Sorafenib	Case reports [24]

Targeted Therapy-Associated DS

DS has also been recognized among those treated with FLT3 and IDH inhibitors. Case reports of DS associated with hypomethylating agents decitabine and azacitidine have been published [16, 17]. Targeted agents like IDH1/2 inhibitors and FLT3 inhibitors induce cell maturation and apoptosis; thus, it is not unexpected that DS may result. In contrast to its ATRA and ATO-associated counterpart, targeted therapy-associated DS is rarely fatal (Table 6.1).

Targeted therapy-associated DS typically occurs within the first 3 weeks of therapy though can occur weeks to months following initiation [18]. In an FDA database of DS associated with ivosidenib and enasidenib, median time to onset of DS was 19 days [19].

DS has been reported in approximately 10–20% of those treated with IDH inhibitors [18].

Clinical Manifestations

Clinical features of targeted agent-associated DS are similar to those noted in APL DS. However, presentation can be more heterogenous.

- Fever.
- Weight gain.
- Dyspnea.
- Hypoxia.
- Pulmonary infiltrates.
- Pleural or pericardial effusion.
- Acute kidney injury.
- Hypotension.
- Rash.

Formal diagnostic criteria and grading of targeted therapy-associated DS have not been established.

Management

Dexamethasone 10 mg q12 h should be initiated at promptly. If clinical improvement is not observed in 12–24 h, then dexamethasone should be increased to 10 mg q6 h. When clinical improvement is sustained for >72 h, steroids may be tapered.

IDH and FLT3 inhibitors should be discontinued, though this is unlikely to result in rapid symptomatic improvement given the agents' prolonged half-lives. Often, targeted-agent DS does not necessitate permanent cessation of targeted therapy. Rather, dose adjustments or schedule modifications may be necessary [18].

Recurrent DS has been reported in 12–15% of patients with IDH-associated DS [19].

References

1. Sanz MA, Montesinos P. How we prevent and treat differentiation syndrome in patients with acute promyelocytic leukemia. Blood. 2014;123(18):2777–82. https://doi.org/10.1182/blood-2013-10-512640.
2. Seale J, et al. All-trans retinoic acid rapidly decreases cathepsin G synthesis and mRNA expression in acute promyelocytic leukemia. Leukemia. 1996;10(1):95–101.
3. Stahl M, Tallman MS. Differentiation syndrome in acute promyelocytic leukaemia. Br J Haematol. 2019;187(2):157–62. https://doi.org/10.1111/bjh.16151.
4. Montesinos P, Sanz MA. The differentiation syndrome in patients with acute promyelocytic leukemia: experience of the pethema group and review of the literature. Mediterr J Hematol Infect Dis. 2011;3(1):e2011059. https://doi.org/10.4084/MJHID.2011.059. Epub 2011 Dec 4. PMID: 22220256; PMCID: PMC3248336

5. Jung J, Choi J, Hahn. Radiologic features of all-trans-retinoic acid syndrome. Am J Roentgenol. 2002;178(2):475–80.
6. Montesinos P, et al. Differentiation syndrome in patients with acute promyelocytic leukemia treated with all-trans retinoic acid and anthracycline chemotherapy: characteristics, outcome, and prognostic factors. Blood. 2009;113(4):775–83. https://doi.org/10.1182/blood-2008-07-168617.
7. Ben El Makki A, Mahtat EM, Kheyi J, Bouzelmat H, Chaib A. A rare case of perimyocarditis induced by all-trans retinoic acid administration during induction treatment of acute promyelocytic leukemia. Med Pharm Rep. 2019;92:418–20. https://doi.org/10.15386/mpr-1229.
8. Klein SK, Biemond BJ, van Oers MH. Two cases of isolated symptomatic myocarditis induced by all-trans retinoic acid (ATRA). Ann Hematol. 2007;86:917–8. https://doi.org/10.1007/s00277-007-0333-3.
9. Choi S, Kim HS, Jung CS, et al. Reversible symptomatic myocarditis induced by all-trans retinoic acid administration during induction treatment of acute promyelocytic leukemia: rare cardiac manifestation as a retinoic acid syndrome. J Cardiovasc Ultrasound. 2011;19:95–8. https://doi.org/10.4250/jcu.2011.19.2.95.
10. Vassilakopoulos TP, Asimakopoulos JV, Plata E, et al. Recurrent acute myopericarditis without effusion during ATRA induction and ATO salvage of APL: a variant form of the differentiation syndrome? Leuk Lymphoma. 2017;58:1743–6. https://doi.org/10.1080/10428194.2016.1253838.
11. Carcelero San Martín E, Riu Viladoms G, Creus Baró N. Severe myopericarditis following induction therapy with idarubicin and transretinoic acid in a patient with acute promyelocytic leukemia. Med Clin (Barc). 2018;22:492–3. https://doi.org/10.1016/j.medcli.2017.10.030.
12. Alyami B, Alharbi AA, Patel B. A rare case of acute pericarditis as a primary presentation of differentiation syndrome. Cureus. 2022;14(4):e24213. https://doi.org/10.7759/cureus.24213.
13. Lo-Coco F, et al. Retinoic acid and arsenic trioxide for acute promyelocytic leukemia. N Engl J Med. 2013;369(2):111–21. https://doi.org/10.1056/NEJMoa1300874.
14. Sanz MA, et al. Risk-adapted treatment of acute promyelocytic leukemia based on all-trans retinoic acid and anthracycline with addition of cytarabine in consolidation therapy for high-risk patients: further improvements in treatment outcome. Blood. 2010;115(25):5137–46. https://doi.org/10.1182/blood-2010-01-266007.
15. Reyhanoglu G, et al. Differentiation syndrome, a side effect from the therapy of acute promyelocytic leukemia. Cureus. 2020;12(12):e12042. https://doi.org/10.7759/cureus.12042.
16. Khalaf D, Al-Jehani F. Pseudo differentiation syndrome. Mediterr J Hematol Infect Dis. 2011;3(1):e2011061. https://doi.org/10.4084/MJHID.2011.061.
17. Laufer CB, Roberts O. Differentiation syndrome in acute myeloid leukemia after treatment with azacitidine. Eur J Haematol. 2015;95(5):484–5. https://doi.org/10.1111/ejh.12598.
18. Fathi AT, et al. Differentiation syndrome with lower-intensity treatments for acute myeloid leukemia. Am J Hematol. 2021;96(6):735–46. https://doi.org/10.1002/ajh.26142.
19. Norsworthy KJ, et al. Differentiation syndrome with Ivosidenib and Enasidenib treatment in patients with relapsed or refractory IDH-mutated AML: a U.S. Food and Drug Administration systematic analysis. Clin Cancer Res. 2020;26(16):4280–8. https://doi.org/10.1158/1078-0432.CCR-20-0834.
20. TIBSOVO® (ivosidenib) Prescribing Information. Agios Pharmaceuticals, Inc. Cambridge, MA. Rev 07/2018. 2018. Accessed October 15, 2023.
21. Perl AE, et al. Gilteritinib or chemotherapy for relapsed or refractory FLT3-mutated AML. N Engl J Med. 2019;381(18):1728–40. https://doi.org/10.1056/NEJMoa1902688.
22. Larrosa-Garcia M, Baer MR. FLT3 inhibitors in acute myeloid leukemia: current status and future directions. Mol Cancer Ther. 2017;16(6):991–1001. https://doi.org/10.1158/1535-7163.MCT-16-0876.

23. Fathi AT, et al. FLT3 inhibitor-induced neutrophilic dermatosis. Blood. 2013;122(2):239–42. https://doi.org/10.1182/blood-2013-01-478172.
24. Fathi AT, et al. Differentiation syndrome associated with Enasidenib, a selective inhibitor of mutant Isocitrate dehydrogenase 2: analysis of a phase 1/2 study. JAMA Oncol. 2018;4(8):1106–10. https://doi.org/10.1001/jamaoncol.2017.4695.

Chapter 7
Cardiovascular Complications After Chemotherapy and Targeted Agents

Lacey Williams, Sarah Mudra, and Gustavo Rivero

Case 1

A 59-years-old obese patient with history of OSA who presents with *P53* acute myelogenous leukemia (AML). He proceeds with workup for induction chemotherapy. Echocardiogram evaluation revealed an EF of 50%.

- Anthracyclines are the primary drug class associated with major cardiotoxicity within the treatment of leukemia, with dose-dependent risk for heart failure at higher cumulative doses.
- Tyrosine kinase inhibitors used in some lymphomas, leukemias, and other solid tumors may demonstrate cardiotoxicity related to arrythmia (Table 7.1).

Definition

- Anthracycline-induced cardiotoxicity is defined as LVEF decrease by >10% points, with a final value <53% [1].

L. Williams (✉) · S. Mudra
Medstar Georgetown University Hospital, Washington, DC, USA

Georgetown University School of Medicine, Washington, DC, USA
e-mail: Lacey.s.williams@medstar.net; Sarah.e.mudra@medstar.net

G. Rivero
Lombardi Cancer Institute, Georgetown University School of Medicine, Washington, DC, USA
e-mail: garivero@bcm.edu

© The Author(s), under exclusive license to Springer Nature Switzerland AG 2024
G. Rivero, I. R. Sosa (eds.), *Consulting Hematology and Oncology Handbook*, https://doi.org/10.1007/978-3-031-75810-2_7

Table 7.1 Anthracyclines used in hematologic malignancy and associated connection with cardiovascular toxicity [2–7]

Agents	Risk factors for toxicity of >5% heart failure incidence	Incidence
Anthracyclines	Age > 65, BMI ≥ 30 kg/m², DM, HTN, RT with heart in treatment field	Up to 25% with doxorubicin doses >550 mg/m²
Daunorubicin	Total cumulative dose of ≥400–550 mg/m² in adults	1.3% of AML patients with treated with 270 mg/m²
Idarubicin	Total cumulative dose of ≥90 mg/m² in adults	5% of AML/MDS patients at >150 mg/m²
CPX compound	Total cumulative dose ≥1000 mg/m² in adults	9% in trial studying CPX-

Treatment-related Cardiovascular Toxicity

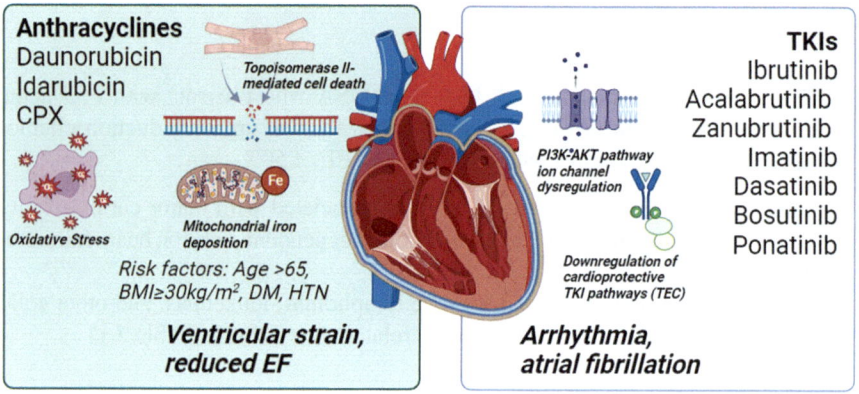

Fig. 7.1 Mechanisms of drug-induced cardiovascular toxicity ("Created with biorender.com")

Pathogenesis

Anthracyclines mediate cardiotoxicity through stabilization of topoisomerase 2-alpha DNA cleavage increasing double-strand breaks and iron accumulation in the mitochondria enhancing reactive oxygen species production (Fig. 7.1) [8].

Investigation in Patients with Suspected Impaired Heart Failure

– Patients with a history or symptoms of cardiac disease and prior exposure to cardiotoxic drugs or thoracic radiation, or those of an older age, should have an echocardiogram completed in pretreatment workup and consideration between cycles of regimens with high cumulative doses of anthracyclines. Patients should have full medical history obtained to screen for risk factors related to

cardiovascular disease, including hypertension, diabetes, dyslipidemia, obesity, and smoking.
- Many treating facilities include baseline echocardiogram for all patients planned to receive anthracyclines.

Additional Investigation in Patients with Suspected Impaired EF

- Consideration of troponin levels, BNP, and global longitudinal strain (GLS) assessment.

Case 1 Cont'd

A 59-year-old obese patient with history of OSA who presents with P53 mutant AML. Evaluation revealed an EF of 50%. He received Vyxeos—10 days later, he complained of SOB. CXR showed pulmonary edema. Repeat echo showed an EF 50%. Lasix at 40 mg IV was administered and patient was recommended to adhere to CPAP machine at night. He reported quick improvement of his breathing.

Clinical Context

Even without EF decrement, OSA exerts cardiovascular stress through changes in thoracic pressure and nocturnal hypoxia/hypercapnia with subsequent rebound oxygenation/hypocapnia. Introduction of anthracycline presented myocyte dysfunction leading to congestion from the left heart, improved with addressing OSA cardiovascular stressor (Fig. 7.2).

Dexrazoxane Dosing

- Recommended dosing at a **10:1 ratio of dexrazoxane:doxorubicin (i.e., dexrazoxane 500 mg/m²:doxorubicin 50 mg/m²)** [10].
- Daunorubicin can be considered at the same ratio as doxorubicin.
- 10:0.3 conversion for idarubicin.
- Do not administer anthracycline before dexrazoxane. Doxorubicin must be administered within 30 minutes of the completion of the dexrazoxane infusion.

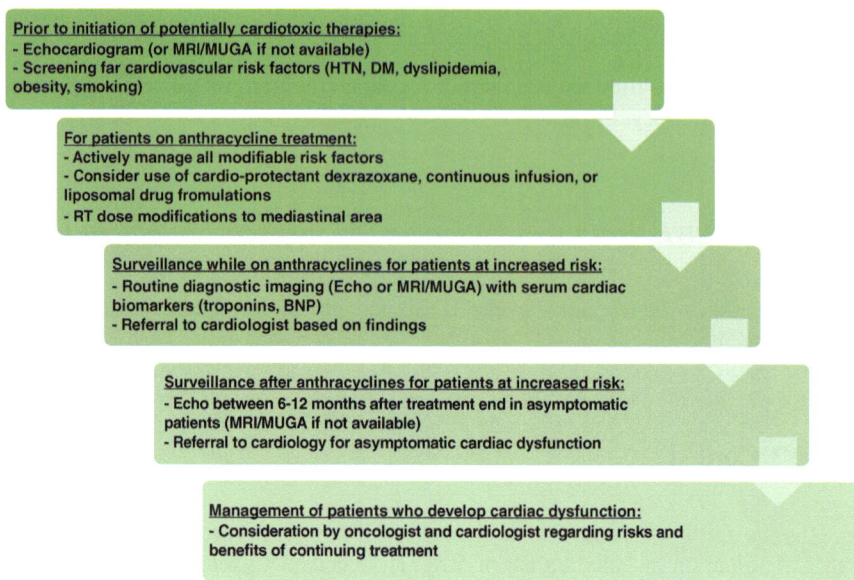

Fig. 7.2 Prevention and management of cardiotoxicity [9]

Case 2

A 68-year-old smoker patient with history of severe left lower extremity femoro-popliteal bypass presented with 128 K/uL WBC and basophilia of 20%. His Hb was 10 g/dL. Splenomegaly was detected 5 cm below left rib border. Bone marrow was hypercellular 90%. Cytogenetic showed t [9;22]-BCR ABL RT PCR was positive.

Cardiovascular Side Effects Initiated by TKI

TKI medications have multikinase targets and make up a heterogenous group of drugs (Table 7.2), some of which result in arrhythmias, including hypertension, QT prolongation, and atrial fibrillation.

Patient Management

For CML, patients with CV risk factor of arterial vascular disease would prefer to avoid ponatinib and agents with more QT prolongation, like nilotinib.

Table 7.2 TKIs used in hematologic malignancy and associated connection with cardiovascular toxicity [11–16]

Agents	Incidence of cardiotoxicity	Risk factors for toxicity
Bruton's TKIs		
Ibrutinib	78% hypertension 10–15% Afib, less frequent ventricular arrythmias	Shorten of QT interval
Acalabrutinib	10% hypertension 5% Afib	Underlying HTN, CAD
Zanubrutinib	2.5% Afib	
BCR-ABL Directed TKIs		
Imatinib	Rare cardiotoxicity	
Dasatinib	Pleuropericardial effusions Rare prolongation of QT	
Nilotinib	6.1% QT prolongation Rare arterial stenosis, vasospasm	Prolongation of QT interval
Ponatinib	9% arrhythmia 7.7% hypertension 3.8% myocardial infarcts	Underlying CV disease (HTN, CAD, DM)
Asciminib	19% hypertension	

Risk Factors

- Cardiovascular diseases (HTN, CAD, DM).
- Electrolyte abnormalities.
- Drug interactions with other drugs utilizing the same CYP enzymes.
- Drug interactions with QT prolonging agents.

Management

- Patients with underlying cardiovascular diseases (HTN, CAD, DM) should be evaluated prior to selecting or starting TKI drugs (Fig. 7.3) [11].
- Drug interactions should be investigated for current drugs that influence CYP metabolism or concurrently affect QT interval.
- When QT interval > 500 ms, or change >60 ms from baseline, consider decreased dose or stopped; consideration to restart TKI once QT <450 ms.
- Patients should be educated to notify their medical team if they have episode of fainting, headache, or irregular heartbeat.
- Consideration of rhythm control for patients, usually preference for beta-blockers.

Selection of TKI based on mutations leading to primary resistance should be considered after careful evaluation of treatment compliance. Mutations shown in Table 7.3 could result in primary TKI failure [16].

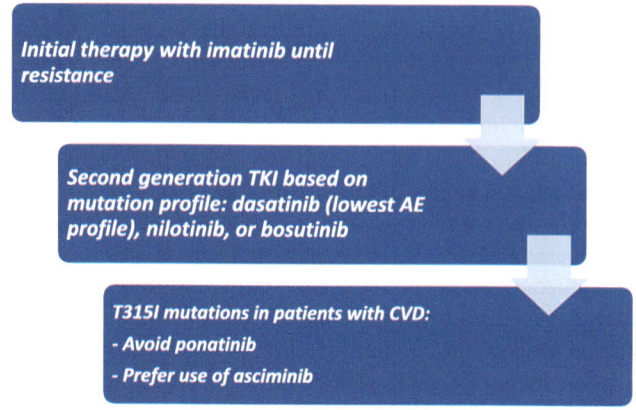

Fig. 7.3 TKI selection considerations based on cardiovascular disease status in CML [17]. *AE* adverse event, *CVD* cardiovascular disease

Table 7.3 Mutations observed in Chronic Myelogenous Leukemia patients inducing drug refractoriness/inferior response

Therapy	Contraindicated mutations [17]
Asciminib	A337T, P465S, or F359V/I/C
Bosutinib	T315I, V299L, G250E, or F317L
Dasatinib	T315I/A, F317L/V/I/C, or V299L
Nilotinib	T315I, Y253H, E255K/V, or F359V/C/I
Ponatinib, Omacetaxine	None

>>Consideration for anticoagulation risks and benefits for patients who develop atrial fibrillation.

- **HAS-BLED score** *estimates risk of major bleeding for patients on anticoagulation to assess risk benefit in atrial fibrillation care*:
  - **Hypertension.**
  - **Renal disease.**
  - **Liver disease.**
  - **Stroke history.**
  - **Prior major bleeding or predisposition to bleeding.**
  - **Labile INR, in therapeutic range < 60%.**
  - **Age > 65.**
  - **Medications that predispose bleeding (aspirin, clopidogrel, NSAIDs).**
  - **Alcohol use.**

- *Scores > 2 indicate significant risk for bleeding with 5.8% risk (detected in study during follow-up ranging 12–26 months)* [18].

References

1. Plana JC, Galderisi M, Barac A, et al. Expert consensus for multimodality imaging evaluation of adult patients during and after cancer therapy: a report from the American Society of Echocardiography and the European Association of Cardiovascular Imaging. Eur Heart J Cardiovasc Imaging. 2014;15(10):1063–93. https://doi.org/10.1093/ehjci/jeu192.
2. Huang W, Xu R, Zhou B, et al. Clinical manifestations, monitoring, and prognosis: a review of cardiotoxicity after antitumor strategy. Front Cardiovasc Med. 2022;9:912329. https://doi.org/10.3389/fcvm.2022.912329.
3. Neuendorff NR, Loh KP, Mims AS, et al. Anthracycline-related cardiotoxicity in older patients with acute myeloid leukemia: a young SIOG review paper. Blood Adv. 2020;4(4):762–75. https://doi.org/10.1182/bloodadvances.2019000955.
4. Swain SM, Whaley FS, Ewer MS. Congestive heart failure in patients treated with doxorubicin: a retrospective analysis of three trials. Cancer. 2003;97(11):2869–79. https://doi.org/10.1002/cncr.11407.
5. Anderlini P, Benjamin RS, Wong FC, et al. Idarubicin cardiotoxicity: a retrospective study in acute myeloid leukemia and myelodysplasia. J Clin Oncol. 1995;13(11):2827–34. https://doi.org/10.1200/JCO.1995.13.11.2827.
6. Fernandez HF, Sun Z, Yao X, et al. Anthracycline dose intensification in acute myeloid leukemia. N Engl J Med. 2009;361(13):1249–59. https://doi.org/10.1056/NEJMoa0904544.
7. Mitchell J, Pfeiffer M, Boehmer J, et al. Cardiotoxicity of CPX-351 vs 7+3 in patients with untreated high-risk acute myeloid leukemia. JCO. 2023;41(16_suppl):7029. https://doi.org/10.1200/JCO.2023.41.16_suppl.7029.
8. Henriksen PA. Anthracycline cardiotoxicity: an update on mechanisms, monitoring and prevention. Heart. 2018;104(12):971–7. https://doi.org/10.1136/heartjnl-2017-312103.
9. Armenian SH, Lacchetti C, Barac A, et al. Prevention and monitoring of cardiac dysfunction in survivors of adult cancers: American Society of Clinical Oncology clinical practice guideline. JCO. 2017;35(8):893–911. https://doi.org/10.1200/JCO.2016.70.5400.
10. Ganatra S, Nohria A, Shah S, et al. Upfront dexrazoxane for the reduction of anthracycline-induced cardiotoxicity in adults with preexisting cardiomyopathy and cancer: a consecutive case series. Cardiooncology. 2019;5:1. https://doi.org/10.1186/s40959-019-0036-7.
11. Cheng M, Yang F, Liu J, et al. Tyrosine kinase inhibitors-induced arrhythmias: from molecular mechanisms, pharmacokinetics to therapeutic strategies. Front Cardiovasc Med. 2021;8:758010. https://doi.org/10.3389/fcvm.2021.758010.
12. Htut TW, Han MM, Thein KZ. Acalabrutinib-related cardiac toxicities in patients with chronic lymphocytic leukemia: a meta-analysis of randomized controlled trials. J Immunother Precis Oncol. 2022;5(2):43–7. https://doi.org/10.36401/JIPO-21-12.
13. Hillmen P, Eichhorst B, Brown JR, et al. Zanubrutinib versus Ibrutinib in relapsed/refractory chronic lymphocytic leukemia and small lymphocytic lymphoma: interim analysis of a randomized phase III trial. J Clin Oncol. 2023;41(5):1035–45. https://doi.org/10.1200/JCO.22.00510.
14. Sharman JP, Egyed M, Jurczak W, et al. Efficacy and safety in a 4-year follow-up of the ELEVATE-TN study comparing acalabrutinib with or without obinutuzumab versus obinutuzumab plus chlorambucil in treatment-naïve chronic lymphocytic leukemia. Leukemia. 2022;36(4):1171–5. https://doi.org/10.1038/s41375-021-01485-x.
15. Shyam Sunder S, Sharma UC, Pokharel S. Adverse effects of tyrosine kinase inhibitors in cancer therapy: pathophysiology, mechanisms and clinical management. Signal Transduct Target Ther. 2023;8(1):262. https://doi.org/10.1038/s41392-023-01469-6.
16. Hughes TP, Mauro MJ, Cortes JE, et al. Asciminib in chronic myeloid leukemia after ABL kinase inhibitor failure. N Engl J Med. 2019;381(24):2315–26. https://doi.org/10.1056/NEJMoa1902328.
17. NCCN Clinical Practice Guidelines in Oncology, Chronic Myeloid Leukemia, Version 1.2024. Published online August 1, 2023.

18. Lip GYH, Frison L, Halperin JL, Lane DA. Comparative validation of a novel risk score for predicting bleeding risk in anticoagulated patients with atrial fibrillation: the HAS-BLED (hypertension, abnormal renal/liver function, stroke, bleeding history or predisposition, labile INR, elderly, drugs/alcohol concomitantly) score. J Am Coll Cardiol. 2011;57(2):173–80. https://doi.org/10.1016/j.jacc.2010.09.024.

Chapter 8
Neutropenic Sepsis: Antibiotic Prophylaxis

Rachel Zemel, Olivia Wilkins, and Grace Park

Case Demonstration Part 1

A 71-year-old patient underwent treatment with liposomal daunorubicin and cytarabine (Vyxeos) induction for secondary acute myeloid leukemia (sAML). On day 14 of the induction cycle, patient had a fever at 39 °C, and her absolute neutrophil count (ANC) was found to be 60 cells/microL.

Clinical Context

Liposomal daunorubicin and cytarabine induction chemotherapy for acute myeloid leukemia is an intensive chemotherapy regimen. Decrease in blood counts is an expected side effect of this therapy. Blood counts are expected to reach the lowest point or nadir at around days 4–14 of a treatment cycle. There are different definitions available for neutropenia, but most definitions agree a value less than 500 cells/microL meets the criteria for neutropenia. In this patient with 60 cells/microL, she meets criteria for neutropenia. Due the functioning of neutrophils in the immune system, this low number of neutrophils puts the patient at an increased risk for developing severe infections. There are many causes of neutropenia; however in this case, the likely cause is the induction chemotherapy.

R. Zemel · O. Wilkins
Medstar Georgetown University Hospital, Washington, DC, USA
e-mail: Rachel.a.zemel@medstar.net; Olivia.Wilkins@medstar.net

G. Park (✉)
Division of Pharmacy, The University of Texas MD Anderson Cancer Center, Houston, TX, USA
e-mail: ghwang1@mdanderson.org

G. Rivero, I. R. Sosa (eds.), *Consulting Hematology and Oncology Handbook*,
https://doi.org/10.1007/978-3-031-75810-2_8

Neutrophils and the Immune System

Neutrophils, also known as polymorphonuclear cells (PMNs), are the largest subset of white blood cells which fight infection and promote healing. Neutrophils control infections through the innate immune system by generating reactive oxygen species, releasing granules that degrade pathogens, creating neutrophil extracellular traps (NETs) of DNA to bind microorganisms, and promoting skin regeneration to bolster the barriers against microbe invasion, including gastrointestinal mucosa and general keratinized skin [1, 2]. Neutrophils also prime the adaptive immune system via their involvement in macrophage recruitment and activation [2]. Through these various mechanisms, neutrophils provide a first line of defense against bacteria and fungi, particularly *Candida* and *Aspergillus* species [3]. When patients have neutropenia, defined as a significantly low number of neutrophils, they become extremely prone to various bacterial and fungal infections.

Definitions of Neutropenia

The unit of measurement for the number of neutrophils in each patient's blood sample is the absolute neutrophil count (ANC), calculated by multiplying the amount of white blood cells in a blood sample by the percentage of which are neutrophils. The ANC provides an overall estimate of the number of neutrophils in a patient's blood sample, after which the presence and severity of neutropenia can be established.

Absolute neutrophil count = (total number of white blood cells) × (percentage of neutrophils). This will provide a decimal, which is then multiplied by 1000.

The formal definition of neutropenia is controversial, as the American Academy of Asthma, Allergy, and Immunology define neutropenia as an ANC under 1500 per microL, while the American Society of Clinical Oncology (ASCO) in conjunction with the Infectious Diseases Society of America (IDSA) recognizes neutropenia as an ANC below 1000 per microL [4]. The National Comprehensive Cancer Network (NCCN) defines neutropenia as ANC < below 500 (or < 1000 with a predicted decline to <500 over the next 48 h). Overall, severe neutropenia and profound neutropenia are defined as ANC under 500 per microL and ANC under 100 per microL, respectively [4]. Neutropenia is considered protracted when the neutropenia is sustained for 7 or more days, while chronic neutropenia implies neutropenia remaining over more than 3 months [4]. Nevertheless, with a lower ANC nadir and longer duration of prolonged neutropenia, it increases likelihood of infection from bacteria and fungi.

Etiologies of Neutropenia

Neutropenia is either congenital or acquired via infectious, oncologic, hematologic, iatrogenic, or nutritional means [1, 4]. Table 8.1 depicts the most frequent etiologies that should be investigated during evaluation of neutropenia.

Neutropenic Fever

- **Febrile Neutropenia** is a medical emergency, defined by ASCO and the IDSA as a temperature elevated to greater than or equal to 38.0 C (100.4 F) or an oral temperature of 38.3 C (101 F) persistent over 1 h in a patient with an ANC of less than 500 per microL [4]. As neutropenic patients have severely compromised immune systems, fever may be the only indicator of impending septic shock and mortality [4]. Unfortunately, most patients will be diagnosed with "fever of unknown origin," while only 30% of patients will have an isolated source of

Table 8.1 Factors and frequent etiologies of neutropenia to consider during consult evaluation [4–6]

Factor	Frequent etiologies
Nutritional deficiencies	• Vitamin B12, folate deficiency
Drug induced	• Antineoplastic medications (cytotoxic chemotherapy) • Immunosuppressive agents (tacrolimus, mycophenolate, among others) • Antibiotics: Chloramphenicol, linezolid • Antiepileptic: Carbamazepine
Viruses	• Influenza • Epstein-Barr virus (EBV) • Cytomegalovirus (CMV) • Parvovirus B19 • Varicella • Rubella • Measles • Hepatitis A • Hepatitis B • Human Immunodeficiency Virus (HIV) • Myelophthisic bacterial or fungal infections
Solid tumors infiltrating bone marrow	• Lung • Gastric • Breast, among others
Hematopoietic malignancies	• Myelofibrosis • Leukemia • Lymphoma • Myeloma
Acquired bone marrow failure	• Aplastic anemia • Myelodysplastic syndrome • Large granular lymphocytosis (LGL)

infection. In patients with profound neutropenia, 20% of the cases will have confirmed bacteremia [4].

- **Microorganism**: The most isolated causative pathogens in patients with febrile neutropenia are gram positive, including Staphylococcus, Streptococcus, and Enterococcus [4, 7]. Historically, the most common source for infections were gram-negative rods. Due to use of fluoroquinolones to cover gram-negative species, gram-positive staph species have been more prevalent. Gram-positive microbes on the skin that infect central venous lines or Mediports can be a culprit. Gram-negative and/or drug-resistant microbes may also be significant etiologies for febrile neutropenia; drug-resistant organisms may include methicillin-resistant *Staphylococcus aureus* (MRSA), vancomycin-resistant *Enterococcus* (VRE), *Pseudomonas aeruginosa*, *Acinetobacter* species, *Stenotrophomonas maltophilia*, extended spectrum beta-lactamase (ESBLE), and *Klebsiella* species [4, 7]. Regardless of known pathogen, approximately one-third of patients with febrile neutropenia develop complications of renal failure, respiratory failure, heart failure, and/or hypotension; the mortality rate in this setting extends to 11%. If febrile neutropenia progresses further to septic shock, the resultant mortality rate can range up to 50% [8].

Risk of Febrile Neutropenia Development

- The likelihood of developing febrile neutropenia depends on three categories of risk factors: those related to the patient's overall clinical status and health, those related to the malignancy itself, and those related to treatment for the malignancy. Such patient-related factors may include those that contribute to patient fragility, such as age over 65 years, clinical performance status, nutrition, and cachexia [9, 10].
- Additionally, with one additional comorbidity, two comorbidities, and greater than or equal to three comorbidities, febrile neutropenia risk is 27%, 67%, and 125%, respectively [9]. Risk factors relating to the overall malignancy include advanced progressive disease, a rise in lactate dehydrogenase (LDH) in patients with lymphoreticular disease, decreased lymphocyte count, and infiltration of the bone marrow with abnormal tissue that ultimately leads to bone marrow failure.
- Some malignancies have substantially higher risk of febrile neutropenia than others. Indeed, acute leukemia and myelodysplastic syndrome have an 85–95% rate of febrile neutropenia; high grade lymphoma's rates of febrile neutropenia range from 35% to 71% [9].
- In contrast, head and neck carcinomas, colorectal cancers, breast cancer, and prostate cancer's rates of febrile neutropenia range from 5.5% to 1.0% [9].
- Chemotherapy treatment-related risk factors for the development of febrile neutropenia include the type of myelosuppressive chemotherapy regimen and the dosage of the treatment [8, 9]. Particularly, high-dose anthracyclines, ifosfamide, cisplatin, cyclophosphamide, cytarabine, and etoposide all increase the risk of

febrile neutropenia [9]. The likelihood of the chemotherapy regimen to induce profound protracted neutropenia and significant Grade 3 or more mucositis both significantly increase febrile neutropenia risk [9].

Environmental Considerations in Reducing Opportunistic Infection in Neutropenic Hosts

Environmental considerations for infection prevention in neutropenic patients include specific attention to hand-hygiene, avoidance of fungal environments such as gardening and construction sites, and a preference for laminar air flow reverse isolation rooms [9, 11, 12]. Out of an abundance of caution, some may recommend the neutropenic diet, which requires an avoidance of uncooked vegetables or fruits without protective outer layers or peels, to further prevent potential infection. However, randomized control trials and meta-analysis have since shown that the neutropenic diet is not correlated with decreased infection or mortality in neutropenic patients with leukemia and other malignancies [13–15].

Case 1 (Continued)

An infectious workup including blood cultures, chest x-ray, and urinalysis are obtained. The initial results show no growth on the blood and urine cultures. Her chest x-ray was negative. The patient is started empirically on broad spectrum antibiotics with cefepime.

Clinical Context

With this patient developing neutropenic fever, the main concern is infection. Due to severe neutropenia, focal symptoms such as pain could be attenuated. Also, with the impaired immune system, neutropenic patients are at a high risk for severe infections. Due to high risk of severe infection, effort should be directed to identify a potential source of infection. The initial evaluation typically includes two sets of blood cultures, a chest radiograph and/or computed tomography, and a urinalysis.

Febrile Neutropenia Evaluation/Investigation

During induction chemotherapy for acute myeloid leukemia, neutrophil count nadirs is observed approximately 2 weeks after. 70% of chemotherapy complications occur within 4–6 weeks of chemotherapy treatment [16]. Table 8.2 summarizes major areas of clinical evaluation for patients exhibiting neutropenic fever after chemotherapy.

Risk Calculations

Both ASCO in conjunction with the IDSA and the National Comprehensive Cancer Network (NCCN) stratify patients by risk of febrile neutropenia complications to determine next steps in care. Both clinical decision-making criteria account for patients' comorbidities, diagnosis, chemotherapy agents, neutropenia duration, and clinical status. However, for more formal guidance, both refer to clinical decision-making tools, such as the Multinational Association for Supportive Care in Cancer Risk (MASCC) index, the Clinical Index of Stable Febrile Neutropenia) CISNE, and Talcott's Rules [8] (Table 8.3).

Prophylaxis for Febrile Neutropenia

Antibacterial Prophylaxis

In patients experiencing prolonged neutropenia, or an absolute neutrophil count <500 cells/microL for 7 days or greater, antimicrobial prophylaxis is indicated. Typically, antibacterial, antifungal, and antiviral are needed. Initiation of antimicrobial prophylaxis relies on careful evaluation of drug adverse effects and resistance [9, 17]. Febrile neutropenia prophylaxis is only recommended for patients who are at high risk for developing profound, protracted neutropenia, specifically those undergoing intense induction chemotherapy for acute leukemia, myeloablative pre-engraftment phase treatment for hematopoietic stem cell transplant, and therapy for myelodysplastic syndrome [9, 17] (Fig. 8.1).

Recommendations

- Per the IDSA-ASCO guidelines, fluoroquinolones, specifically levofloxacin, are antibiotics of choice for prophylaxis [9, 17]. Prophylaxis with levofloxacin has been found to reduce febrile neutropenia hospital admission rates in acute myeloid leukemia patients after first consolidation therapy from 72% to 42%

Table 8.2 Diagnostic evaluation of neutropenic fever

Evaluation	Components/specific areas of focus
General evaluation	
History	Chemotherapy regimen
	Date of the most recent treatment
	History of complications from chemotherapy
	History of neutropenia
	History of antibiotic resistant infections
Review of systems	Urinary
	Skin
	Neurologic
	Respiratory
	Gastrointestinal
	Skin
	Constitutional
Physical exam	Invasive/central lines
	Mediports
	Indwelling Foley catheters
	Skin (specific focus on areas of pressure ulcers, skin breakdown, sites of invasive lines, and catheters)
	*Avoid rectal exams
Laboratory	CBC with Differential
	Comprehensive metabolic panel
Fungal markers	Beta-D-glucan serum assay (nonspecific fungal marker)
	Serum *Aspergillus* galactomannan antigen (specific for *Aspergillus* fungal infections)
	*Procalcitonin serum levels are not recommended
Blood cultures	Two sets of blood cultures (including a peripheral venous puncture and a central venous catheter)
	Repeat blood cultures every 48 h until negative
Evaluation driven by symptoms	
Urinary	Urinalysis with urine culture
Skin	Skin biopsy
	Wound culture
	Swab of vesicular lesions (For HSV and VZV)
Neurologic	LP (with analysis including cytology, glucose, protein, bacterial culture)
	Cryptococcal antigen on CSF
	HSV, VZV, CMV, and even Human Herpes Virus 6 (HHV6) on CSF
	West Nile Virus, Eastern Equine encephalitis on CSF
	CT head
Respiratory	Sputum culture
	Chest X-ray
	Respiratory viral panel
	CT chest
	CT maxillofacial
Gastrointestinal	Stool culture
	C. difficile testing
	CT abdomen

*important

Table 8.3 Risk stratification tool used in febrile neutropenia

	Risk stratification based on	Target population	Score interpretation
MASCC (Multinational Association for Supportive Care in Cancer)	Symptom severity Hypotension Active COPD Prior fungal infection Fluid status Inpatient/ outpatient Age	Not used in patients with acute leukemia undergoing induction or allogeneic HSCT conditioning	<21: high risk (recommend admission for empiric antibiotics) 21–26: low risk (consider outpatient management)
CISNE (Clinical Index of Stable Febrile Neutropenia)	Performance status Hyperglycemia COPD Cardiovascular disease Mucositis Monocyte number	Used in hemodynamically stable patients with solid organ malignances in the outpatient setting	Low risk (1.1% risk of complications, consider discharge/ outpatient management) Intermediate risk (6.2% risk of complications) High risk (36% risk of complications, admit to the hospital)
Talcott's rules	Inpatient/ outpatient status Status of cancer (controlled vs. progressive) Comorbidities	N/A	Group I inpatients Group II outpatients with comorbidity requiring hospitalization Group III outpatient with uncontrolled cancer Group IV outpatient, controlled cancer, no comorbidities

[18]. As there are risks for every medical intervention, fluoroquinolones do retain a "Black Box Warning" for orthopedic and nervous system injuries [9] (Table 8.4).

Antifungal Prophylaxis

Antifungal prophylaxis is recommended primarily for those with risk of profound protracted neutropenia; as such, it is generally not used for patients with solid malignancy [9]. Since mucositis further increases risk for invasive candidiasis, antifungal prophylaxis is especially recommended in patients with profound protracted neutropenia who concomitantly suffer from severe mucositis [9]. History of prior fungal infection, chimeric antigen receptor (CAR)-T-cell therapy, treatment for cytokine release syndrome (CRS), and immunomodulatory monoclonal antibody

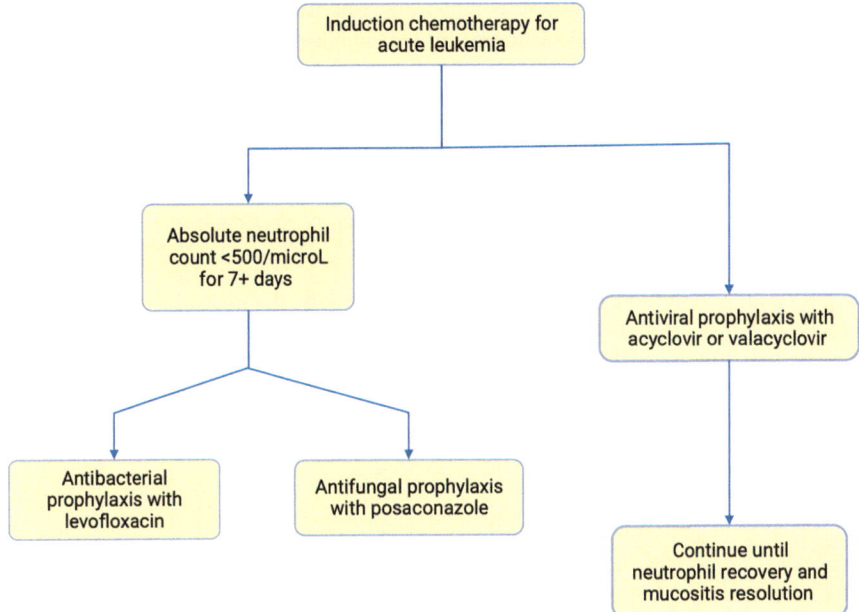

Fig. 8.1 Indications for prophylaxis

Table 8.4 Antimicrobial prophylaxis indication, medication, dosing

	Indication	Agents	Dose	Pathogens
Antiviral prophylaxis	Hematopoietic stem cell transplant, chemotherapy for acute leukemia, seropositive for VZV or HSV	Acyclovir Valacyclovir	800 mg 2×/ day 500 mg 2×/ day	VZV HSV
Antifungal prophylaxis	Prolonged neutropenia [ANC < 500 for 7+ days]	Posaconazole	300 mg 2×/ day for 2 doses then 300 mg daily	*Candida* spp. *Aspergillus* spp.
Antibacterial prophylaxis	Prolonged neutropenia [ANC <500 for 7+ days]	Levofloxacin	500 mg once daily	*P. aeruginosa* *S. epidermidis* *S. aureus*
PJP prophylaxis	Prolonged leukopenia	Bactrim Atovaquone Aerosolized pentamidine	1 DS tablet 3×/week 1500 mg daily 300 mg monthly	*Pneumocystis jirovecii*

therapy for multiple myeloma are also all risk factors for invasive fungal infections [9].

Bruton Tyrosine Kinase (BTK) inhibitors used to treat relapsed/refractory B-cell lymphoproliferative disorders and primary CNS lymphoma have increased invasive fungal infection rates of 3–12% and 5–44%, respectively [9]. Of those relapsed/

refractory B-cell lymphoproliferative disorder patients treated with BTK inhibitors, 40% of the invasive fungal infections are invasive aspergillosis with CNS infiltration [9].

Recommendations

- In choosing antifungal prophylaxis, it is important to determine if the goal is to target yeast, such as *Candida*, or mold, such as *Aspergillus*. While fluconazole is primarily effective against yeast, echinocandins and other triazoles in the form of posaconazole, voriconazole, and isavuconazole are effective against both [9].
- The first-line agent for yeast and mold antifungal prophylaxis is posaconazole. Posaconazole was found to reduce invasive fungal infections and infection-related mortality in patients with hematologic malignancies and immunosuppression [19]. Posaconazole also has the additional benefit that it can be administered orally or parenterally, which can be helpful for patients who cannot tolerate oral intake or having defects in gastrointestinal absorption. Voriconazole is an effective agent; however, it remains second line due to its elevated risk of hepatotoxicity [9].
- Isavuconazole is alternative for patients with QTc prolongation. it is generally not recommended as a prophylactic agent because of studies showing increased risk of breakthrough invasive fungal infections [9].
- The echinocandin drug class including micafungin and caspofungin are options for patients who cannot tolerate triazoles and/or require parenteral treatment [9].
- Amphotericin B deoxycholate is an effective antifungal option, but has significant adverse effects including nephrotoxicity, infusion-reactions, and gastrointestinal upset [9, 20, 21]. Thus, lipid formulations of Amphotericin B, including Liposomal Amphotericin B, have been more utilized for its equivalent efficacy and improved safety profile, particularly less nephrotoxicity and infusion reactions [9, 20] (Table 8.4).

Additional Microorganism to Consider

- *Pneumocystis jirovecii* (PJP) prophylaxis is also included within the scope of antifungal prophylaxis. Per the IDSA-ASCO guidelines, *Pneumocystis jirovecii* (PJP) prophylaxis is generally indicated for patients with over 3.5% risk of PJP pneumonia development due to chronic high dose systemic steroids, defined as 20 or more mg of prednisone equivalents daily for greater than or equal to 1 month [9].
- T-cell suppression by chemotherapy regimen is also a consideration, if lymphodepleting agents are used and CD4 count <200 cells/mm^3. In addition, if chemotherapy regimen includes a purine analog, PJP prophylaxis is also indicated. While Bactrim is considered first line, alternative agents include dapsone,

primaquine, atovaquone, and aerosolized pentamidine [9]. However, in patients with Glucose-6-Phosphate-Dehydrogenase (G6PD) deficiency, PJP prophylaxis must be chosen with caution, as sulfanilamide, dapsone, and primaquine may lead to severe hemolytic anemia in this population [22]. Thus, in patients with G6PD deficiency, it is recommended to utilize atovaquone or aerosolized pentamidine as the PJP prophylaxis of choice [17].

Antiviral Prophylaxis

- Antiviral prophylaxis may be considered in patients who are serologically positive. For example, in acute leukemia and hematopoietic stem cell transplant patients with positive HSV serologies, it may be necessary to consider antiviral prophylaxis in the form of acyclovir, a nucleoside analogue [9]. Patient populations who benefit from viral prophylaxis include those expected to experience prolonged neutropenia, patients who are seropositive for Herpes simplex virus (HSV) or Varicella zoster virus (VZV), and patients with a history of HSV or VZV infection. Viral infections can be a cause of significant mucositis, oral ulcers, and vesicular dermatologic findings. Viral prophylaxis should be considered in all patients expected to experience prolonged neutropenia and have a history of HSV or VZV seropositivity, or those that are experiencing mucositis, oral ulcers, or rash. Treatment options for common viral infections in patients receiving chemotherapy for hematologic malignancy include acyclovir or valacyclovir. Valacyclovir is a prodrug of acyclovir. Valacyclovir is generally preferred over acyclovir due to better prevention of VZV. One significant side effect with acyclovir is crystalline nephropathy, so caution and consideration of use of IV fluids with administration is advised. If infection is confirmed, treatment dosing of antiviral medications should be used.
- For those with evidence of chronic Hepatitis B, they may be at risk for Hepatitis B reactivation, requiring entecavir or tenofovir for preventing reactivation [9].
- While not technically a form of prophylaxis, non-live vaccines, especially flu and COVID vaccines serve a significant purpose in preventing complications from those viruses [9] (Table 8.4).

Treatment of Neutropenic Fever

Case 1 (Continued)

Our patients developed fever of 39 °C despite antimicrobial, antiviral, and antifungal prophylaxis. Her vital signs remain stable with a blood pressure of 118/75, pulse of 76, and oxygen saturation of 99% on room air. Beta-D-glucan serum assay and serum *Aspergillus* galactomannan antigen testing are obtained and return to be negative. Respiratory viral panel including influenza, parainfluenza, and respiratory syncytial virus was negative.

Clinical Context

This patient with persistent fevers. Broadening antimicrobial treatment would also be appropriate. It is important to repeat blood cultures while the patient remains febrile.

Empiric Antibiotic Treatment

- Given high risk of complications, prompt investigation must be performed concurrently with immediate empiric treatment for patients with febrile neutropenia.
- Specifically, parenteral broad-spectrum antibiotics must be administered within 1 h of presentation. First-line agents recommended as monotherapy are all antipseudomonal beta-lactam antibiotics, including Cefepime, Piperacillin-Tazobactam, and antipseudomonal carbapenems in the form of Meropenem or Imipenem-Cilastatin [8].
- As Ertapenem is one of the few carbapenems that does not provide coverage for pseudomonal infections, it would not be recommended as a first-line agent [17].
- Additional coverage with aminoglycosides, fluoroquinolones, or vancomycin may be indispensable in the setting of hemodynamic instability or antibiotic resistance [17].
- Risk factors for high likelihood of antibiotic resistance include prior exposure to broad-spectrum antibiotics, prolonged hospitalization, and prior infection with antibiotic-resistant organisms [23].
- Adding vancomycin to the empiric treatment may be necessary in the setting of gram-positive bacterial infections, including central venous catheter infections and skin or soft tissue infections. If concerned for strep viridians infection or bacteremia, especially in patients with mucositis and hypotension, it is recommended to also introduce vancomycin. Starting with vancomycin rather than penicillin is now the standard of care because of increasing rates of resistance to penicillins and even cephalosporins [17, 24, 25].
- It is ultimately imperative to consider clinical indication, renal injury, and hepatic function to treat the infection with the appropriate medications and doses while avoiding further organ injury. Lastly, empiric antibiotics may be ceased when resolution of the infection or neutropenia recovery to an ANC is over 500 [4, 17].
- When starting empiric treatment, it is important to cease prophylactic antimicrobials that redundantly prevent the same pathogens. However, if prophylactic antimicrobials are not treating the same pathogens as the empiric treatment, they should be continued. For example, if a patient with febrile neutropenia is starting empiric cefepime, the prophylactic Levofloxacin should be held and only

restarted when the cefepime is discontinued. In contrast, because cefepime does not treat viral or fungal infections, it is necessary to continue the prophylactic acyclovir and posaconazole with the cefepime.

- Of note, if there is resolution of the infection but the patient remains neutropenic, it would be vital to immediately restart all indicated antimicrobial prophylaxis upon discontinuation of empiric therapeutic antibiotics.

Case 1 (Continued)

After 3 days of intravenous antibiotic, the patient develops severe mucositis with ulceration in the oral cavity. Her blood cultures are reported positive for gram-positive organisms. The patient is started on vancomycin. Her fevers subsided after 24 h of therapy. On day 25 of induction, her absolute neutrophil increases to 1600 cells/microL. As her neutrophil count continues to improve, her oral mucositis resolves.

Clinical Context

Mucositis is a common side effect of induction chemotherapy. It is common to observe neutropenia and mucositis in patients receiving leukemia induction therapy. Alpha *Streptococcus* or methicillin-resistant *Staphylococcus aureus* (MRSA) infection are important to consider since cefepime would not cover for MRSA bacteria.

In our patient, blood cultures finally identified MRSA. Other resistant microbes to consider in a patient with persistent fever despite broad spectrum antibiotics include vancomycin-resistant *Enterococcus* (VRE), extended spectrum beta-lactamase (ESBL)-producing gram-negative bacteria, and carbapenemase-producing organisms.

Persistent Fevers in Neutropenic Patient

- When neutropenic patients continue to fever for over 48 h despite empiric antibiotics, the next steps must account for other untreated bacteria, antimicrobial resistance, and potential fungal infections.
- The workup would include continuing with two blood cultures daily to monitor for new or continued presence of bacteremia, the pathogen's antibiotic sensitivities, and when the pathogen is successfully cleared. Additionally, monitoring fungal markers such as D-glucan, galactomannan, and aspergilus antigen in addition to obtaininng CT imaging of the chest, abdomen, and pelvis are recommened to uncover potential source of infection [26].
- Empiric antibiotic treatment should be further broadened to target resistant organisms, including methicillin-resistant *Staph aureus* (MRSA),

vancomycin-resistant *Enterococcus* (VRE), extended spectrum beta-lactamase (ESBL)-producing gram-negative bacteria, and carbapenemase-producing organisms. Vancomycin, linezolid, and daptomycin are effective against MRSA, while just linezolid and daptomycin are used to target VRE. Carbapenems can treat ESBL infections; polymyxin or tigecycline is employed for *Klebsiella pneumoniae* carbapenemase infections [27] (Fig. 8.2).

Caveats

In certain situations, such as those involving abscesses, wounds, and osteomyelitis, infection may be severe requiring weeks of parenteral antibiotics. Unfortunately, because neutropenic patients have a significantly impaired adaptive immune system, invasive procedures are challenging. During this time, patient safety depends on supportive care, close monitoring, and antimicrobial medications.

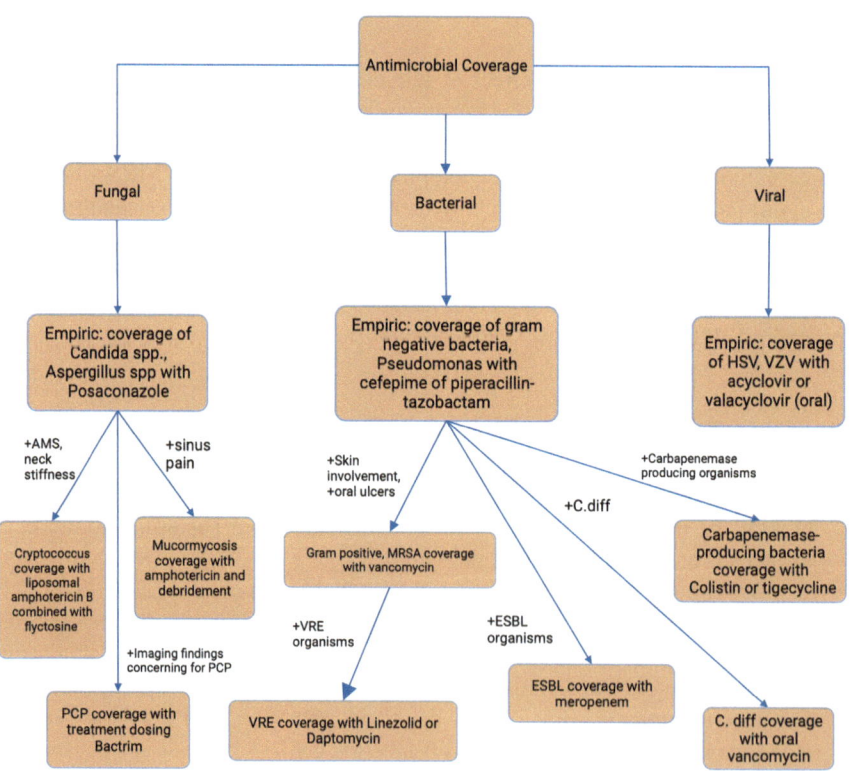

Fig. 8.2 Treatment escalation and antimicrobial coverage in neutropenic infections

Antifungal Treatment

- Empiric antifungal treatment should be initiated as soon as possible in high-risk neutropenic patients who continue to fever despite 4–7 days of appropriate antibiotic treatment [4, 7, 27]. Invasive fungal infections are extremely common in patients with acute leukemia such that risk of developing invasive fungal infection (IFI) is approximately 11.1% at 100 days of acute leukemia diagnosis. Those patients with acute leukemia and other hematologic malignancy have a 35-38% risk of mortality due to IFI. Thus, IFI are treated aggressively [7] (Table 8.5).
- If there is sufficient clinical suspicion or very early diagnosis of a particular fungus causing the infection, it is recommended to administer antifungals targeting the specific fungal pathogen.
- As mucositis, central venous catheter irritation, or esophagitis may suggest *Candida* infections, echinocandin antifungals would be first-line treatment. For potential *Candida* infections, fluconazole or voriconazole may also be effective alternatives.
- If potential *Aspergillus* is ascertained on CT chest or bronchoalveolar lavage laboratory studies, voriconazole would be an appropriate first-line agent given its mold coverage. For patients with altered mental status, neck stiffness, and neurologic symptoms concerning for meningoencephalitis, first-line treatment for *Cryptococcus* would be liposomal amphotericin B combined followed by maintenance fluconazole. However, voriconazole, isavuconazole, and posaconazole also maintain efficacy against *Cryptococcus*, especially in non-CNS *Cryptococcus* (Fig. 8.2).
- Additionally, with clinical signs and symptoms of sino-orbital involvement concerning for mucormycosis infection, first-line treatment would be the combination of debridement with one of the following: liposomal amphotericin B, posaconazole, or isavuconazole suspicion should be raised for mucormycosis infection, for which first-line treatment would be amphotericin B, posaconazole, or isavuconazole.

Table 8.5 Fungal markers in evaluation of infection in the neutropenic host

	Pathogens	Sample Type	Infections in which this test will be negative	Type of test
Beta-D-Glucan (Fungitell)	*Candida* spp. *Aspergillus* spp. *Pneumocystis jirovecii* *Fusarium* spp.	Blood BAL	Mucormycosis *Cryptococcus*	PCR
Galactomannan antigen	*Aspergillus* spp.	Blood BAL	Specific test	Enzyme immunoassay (EIA)
Cryptococcus antigen	*Cryptococcus* spp.	Blood CSF	Specific test	Antigen testing
Histoplasma antigen	*Histoplasma capsulatum*	Blood Urine	Specific test	Antigen testing

- For patients with signs and symptoms of PJP pneumonia ascertained clinically, via imaging, or via BAL, the first-line treatment is trimethoprim-sulfamethoxazole [28].
- In many cases of neutropenic fever, there may not be clinical signs or symptoms suggesting a particular fungal pathogen. As such, the first line for purely empiric antifungal treatment would be either voriconazole or posaconazole, irrespective of patient history with any prior antifungal prophylaxis with triazoles. It can be especially challenging to ensure efficacy and safety of therapeutic triazole treatment given their variable pharmacokinetics from the often-polymorphic Cytochrome P450 metabolism enzymatic system [29]. Thus, it is imperative to administer voriconazole or posaconazole antifungal treatment under the protocol of Therapeutic Drug Monitoring (TDM), a system of monitoring drug levels and adjusting dosage and frequency to ensure therapeutic but nontoxic antifungal treatment [29, 30]. Given the complexities of TDM, it is recommended to confer with clinical pharmacist and Infectious Disease colleagues to ensure proper clinical care.

Antiviral Treatment

- One consideration in patients presenting with neutropenic fever are viral causes of infection. Neutropenic patients are susceptible to COVID-19 infections. Patients are at risk for severe complications of COVID-19 infection. The core treatment of COVID-19 infection includes oxygen support and steroid treatment. In hospitalized patients with COVID-19 infection who are not on mechanical ventilation, treatment with Remdesivir can be considered.
- Other viral causes of severe infection include Herpes simplex virus (HSV) and Varicella zoster virus (VZV). Viral infections can be a cause of significant mucositis, oral ulcers, and vesicular dermatologic findings. Treatment options for common viral infections in patients receiving chemotherapy for hematologic malignancy include acyclovir or valacyclovir. While many patients are treated with antiviral prophylaxis, if a confirmed viral infection is diagnoses, dosing of antiviral medications is altered for treatment dosing rather than prophylactic dosing.

Therapeutic Drug Monitoring

- Therapeutic drug monitoring for voriconazole consists of checking a trough 10–12 h after the last dose on day 4 of voriconazole treatment or later [29, 31]. For therapeutic treatment, the goal trough would be above 1 mg/L, albeit occasional case may require above 2 mg/L. However, it is crucial to maintain the trough level below 5.5 to minimize risk of hepatotoxicity, QTc prolongation, and visual hallucinations [29, 31, 32].

- If the voriconazole trough level is under 1 mg/L and consequently considered subtherapeutic, the daily dose should be raised by 50 to 100 mg, and another trough should be rechecked in 4–7 days. If the trough level is above 5.5 and considered supratherapeutic, the daily dose should be lowered by 50–100 mg and another trough should be rechecked in 4–7 days [29, 31]. Other troughs may be necessary in the future with potential medication interactions, concern for toxicity, dose changes, and more.
- For posaconazole, the TDM levels are obtained via troughs 7 days after posaconazole initiation or dosage adjustment. The goal for therapeutic antifungal treatment is above 1–1.5 mg/L, but it is recommended to avoid troughs above 3–3.75 mg/L due to concern for toxicities including QTc prolongation, hepatotoxicity, and GI upset [29–31].
- Dose adjustments are dependent on posaconazole formulation [31]. For subtherapeutic posaconazole levels with direct release tablets and parenteral formulations, doses should be raised by 100 mg daily, with the next level obtained in 5–7 days [31]. In the case of the oral suspension formulation, subtherapeutic levels are adjusted by increasing the daily dose by 200 mg such that instead of 200 mg TID it is 200 mg QID and rechecking levels in 5–7 days [31]. More additional monitoring levels may be needed in the cases of patients with dose changes, morbid obesity, lack of antifungal efficacy, and concern for toxicity [29] (Fig. 8.3).
- Due to moderate to strong cytochrome 3A4 (CYP3A4) inhibition, dose of concomitant CYP3A4 substrates including oral oncolytics needs to be adjusted to prevent toxicity and overdosing.

Key Points
- Patients with hematologic malignancies including acute leukemia are at an increased risk for neutropenia due to treatment with regimens that are cytotoxic and myeloablative. These regiments lead to pancytopenia including leukopenia and neutropenia. Common regimens implicated in neutropenia include anthracyclines, cytarabine, gemcitabine, and venetoclax, among others.
- Fever is defined as a one-time temperature greater than 38.3 °C or greater than 38 °C that persists over a 1-h period.
- Neutropenic patients have less effective mucosal barriers due to mucositis and decreased healing of these injured barriers. This in combination with decreased number and function of circulating granulocytes places them at an increased risk for infection.
- Initiate antibacterial and antifungal prophylaxis when absolute neutrophil count is less than 500 cells/microL for a prolonged period of 7 days or more.
- Antiviral prophylaxis is indicated in all patients with prolonged neutropenia.
- Consider *Pneumocystis jirovecii* prophylaxis with trimethoprim-sulfamethoxazole in all patients with acute lymphocytic leukemia, patients receiving purine analogs, t-cell-depleting agents, Alemtuzumab, or CAR-T therapy. Prophylaxis should be continued until CD4 count is >200 cells/microL.

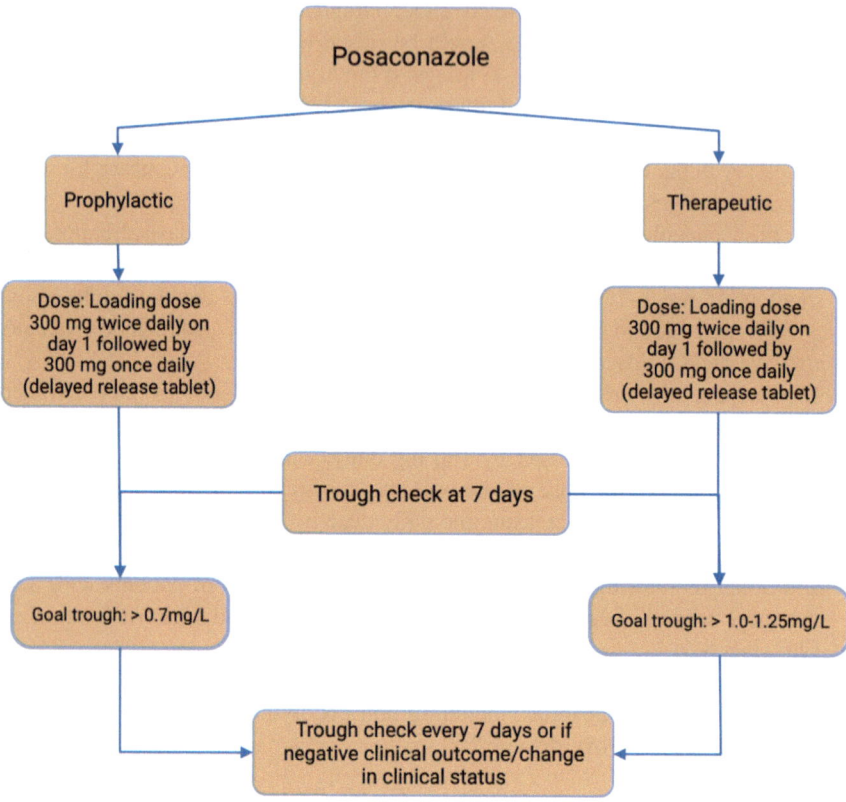

Fig. 8.3 Therapeutic drug monitoring in posaconazole

- If fever develops during a period of neutropenia, initiate infectious workup, and start empiric antibiotics with broad spectrum antipseudomonal treatment within 60 min of fever.
- If a patient develops persistent fevers, repeat blood cultures every 48 h while still febrile. Expand infectious evaluation to include resistant organisms and fungal organisms.
- Beta-D-glucan and *Aspergillus* galactomannan antigen testing can be helpful in identifying fungal causes of infection.
- Indications for antimicrobial escalation in neutropenic fever include skin involvement, concern for resistant bacteria (MRSA, VRE, ESBL, carbapenemase-producing bacteria), concern for invasive fungal infection (sinus involvement, neck stiffness, travel to endemic areas, positive fungal markers), changes in clinical status, and persistent fevers despite treatment.

References

1. Lehman HK, Segal BH. The role of neutrophils in host defense and disease. J Allergy Clin Immunol. 2020;145(6):1535–44. https://doi.org/10.1016/j.jaci.2020.02.038.
2. Selders GS, Fetz AE, Radic MZ, Bowlin GL. An overview of the role of neutrophils in innate immunity, inflammation and host-biomaterial integration. Regen Biomater. 2017;4(1):55–68. https://doi.org/10.1093/rb/rbw041.
3. Neth OW, Bajaj-Elliott M, Turner MW, Klein NJ. Susceptibility to infection in patients with neutropenia: the role of the innate immune system. Br J Haematol. 2005;129(6):713–22. https://doi.org/10.1111/j.1365-2141.2005.05462.x.
4. Punnapuzha S, Edemobi PK, Elmoheen A. Febrile neutropenia. *StatPearls*. StatPearls Publishing. Copyright © 2023, StatPearls Publishing LLC.; 2023.
5. Munshi HG, Montgomery RB. Severe neutropenia: a diagnostic approach. West J Med. 2000;172(4):248–52. https://doi.org/10.1136/ewjm.172.4.248.
6. Moore DC. Drug-induced neutropenia: a focus on rituximab-induced late-onset neutropenia. P T. 2016;41(12):765–8.
7. Hansen BA, Wendelbo Ø, Bruserud Ø, Hemsing AL, Mosevoll KA, Reikvam H. Febrile neutropenia in acute leukemia. epidemiology, etiology, pathophysiology and treatment. Mediterr J Hematol Infect Dis. 2020;12(1):e2020009. https://doi.org/10.4084/mjhid.2020.009.
8. Taplitz RA, Kennedy EB, Bow EJ, et al. Outpatient management of fever and neutropenia in adults treated for malignancy: American Society of Clinical Oncology and Infectious Diseases Society of America Clinical Practice Guideline Update. J Clin Oncol. 2018;36(14):1443–53. https://doi.org/10.1200/jco.2017.77.6211.
9. Taplitz RA, Kennedy EB, Bow EJ, et al. Antimicrobial prophylaxis for adult patients with cancer-related immunosuppression: ASCO and IDSA Clinical Practice Guideline Update. J Clin Oncol. 2018;36(30):3043–54. https://doi.org/10.1200/jco.18.00374.
10. Lyman GH, Abella E, Pettengell R. Risk factors for febrile neutropenia among patients with cancer receiving chemotherapy: a systematic review. Crit Rev Oncol Hematol. 2014;90(3):190–9. https://doi.org/10.1016/j.critrevonc.2013.12.006.
11. Buckner CD, Clift RA, Sanders JE, et al. Protective environment for marrow transplant recipients: a prospective study. Ann Intern Med. 1978;89(6):893–901. https://doi.org/10.732 6/0003-4819-89-6-893.
12. Masaoka T. Infection prevention for patients with acute leukemia using laminar air flow rooms. Tokai J Exp Clin Med. 1986;11(Suppl):9–14.
13. Ball S, Brown TJ, Das A, Khera R, Khanna S, Gupta A. Effect of neutropenic diet on infection rates in cancer patients with neutropenia: a meta-analysis of randomized controlled trials. Am J Clin Oncol. 2019;42(3):270–4. https://doi.org/10.1097/coc.0000000000000514.
14. Ma Y, Lu X, Liu H. Neutropenic diet cannot reduce the risk of infection and mortality in oncology patients with neutropenia. Front Oncol. 2022;12:836371. https://doi.org/10.3389/fonc.2022.836371.
15. Radhakrishnan V, Lagudu PBB, Gangopadhyay D, et al. Neutropenic versus regular diet for acute leukaemia induction chemotherapy: randomised controlled trial. BMJ Support Palliat Care. 2022;12(4):421–30. https://doi.org/10.1136/spcare-2022-003833.
16. McKenzie H, Hayes L, White K, et al. Chemotherapy outpatients' unplanned presentations to hospital: a retrospective study. Support Care Cancer. 2011;19(7):963–9. https://doi.org/10.1007/s00520-010-0913-y.
17. Segal BH, Freifeld AG. Antibacterial prophylaxis in patients with neutropenia. J Natl Compr Cancer Netw. 2007;5(2):235–42. https://doi.org/10.6004/jnccn.2007.0023.
18. Lee SSF, Fulford AE, Quinn MA, Seabrook J, Rajakumar I. Levofloxacin for febrile neutropenia prophylaxis in acute myeloid leukemia patients associated with reduction in hospital admissions. Support Care Cancer. 2018;26(5):1499–504. https://doi.org/10.1007/s00520-017-3976-1.

19. Wong TY, Loo YS, Veettil SK, et al. Efficacy and safety of posaconazole for the prevention of invasive fungal infections in immunocompromised patients: a systematic review with meta-analysis and trial sequential analysis. Sci Rep. 2020;10(1):14575. https://doi.org/10.1038/s41598-020-71571-0.
20. Hamill RJ. Amphotericin B formulations: a comparative review of efficacy and toxicity. Drugs. 2013;73(9):919–34. https://doi.org/10.1007/s40265-013-0069-4.
21. Laniado-Laborín R, Cabrales-Vargas MN. Amphotericin B: side effects and toxicity. Rev Iberoam Micol. 2009;26(4):223–7. https://doi.org/10.1016/j.riam.2009.06.003.
22. Zhang Z, Li Q, Shen X, et al. The medication for pneumocystis pneumonia with glucose-6-phosphate dehydrogenase deficiency patients. Front Pharmacol. 2022;13:957376. https://doi.org/10.3389/fphar.2022.957376.
23. Rao GG. Risk factors for the spread of antibiotic-resistant bacteria. Drugs. 1998;55(3):323–30. https://doi.org/10.2165/00003495-199855030-00001.
24. Tunkel AR, Sepkowitz KA. Infections caused by viridans streptococci in patients with neutropenia. Clin Infect Dis. 2002;34(11):1524–9. https://doi.org/10.1086/340402.
25. Marron A, Carratalà J, González-Barca E, Fernández-Sevilla A, Alcaide F, Gudiol F. Serious complications of bacteremia caused by Viridans streptococci in neutropenic patients with cancer. Clin Infect Dis. 2000;31(5):1126–30. https://doi.org/10.1086/317460.
26. Zimmer AJ, Freifeld AG. Optimal management of neutropenic fever in patients with cancer. J Oncol Pract. 2019;15(1):19–24. https://doi.org/10.1200/jop.18.00269.
27. Freifeld AG, Bow EJ, Sepkowitz KA, et al. Clinical practice guideline for the use of antimicrobial agents in neutropenic patients with cancer: 2010 update by the infectious diseases society of America. Clin Infect Dis. 2011;52(4):e56–93. https://doi.org/10.1093/cid/cir073.
28. Ibrahim A, Chattaraj A, Iqbal Q, et al. Pneumocystis jiroveci pneumonia: a review of management in human immunodeficiency virus (HIV) and non-HIV immunocompromised patients. Avicenna J Med. 2023;13(1):23–34. https://doi.org/10.1055/s-0043-1764375.
29. McCreary EK, Davis MR, Narayanan N, et al. Utility of triazole antifungal therapeutic drug monitoring: insights from the Society of Infectious Diseases Pharmacists: endorsed by the mycoses study group education and research consortium. Pharmacotherapy. 2023;43(10):1043–50. https://doi.org/10.1002/phar.2850.
30. Dekkers BGJ, Bakker M, van der Elst KCM, et al. Therapeutic drug monitoring of posaconazole: an update. Curr Fungal Infect Rep. 2016;10:51–61. https://doi.org/10.1007/s12281-016-0255-4.
31. Gómez-López A. Antifungal therapeutic drug monitoring: focus on drugs without a clear recommendation. Clin Microbiol Infect. 2020;26(11):1481–7. https://doi.org/10.1016/j.cmi.2020.05.037.
32. Yi WM, Schoeppler KE, Jaeger J, et al. Voriconazole and posaconazole therapeutic drug monitoring: a retrospective study. Ann Clin Microbiol Antimicrob. 2017;16(1):60. https://doi.org/10.1186/s12941-017-0235-8.

Chapter 9
Diagnosis and Management of Diffuse Large B-Cell Lymphoma

Sravanti Teegarapavu

Case Demonstration

A 54 years old male presented to the ER with worsening abdominal pain and constipation. CT abdomen/pelvis showed extensive bulky intra-abdominal and retroperitoneal adenopathy, including a conglomerated mass of lymph nodes in the small bowel mesentery measuring $15.7 \times 10.5 \times 15.1$ cm. Biopsy of the abdominal mass showed diffuse large B-cell lymphoma and germinal center subtype with high grade features. FISH studies were negative for re-arrangement of myc and bcl-6. Staging scans showed him to be stage III DLBCL. He was started on therapy with Rituximab-Cyclophosphamide +Vincristine +Doxorubicin + Prednisone (R-CHOP) and completed six cycles achieving complete remission.

Definition

DLBCL is the most common histologic subtype of non-Hodgkin's lymphoma accounting for 25–30% of cases and displays significant molecular and genetic heterogeneity. DLBCL is an aggressive disease and diagnosis is typically made by core or excisional biopsy of a suspicious lymph node. It arises from large B cells and expresses CD19, CD20, CD22, and CD79a. Standard treatment of DLBCL is chemoimmunotherapy with R-CHOP with response rates of 55–60%. About 35–40%

S. Teegarapavu (✉)
Dan L Duncan Comprehensive Cancer Center at Baylor College of Medicine,
Houston, TX, USA

Baylor College of Medicine, Houston, TX, USA
e-mail: teegavar@bcm.edu

© The Author(s), under exclusive license to Springer Nature
Switzerland AG 2024
G. Rivero, I. R. Sosa (eds.), *Consulting Hematology and Oncology Handbook*,
https://doi.org/10.1007/978-3-031-75810-2_9

101

relapse or remain refractory to first-line chemoimmunotherapy requiring the use salvage chemotherapy and other novel treatment combinations. In this chapter, we aim to discuss molecular and genomic landscape of DLBCL and explore novel treatment regimens available for relapsed setting.

Clinical Context

DLBCL usually presents as a rapidly enlarging mass, nodal enlargement in the neck and abdomen, or mediastinum or extranodal disease which can occur in up to 40% of cases. Common extranodal sites include the stomach, gastrointestinal tract, lung, skin, bone, testis, thyroid, tonsil, liver, breast, adrenals, kidney, nasal cavity, paranasal sinuses, central nervous system, uterine cervix, and vagina. 40% of patients present with localized disease, whereas 60% of patients present with advanced stage DLBCL. Bone marrow involvement may be seen in up to 30% of cases. B symptoms consisting of fever, drenching night sweats, and weight loss can be observed in up to 30% of patients.

Investigation/Workup

Diagnosis of DLBCL requires core or excisional(preferred) biopsy of suspicious lymph node or extranodal mass. Diagnosis is best made by morphology and immunophenotyping with additional evaluation of cytogenetics and molecular studies.

Morphology

Complete effacement of the lymph node architecture is seen with medium to large cells which have large nucleoli and abundant cytoplasm. Most common variants of DLBCL include centroblastic, immunoblastic, and anaplastic. Centroblastic variants represent 80% of all DLBCL cases, while immunoblastic variant comprises 8–10% and anaplastic about 3%.

Immunophenotyping

The neoplastic cells of DLBCL express pan B-cell antigens such as CD19, CD20, CD22, CD79a, and CD45 and B-cell transcription factors such as PAX5. About 5–10% of cases have aberrant expression of CD5, while 10–15% of cases express CD30. BCL-2 is seen in 25–80% of DLBCL, BCL-6 in 70%, and MUM/IRF4 in 35–65% of cases.

Cytogenetics/FISH

- t(14;18) (q21;q32)/IGH-BCL-2.
- MYC at 8q24.
- Assess for rearrangements of BCL6, BCL2, and MYC.

Others

- EBV Epstein-Barr virus (EBV)-encoded RNA (EBER) in situ hybridization (EBER-ISH).
- HHV-8.

Next-Generation Sequencing [1]

Classification: DLBCL NOS

Cell of Origin

Gene expression profiling [2] is the gold standard for determining cell of origin though in routine practice immunohistochemistry using Tally & Hans algorithm [3] is commonly used. Two major groups identified by GEP are as follows:

GCB: CD10+ or BCL6+ CD10−, MUM1/IRF4− 60%.
Non-GCB (ABC): CD10−, MUM1/IRF+, BCL6+/− 25–30%.
Unclassifiable—10–15%.

Immunophenotypic subclassification is illustrated in Fig. 9.1.

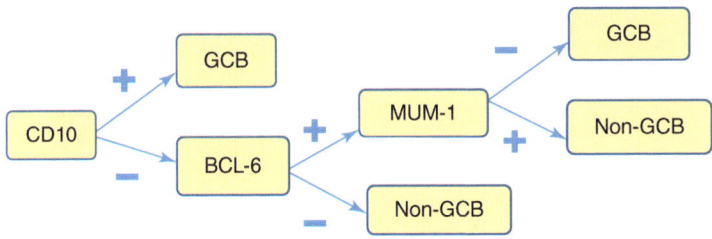

Fig. 9.1 Han's algorithm

Molecular (Fig. 9.2)

Cytogenetic abnormalities involving oncogenes BCL-2, BCL-6, and MYC.

High grade B-cell lymphoma with MYC, BCL-2, and/or BCL-6 rearrangements. DH typically contains MYC rearrangement along with BCL-2 and/or BCL-6 (triple hit). All DHT and triple hit DLBCL retain GCB cell of origin [4].

Double Expressor (DE): Overexpression of MYC (40%) and BCL-2(50%), far more common in ABC/non-GCB subgroup of DLBCL.

Genetic

Whole exome sequencing has identified distinct genetic subtypes characterized by recurring genetic mutations which hold the potential to provide specific groups enriched for patients who, albeit not approved, may benefit from targeted agents and other novel therapies [5–7] (Table 9.1).

- MCD (MYD88 and CD79).
- BN2 (BCL-6 and NOTCH2).
- N1 (NOTCH1).
- EZB (EZH2 and BCL-2).
- DLBCL Clusters: C1,C2,C3,C4,C5.

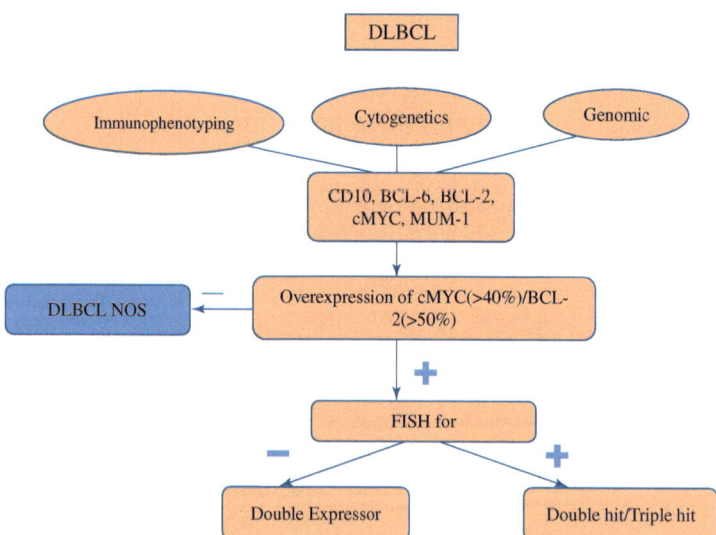

Fig. 9.2 Molecular classification of diffuse large B-cell lymphoma

Table 9.1 Common mutations observed in DLBCL according to cell of origin

Cell of origin	Signaling pathway/process	Recurring genes
GCB[a]	Histone methylation/acetylation	EZH EP300 CREBBP KMT2D GNA13 GNAI2 SIPR2 PI3K JAK-STAT
ABC[b]	NF-kB	MYD88 CD79A/B CARD11 MALT1 BCL-10 MYD88 TNFAIP3

[a]*GCB* germinal center B cell
[b]*ABC* Activated B-cell like

Prognostic Index

Clinical: International Prognostic Index (IPI) [8].

- Age > 60 years.
- Serum lactate dehydrogenase (LDH) concentration greater than normal.
- Eastern Cooperative Oncology Group (ECOG) performance status ≥ 2.
- Clinical stage III or IV.
- >1 extranodal disease site.

  1. Low risk—IPI score of zero or one.
  2. Low-intermediate risk—IPI score of two.
  3. High-intermediate risk—IPI score of three.
  4. High risk—IPI score of four or five.

Cell of Origin: ABC subtype has poorer outcomes compared to GCB.
Molecular: MYC rearrangements, DEL, and DH/THL have worse prognosis compared to DLBCL NOS.

Pretreatment Evaluation

History and physical with special attention to underlying heart disease, nodal areas, liver, and spleen.

Laboratory Studies

- Complete blood count.
- Baseline chemistries (i.e., liver function, uric acid, calcium, renal function).
- Hepatitis and HIV viral panel.
- LDH, Beta-2 microglobulin.
- Pregnancy test in patients of child-bearing age.

Other

- 2D echocardiogram or MUGA.
- PET-CT or CT CAP with contrast.
- Bone marrow biopsy, not needed if PET-CT demonstrates bone disease.
- Neurological evaluation with lumbar puncture for patients with high risk of CNS disease/relapse and high IPI.
- Fertility counseling for men and women with child-bearing potential.

CNS Prophylaxis

For patients with high risk of CNS recurrence:
  CNS-IPI [9]: score of 4 or more:

- Age > 60 years.
- Serum LDH > normal.
- Performance status >1.
- Ann Arbor stage III–IV disease.
- Involvement of >1 extranodal site.
- Kidney of adrenal gland involvement.
- Additionally, extranodal site such as testes, breast.
- Risk factors such as HIV.
- Double/triple hit lymphoma.

Commonly used regimens include intrathecal methotrexate and/or cytarabine or systemic high dose methotrexate.

Management (Fig. 9.3)

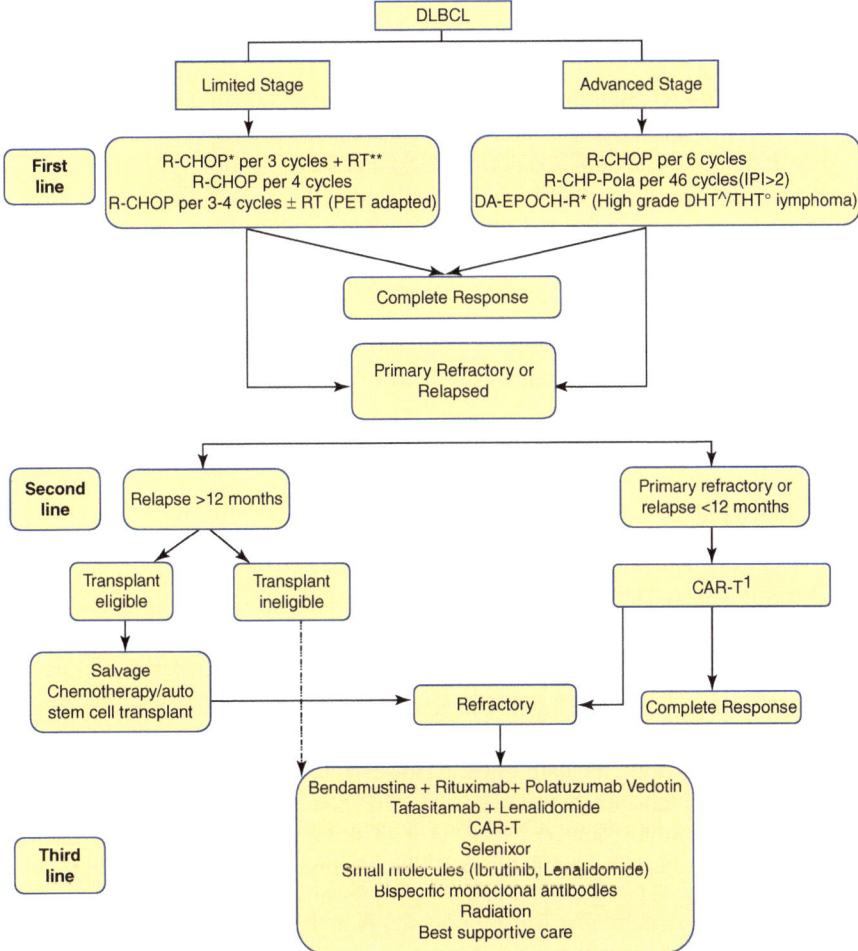

Fig. 9.3 Management of DLBCL. *R-CHOP* Rituximab+ Cyclophosphamide+ Doxorubicin+ Vincristine+ Prednisone, **RT* radiation, *DA-EPOCH* dose adjusted Etoposide+ Prednisone+ Vincristine+ Cyclophosphamide+ Doxorubicin, ^DH double hit, °TH triple hit; [1] *CD19 CAR-T* Anti CD19 Chimeric Antigen receptor T cell

Upfront Therapy

Limited Stage DLBCL

Options include the following:

- R-CHOPx3 + RT. Based on SWOG S0014 which showed a 2-year progression-free survival (PFS) of 92% and a 4-year overall-survival (OS) of 92% [10].
- For limited stage, non-bulky, normal LDH and ECOG:
- R-CHOPx4 based on FLYER study which showed a 3-year PFS 96% [11].
- PET-adapted approach—R-CHOPx3, negative iPET—one more cycle of R-CHOP, positive PET-involved field radiation therapy followed by ibritumomab tiuxetan radioimmunotherapy (INCTN S1001) [12].

Advanced Stage DLBCL

Standard NOS DLBCL

RCHOP x 6 [13]

- Cyclophosphamide (Cytoxan) 750 mg/m^2 IV once on day 1.
- Doxorubicin (Adriamycin) 50 mg/m^2 IV once on day 1.
- Vincristine (Oncovin) 1.4 mg/m^2 (maximum dose of 2 mg) IV once on day 1.
- Prednisone (Sterapred) 40 mg/m^2 PO once per day on days 1 to 5.

Despite multiple studies looking at improving outcomes in front-line DLBCL treatment including intensification of rituximab, addition of drug x, etc., R-CHOP continues to remain the standard of care. However, a recent phase III study looking at addition of polatuzumab vedotin to R-CHP compared to R-CHOP produced superior 2-year progression-free survival with similar overall survival and safety profile and may be considered for first-line treatment in DLBCL patients with IPI ≥ 2 [14].

Double Expressor Lymphoma

R-CHOP x6. Given lack of randomized data with intense regimens in double expressor lymphomas, R-CHOP is still widely used.

High Grade Lymphoma with MYC, BCL-2, BCL-6 Rearrangements (Double Hit/Triple Hit)

DA-EPOCH-R x6. Several retrospective studies have shown superior PFS and OS with intense regimens such as DA-EPOCH-R compared to R-CHOP [15].

Relapsed/Refractory Disease

Salvage chemotherapy followed by autologous stem cell transplant has been the standard of care for chemosensitive disease in transplant eligible patients as established by PARMA trial [16]. In the rituximab era, the curative effect of auto-SCT remains questionable given that a 3-year PFS of patients previously treated with rituximab who received either R-ICE or R-DHAP prior to ASCT was only 21% as per the CORAL study [17].

In patients eligible for transplant with chemosensitive disease, salvage chemotherapy with R-DHAP/R-ICE is commonly used followed by autologous stem cell transplant. Outcomes of patients with primary refractory disease have been historically poor with median OS of 6.3 months.

Chimeric Antigen Receptor T-Cell Therapy

CARs represent genetically engineered T cell designed to recognize and eliminate cancerous cells by targeting tumor-associated antigens. Axicabtagene ciloleucel (Axicel), Tisagenlecleucel, and Lisocabtagene maraleucel have been approved by FDA following two lines of systemic therapy for relapsed/refractory DLBCL [18–20] (Fig. 9.3). The studies involving approval of Axicel, Tisacel, and Lisocel are summarized in the table below. The main toxicities of CAR-T include cytokine release syndrome (CRS) and immune effector cell-associated neurotoxicity syndrome (ICANS). Risk factors recognized for early progression after CAR-T include involvement of ≥ two extranodal sites, elevated CRP, and high total metabolic tumor volume at the time of treatment. More recently, CARs were compared to standard of care in second-line setting for primary refractory or early relapse (within 12 months of frontline therapy). Zuma-7 [21] showed improved event free survival with Axicabtagene ciloleucel compared to standard of care. Similarly, TRANSFORM [22] evaluating Lisocabtagene maraleucel also demonstrated improved event-free, complete, and overall response rate. BELINDA [23] study, on the other hand, showed similar response rates and outcomes with Tisagenlecleucel when compared to standard of care therapy in second-line setting. The above studies have led to FDA approval of Axixel and Lisocel for second-line therapy in primary refractory or early relapse (<12 months after first-line systemic therapy) DLBCL patients (Table 9.2).

Table 9.2 CD19 CART studies demonstrating best response rate, cytokine release syndrome incidence, and proportion of neurotoxicity (ICANS)

	Axicel ZUMA-1	Tisacel JULIET	Lisocel TRANSCEND
Pt number	112	165	134
Median turnaround time(days)	17	54	24
CAR-T dose	2×10^6 kg	$1-5 \times 10^8$ kg	DL1: 5×10^7 cells DL2: 1×10^8 cells
Best response rate(ORR/CR)	83%/58%	52%/40%	73%/53%
Median follow-up duration ORR/CR	27.1 months 39%/37%	14 months 33%/29%	8 months 49%/46%
CRS			
Overall/>Grade 3	94%/13%	74%/23%	42%/2%
Median time to onset(days)	2 (1–12)	3 (1–51)	5 (1–14)
Median duration(days)	7 (2–58)	8 (1–36)	5 (1–17)
Neurotoxicity (ICANS)			
Overall/>Grade 3	87%/31%	58%/18%	30%/10%
Median time to onset(days)	4 (1–43)	6 (1–359)	9 (1–66)
Median duration(days)	17	14	11

In patients ineligible for transplant, various options which can be availed include chemotherapy; antibody drug conjugates such as polatuzumab vedotin in combination with BR, Tafasitamab and lenalidomide, loncastuximab tesirine, and brentuximab vedotin (for CD expressing DLBCL); and small molecules such as ibrutinib and lenalidomide especially in non-GCB DLBCL. Other available options include small molecules such as selinexor and antibody drug conjugates such as loncastuximab tesirine.

Agents Available for Relapsed/Refractory Disease

Antibody Drug Conjugates (ADCs)

Antibody drug conjugates combine monoclonal antibodies specific to surface antigens present on particular tumor cells with highly potent anticancer agents linked via a chemical linker.

1. Polatuzumab vedotin anti-CD79b monoclonal antibody also conjugated to MMAE. Phase II study looking at addition of polatuzumab vedotin to rituximab-bendamustine (BR) showed ORR rate of 45% with a CR of 40% and a median DOR of 12.6 months [24].
2. Tafasitamab is an Fc-enhanced monoclonal antibody against CD19 with direct cytotoxicity and enhanced antibody-dependent cell-mediated toxicity. A phase II study of 81 patients with RR DLCBL evaluated the combination of Tafasitamab

with lenalidomide and showed that the ORR was 60% (43% CR, 14% PR) with a median DOR of 21.7 months and median PFS was 12.1 months [25].

3. Loncastuximab tesirine (ADCT-402) is a humanized anti-CD19 monoclonal antibody conjugated to a pyrrolobenzodiazepine dimer (PBD) toxin; phase II study of single-agent loncastuximab tesirine showed ORR of 42.3% with a median DOR of 4.5 months [26].

Small Molecules

Selinexor is an oral selective inhibitor of exportin 1 (XPO1) phase II trial of 267 RR DLBCL patients after at least two prior lines of therapy; at a median follow-up of 27 months, the study reported an ORR rate of 28% with a CR of 12% and a median DOR of 9.3 months [27].

Ibrutinib and Lenalidomide: Single-agent ibrutinib and lenalidomide showed better activity in non-GCB subtypes than GCB in DLBCL patients who had received >2 lines of therapy and could be considered in transplant ineligible DLBCL [28, 29].

BiTEs (Bispecific Antibodies)

Bispecific antibodies targeting CD3/CD20 such as Mosunetuzumab [30], Glofitamab [31], and Epcoritamab [32] provide a promising off-the-shell treatment for relapsed/refractory DLBCL. Ongoing studies will shed more light on the use of these T-cell therapies.

Specific Considerations

1. R-CHOP remains the standard of care for frontline treatment of DLBCL though R-CHP-Pola should be considered in those with IPI > 2.
2. End of treatment delivery of high-dose methotrexate after completion of R-CHOP did not compromise the outcome nor did it increase the risk of CNS events.
3. In older adults with significant comorbidities, R-mini-CHOP is an acceptable alternative.
4. In advanced DLBCL with underlying cardiac disease, data is limited. R-CVP and R-CEOP are reasonable alternative options which can be used.
5. Transplant eligible and chemosensitive disease should be treated with salvage chemotherapy and auto-SCT. However, in early relapse (<12 months) and primary refractory DLBCL, referral to CAR-T should be considered.
6. BiTEs have shown promising activity in multiply relapsed disease including relapse following CAR-T.

Useful Tools

NCCN Guidelines on B-cell lymphomas.
https://www.nccn.org/professionals/physician_gls/pdf/b-cell.pdf

References

1. Li S, Young KH, Medeiros LJ. Diffuse large B-cell lymphoma. Pathology. 2018;50(1):74–87. https://doi.org/10.1016/j.pathol.2017.09.006. Epub 2017 Nov 20
2. Alizadeh AA, Eisen MB, Davis RE, et al. Distinct types of diffuse large B-cell lymphoma identified by gene expression profiling. Nature. 2000;403(6769):503–11.
3. Hans CP, Weisenburger DD, Greiner TC, Gascoyne RD, Delabie J, Ott G, Müller-Hermelink HK, Campo E, Braziel RM, Jaffe ES, Pan Z, Farinha P, Smith LM, Falini B, Banham AH, Rosenwald A, Staudt LM, Connors JM, Armitage JO, Chan WC. Confirmation of the molecular classification of diffuse large B-cell lymphoma by immunohistochemistry using a tissue microarray. Blood. 2004;103(1):275–82. https://doi.org/10.1182/blood-2003-05-1545.
4. Aukema SM, Siebert R, Schuuring E, et al. Double-hit B-cell lymphomas. Blood. 2011;117(8):2319–31.
5. Schmitz R, Wright GW, Huang DW, et al. Genetics and pathogenesis of diffuse large B-cell lymphoma. N Engl J Med. 2018;378(15):1396–407.
6. Chapuy B, Stewart C, Dunford AJ, Kim J, Kamburov A, Redd RA, et al. Molecular subtypes of diffuse large B cell lymphoma are associated with distinct pathogenic mechanisms and outcomes. Nat Med. 2018;24:679–90.
7. Lacy SE, Barrans SL, Beer P, Painter D, Smith A, Roman E, et al. Targeted sequencing in DLBCL, molecular subtypes, and outcomes: a haematological malignancy research network report. 2020;135(20);1759–71.
8. International Non-Hodgkin's Lymphoma Prognostic Factors Project. A predictive model for aggressive non-Hodgkin's lymphoma. N Engl J Med. 1993;329(14):987–94. https://doi.org/10.1056/NEJM199309303291402.
9. Schmitz N, Zeynalova S, Nickelsen M, et al. CNS international prognostic index: a risk model for CNS relapse in patients with diffuse large B-cell lymphoma treated with R-CHOP. J Clin Oncol. 2016;34(26):3150–6. https://doi.org/10.1200/JCO.2015.65.6520.
10. Stephens DM, Li H, LeBlanc ML, et al. Continued risk of relapse independent of treatment modality in limited-stage diffuse large B-cell lymphoma: final and long-term analysis of southwest oncology group study S8736. J Clin Oncol. 2016;34(25):2997–3004.
11. Poeschel V, Held G, Ziepert M, et al. Four versus six cycles of CHOP chemotherapy in combination with six applications of rituximab in patients with aggressive B-cell lymphoma with favourable prognosis (FLYER): a randomised, phase 3, non-inferiority trial. Lancet. 2019;394(10216):2271–81.
12. Persky DO, Li H, Stephens DM, et al. Positron emission tomography-directed therapy for patients with limited-stage diffuse large B-cell lymphoma: results of intergroup national clinical trials network study S1001. J Clin Oncol. 2020;38(26):3003–11.
13. Coiffier B, Lepage E, Briere J, Herbrecht R, Tilly H, Bouabdallah R, Morel P, Van Den Neste E, Salles G, Gaulard P, Reyes F, Lederlin P, Gisselbrecht C. CHOP chemotherapy plus rituximab compared with CHOP alone in elderly patients with diffuse large-B-cell lymphoma. N Engl J Med. 2002;346(4):235–42. https://doi.org/10.1056/NEJMoa011795.
14. Tilly H, Morschhauser F, Sehn LH, et al. Polatuzumab Vedotin in previously untreated diffuse large B-cell lymphoma. N Engl J Med. 2021; https://doi.org/10.1056/NEJMoa2115304.

15. Howlett C, Snedecor SJ, Landsburg DJ, Svoboda J, Chong EA, Schuster SJ, Nasta SD, Feldman T, Rago A, Walsh KM, Weber S, Goy A, Mato A. Front-line, dose-escalated immunochemotherapy is associated with a significant progression-free survival advantage in patients with double-hit lymphomas: a systematic review and meta-analysis. Br J Haematol. 2015;170(4):504–14. https://doi.org/10.1111/bjh.13463. Epub 2015 Apr 24

16. Philip T, Guglielmi C, Hagenbeek A, et al. Autologous bone marrow transplantation as compared with salvage chemotherapy in relapses of chemotherapy-sensitive non-Hodgkin's lymphoma. N Engl J Med. 1995;333:1540–5.

17. Gisselbrecht C, Glass B, Mounier N, et al. Salvage regimens with autologous transplantation for relapsed large B-cell lymphoma in the rituximab era. J Clin Oncol. 2010;28(27):4184–90.

18. Neelapu SS, Locke FL, Bartlett NL, et al. Axicabtagene Ciloleucel CAR T-cell therapy in refractory large B-cell lymphoma. N Engl J Med. 2017;377(26):2531–44.

19. Schuster SJ, Bishop MR, Tam CS, et al. Tisagenlecleucel in adult relapsed or refractory diffuse large B-cell lymphoma. N Engl J Med. 2019;380(1):45–56.

20. Abramson JS, Palomba ML, Gordon LI, et al. Lisocabtagene maraleucel for patients with relapsed or refractory large B-cell lymphomas (TRANSCEND NHL 001): a multicenter seamless design study. Lancet. 2020;396(10254):839–52.

21. Locke FL, Miklos DB, Jacobson CA, et al. All ZUMA-7 investigators and contributing Kite members. Axicabtagene ciloleucel as second-line therapy for large B-cell lymphoma. N Engl J Med. 2022;386:640–54.

22. Kamdar M, Solomon SR, Arnason J, Johnston PB, Glass B, Bachanova V, Ibrahimi S, Mielke S, Mutsaers P, Hernandez-Ilizaliturri F, Izutsu K, Morschhauser F, Lunning M, Maloney DG, Crotta A, Montheard S, Previtali A, Stepan L, Ogasawara K, Mack T, Abramson JS, Investigators TRANSFORM. Lisocabtagene maraleucel versus standard of care with salvage chemotherapy followed by autologous stem cell transplantation as second-line treatment in patients with relapsed or refractory large B-cell lymphoma (TRANSFORM): results from an interim analysis of an open-label, randomised, phase 3 trial. Lancet. 2022;399(10343):2294–308. https://doi.org/10.1016/S0140-6736(22)00662-6.

23. Bishop MR, Dickinson M, Purtill D, et al. Second-line tisagenlecleucel or standard care in aggressive B-cell lymphoma. N Engl J Med. 2022;386:629–39.

24. Sehn LH, Herrera AF, Flowers CR, et al. Polatuzumab Vedotin in relapsed or refractory diffuse large B-cell lymphoma. J Clin Oncol. 2020;38(2):155–65.

25. Salles G, Duell J, González Barca E, et al. Tafasitamab plus lenalidomide in relapsed or refractory diffuse large B-cell lymphoma (L-MIND): a multicentre, prospective, single-arm, phase 2 study. Lancet Oncol. 2020;21(7):978–88.

26. Hamadani M, Radford J, Carlo-Stella C, et al. Final results of a phase 1 study of Loncastuximab Tesirine in relapsed/refractory B-cell non-Hodgkin lymphoma. Blood. 2020; https://doi.org/10.1182/blood.2020007512.

27. Kalakonda N, Maerevoet M, Cavallo F, et al. Selinexor in patients with relapsed or refractory diffuse large B-cell lymphoma (SADAL): a single-arm, multinational, multicentre, open-label, phase 2 trial. Lancet Haematol. 2020;7(7):e511–22.

28. Wilson WH, Young RM, Schmitz R, Yang Y, Pittaluga S, Wright G, Lih CJ, Williams PM, Shaffer AL, Gerecitano J, de Vos S, Goy A, Kenkre VP, Barr PM, Blum KA, Shustov A, Advani R, Fowler NH, Vose JM, Elstrom RL, Habermann TM, Barrientos JC, McGreivy J, Fardis M, Chang BY, Clow F, Munneke B, Moussa D, Beaupre DM, Staudt LM. Targeting B cell receptor signaling with ibrutinib in diffuse large B cell lymphoma. Nat Med. 2015;21(8):922–6.

29. Czuczman MS, Trněný M, Davies A, Rule S, Linton KM, Wagner-Johnston N, Gascoyne RD, Slack GW, Brousset P, Eberhard DA, Hernandez-Ilizaliturri FJ, Salles G, Witzig TE, Zinzani PL, Wright GW, Staudt LM, Yang Y, Williams PM, Lih CJ, Russo J, Thakurta A, Hagner P, Fustier P, Song D, Lewis ID. A phase 2/3 multicenter, randomized, open-label study to compare the efficacy and safety of lenalidomide versus Investigator's choice in patients wih relapsed or refractory diffuse large B-cell lymphoma. Clin Cancer Res. 2017;23(15).

30. Budde LE, Assouline S, Sehn LH, et al. Single-agent mosunetuzumab shows durable complete responses in patients with relapsed or refractory B-cell lymphomas: phase I dose-escalation study. J Clin Oncol. 2022;40:481–91.
31. Hutchings M, Carlo-Stella C, Bachy E, et al. Glofitamab step-up dosing induces high response rates in patients with hard-to-treat refractory or relapsed non-Hodgkin lymphoma. Blood. 2020;136(Suppl. 1):46–8.
32. Subcutaneous Epcoritamab induces complete responses with an encouraging safety profile across relapsed/refractory B-cell non-Hodgkin lymphoma subtypes, including patients with prior CAR-T therapy: updated dose escalation data. Blood. 2020;136(Suppl. 1):45–6.

Chapter 10
Supportive Care for Treatment of Hematologic Malignancies

Grace Park

Case Demonstration

TK is a 32 yo male with past medical history of acute lymphoblastic leukemia, DM Type II, HTN, and anemia who presented for consolidation cycle of hyper CVAD. Patient reports having several days of nausea and vomiting after induction cycle. Patient received NK1 receptor antagonist, HT3 receptor antagonist, and corticosteroids as premedication last time.

Definition [1–4]

- *Acute chemotherapy-induced nausea and vomiting* usually begin within minutes to hours after chemotherapy and lasts up to 24 h. It generally peaks within 5–6 h of administration.
- *Delayed nausea and vomiting* develop more than 24 h after chemotherapy and may last several days. It usually occurs 1–5 days after chemotherapy, especially with administration of platinum, cyclophosphamide, and anthracycline.
- *Anticipatory nausea and vomiting* begin before chemotherapy and is often associated with poorly controlled acute and delayed nausea and vomiting. It occurs in 25–50% of patients.
- *Breakthrough nausea and vomiting* occurs despite prophylactic therapy and is treated with an as needed regimen. It requires rescue therapy often different from prophylactic agent.

G. Park (✉)
Division of Pharmacy, The University of Texas MD Anderson Cancer Center, Houston, TX, USA
e-mail: ghwang1@mdanderson.org

© The Author(s), under exclusive license to Springer Nature Switzerland AG 2024
G. Rivero, I. R. Sosa (eds.), *Consulting Hematology and Oncology Handbook*, https://doi.org/10.1007/978-3-031-75810-2_10

- *Refractory nausea and vomiting* occur when antiemetic prophylaxis and/or rescue has failed.

Emetogenicity is based on the percentage of patients who experienced emesis in the absence of effective antiemetic prophylaxis. It is graded by minimal (<10%), low (10–30%), moderate (30–90%), and high (>90%).

Clinical Context [1, 2, 4, 5]

Etiology

- Chemical/metabolic: Chemotherapy, radiation, electrolyte imbalance, and opioid induced.
- CNS/pscyhoemotional: Increased intracranial pressure, brain tumors, brain metastasis, and anxiety induced.
- Vestibular: Motion sickness or movement related.
- Abdominal/visceral: Gastroesophageal reflux disease (GERD), indigestion, constipation, gastroparesis, ileus, functional obstruction, small bowel obstruction, graft-versus-host disease (GVHD).
- Miscellaneous: Cyclic vomiting syndrome.

Pathophysiology

A complex interaction between gastrointestinal tract, the central, peripheral, and enteric nervous systems. Acute chemotherapy-induced nauseas and vomiting (CINV) developing within 24 h is initiated by serotonin receptors in the gastrointestinal tract (Fig. 10.1). However, CINV developing after 24 h of chemotherapy administration is initiated by NK_1 receptors after stimulation by substance P. This neurotransmitter widely controls sensory, nociceptive, and inflammatory pathways [1].

Risk Factors

- Patient related.

  - Previous episodes of CINV.
  - Age < 50 years.
  - Female gender.
  - History of pregnancy associated nausea and vomiting.

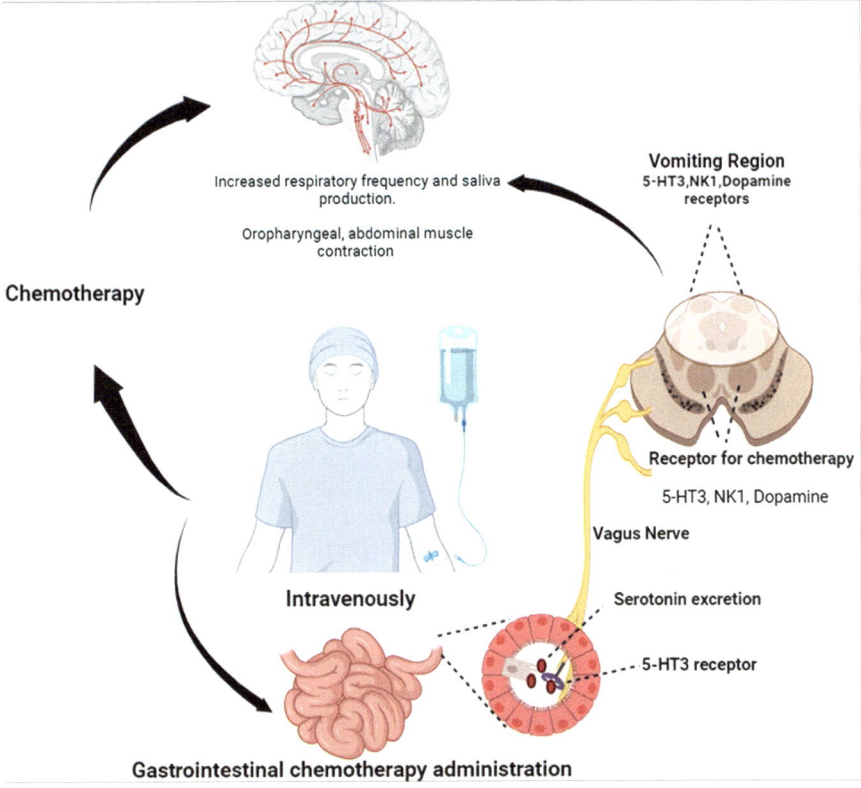

Fig. 10.1 Pathophysiology of chemotherapy induced vomiting

- – History of motion sickness.
- – History of limited/minimal alcohol intake.
- – History of anxiety.
- – Brain metastasis.
- – History of gastritis or GERD.
- Treatment related.

  - – Emetogenicity of cytotoxic regimen.
  - – Chemotherapy dose.
  - – Route and administration of chemotherapy.
  - – First cycle of chemotherapy.
  - – Vomiting during a previous chemotherapy cycle.
- Self-medication with non-prescribed treatments (e.g., dimenhydrinate, bismuth subsalicylate, antacids, cannabis products, and herbal supplements).

Clinical Manifestation [1–4, 6]

Patients can present with acute CINV, delayed CINV, breakthrough CINV, or refractory CINV.

Acute CINV
- Within 24 h of chemotherapy administration.
- Primarily mediated by 5-HT3.
- May occur up to 35% of time despite prophylactic antiemetic.

Delayed CINV
- Between 24 h and 5 days of chemotherapy administration.
- Predominantly mediated by substance P binding to NK1 receptors in the central nervous system.
- May occur 20–50% of time despite prophylactic antiemetic.

Breakthrough CINV
- Within 5 days of chemotherapy administration.
- May occur despite guideline directed prophylactic antiemetic agents.
- Require additional antiemetic agents added to control immediate symptoms.

Refractory CINV
- Occur during the subsequent chemotherapy cycle.
- Primarily due to inadequate control by prophylactic antiemetic agents.

Assessment [1, 2, 5, 6]

- Use visual analog scale (0 to 10, with 0 signifying no nausea and 10 maximum nausea).
- Assessment of the severity and the context such as frequency, time of day, and any associated activities (meals, medications, exertion).
- Physical exam to assess abdominal pain or tenderness for bowel obstruction or gastroparesis and abdominal distention for ascites, hepatomegaly, or splenomegaly.
- Neurologic examination for focal neurologic signs or papilledema suggestive of elevated intracranial pressure or CNS metastasis or any vestibular dysfunction.
- History of weight loss, appetite, anorexia, cachexia, depression, or anxiety.
- Rule out other potential causes of emesis such as bowel obstruction, electrolyte imbalances, dyspepsia, or vestibular dysfunction.
- History of using any prescription or over-the-counter medications.

    - Potential causes of nausea: Nonsteroidal anti-inflammatory drugs, selective serotonin reuptake inhibitors, antibiotics, opioid analgesics, and oral iron.
    - Recent cancer treatment with chemotherapy and/or radiation.
    - Remedies to relieve nausea and vomiting.

Laboratory Investigation [1, 2, 6]

Diagnostic testing for nausea and vomiting should be targeted at finding the etiology suggested by a thorough history and physical examination. Testing should be directed by the history and physical examination to determine underlying cause or consequences of nausea and vomiting.

- Complete blood count.
- Complete metabolic panel.

  - Electrolytes.
  - Protein/albumin.

- Erythrocyte sedimentation rate to assess inflammatory process.
- Pancreatic or liver enzymes.
- Pregnancy test for any female of childbearing age.
- Specific toxins or drug use.
- Thyroid stimulating hormone.
- Imaging or ultrasound of abdomen to assess mechanical obstruction.
- Esophagogastroduodenoscopy if needed.
- MRI of brain for any intracranial mass or lesion if suspected.

Management [2–6]

- Goal is to prevent CINV. Give agents that are effective for the highest emetogenic risk level of any single agent in the regimen each day except for anthracycline and cyclophosphamide combination. Refer to NCCN Guideline on Antiemesis to determine emetogenic potential.
- Risk of acute and delayed nausea is based on the risk of each agent.
- Combination therapy has been shown to improve the efficacy of primary antiemetic. However, it is NOT recommended to use two agents from the same class of antiemetics in combination (e.g., ondansetron and granisetron). This can significantly increase the side effects and does not increase efficacy (Table 10.1).
- Olanzapine should be used with caution in combination with other dopamine antagonists and other CNS depressants.
- Antiemetic prophylaxis for a given day should be based on the agent with the highest emetogenicity administered on that day (Fig. 10.2).
- In addition to medical management, clinician may consider complementary and alternative medicine such as behaviroal therapy, acupuncture, and anxiolytic therapy.

Table 10.1 Classes of commonly used antiemetic

	Dose/routes	Side effects/management
Serotonin antagonist		
Ondansetron (Zofran)	8–24 mg IV/PO/day Max single dose is 16 mg Max daily dose is 32 mg	Constipation QT prolongation Headaches
Palonosetron (Aloxi)	0.25 mg IV once May repeat 48–72 h with multi-day chemotherapy regimen	
Granisetron (Kytril)	10 mcg/kg max (1 mg) IV or 2 mg PO daily	
Dolasetron (Anzemet)	100 mg PO daily	
Substance P (NK1) antagonist		
Netupitant and Palonosetron (Akynzeo)	Netupitant 300 mg / palonosetron 0.5 mg PO once	
Fosnetupitant and Palonosetron (Akynzeo)	Fosnetupitant 235 mg / palonosetron 0.25 mg IV once	
Aprepitant (Emend)	125 mg PO on day 1 80 mg PO on days 2–3	Infusion site reactions (polysorbate 80)
Fosaprepitant (Emend IV)	150 mg IV on day 1	Increase dexamethasone level Decrease warfarin level (monitor INR)
Aprepitant injectable emulsion (Cinvanti)	130 mg IV on day 1 for highly emetogenic regimen	Does not contain polysorbate 80 Followed by aprepitant 80 mg on days 2 and 3
Rolapitant (Varubi)	180 mg PO on day 1 IV form has been discontinued	Monitor digoxin and warfarin levels Monitor ADE related to Methotrexate, Topotecan, and Irinotecan
Dopamine antagonists		
Prochlorperazine (Compazine)	5–10 mg PO TID-QID (max 40 mg/day) 25 mg PR BID	EPS QT prolongation
Perphenazine (Triafon)	2–8 mg PO q2-6h (max 24 mg/day)	
Metoclopramide (Reglan)	10–20 mg PO.IV TID-QID	
Haloperidol (Haldol)	0.5–2 mg IV/PO q4–8 h	
Droperidol (Inapsine)	2.5–5 mg IV q3–4 h	EKG monitoring required
Corticosteroids		
Dexamethasone	4–20 mg PO/IV daily (or BID)	Delirium, anxiety, insomnia, hyperglycemia, and hypertension
Methylprednisolone	50–100 mg IV daily	

(continued)

Table 10.1   (continued)

	Dose/routes	Side effects/management
Atypical antipsychotics		
Olanzapine	2.5–10 mg daily	Sedation, orthostatic hypotension, and weight gain
Antihistamines		
Dimenhydrinate	50–100 mg PO/IV q4–6 h	Sedation and confusion in elderly
Meclizine	25–50 mg PO daily	Avoid use of promethazine and dopamine antagonists due to similar MOA
Promethazine	12.5–25 mg PO/PR q4 h	
Anticholinergics		
Scopolamine	1.5–3 mg TD q72 h	Dry mouth, blurred vision, delirium
Cannabinoids		
Dronabinol	2.5–10 mg BID-TID	Confusion, ataxia
Nabilone	1–2 mg BID	
Dronabinol	5–10 mg PO or 2.1–4.2 mg/m2 PO q6-8 h	
Anxiolytics		
Lorazepam	0.5–2 mg PO/IV q4–6 h	Confusion, sedation

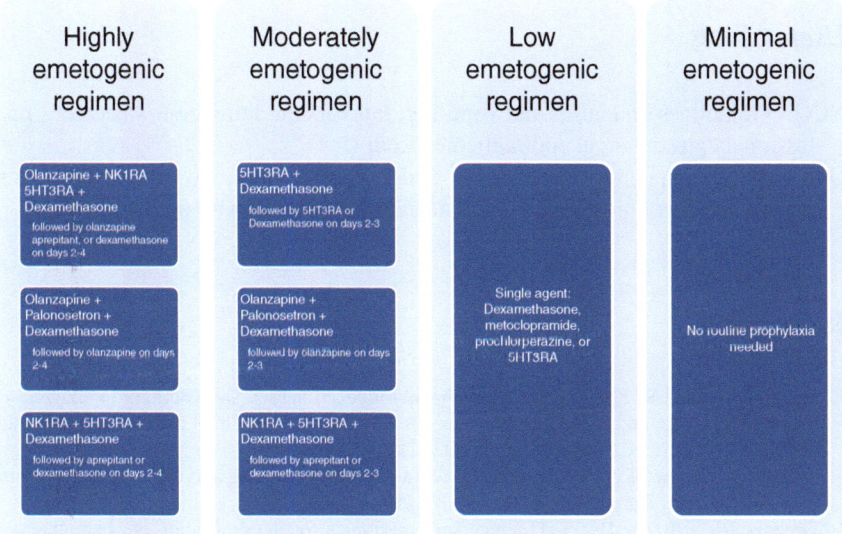

Fig. 10.2   Emesis prevention based on emetic risk of parenteral regimen
NK1RA: NK1 receptor antagonists; 5HT3RA: serotonin receptor antagonists

Specific Considerations [3, 5, 6]

1. NK1 receptor antagonists and dexamethasone: NK1 receptor antagonists may increase the serum concentration of systemic corticosteroids like dexamethasone.

2. NK1 receptor antagonists and ifosfamide: NK1 receptor antagonists may increase the serum concentration of Ifosfamide. Monitor for any possible neurotoxicity (somnolence, confusion, and delirium).
3. NK1 receptor antagonists and the following drugs may lead to adverse events: alcohol (impaired cognition), oxycodone (decreased respiratory rate, increased feeling of a "high"), quetiapine (somnolence), SSRI/SNRIs (vomiting), and warfarin (INR changes).
4. Dexamethasone may have a negative impact on outcomes of immunotherapies (e.g. CAR T cell therapy) due to its immunosuppressive effect. Clinician should consider use of alternative antiemetic agents for CINV prophylaxis and management.
5. After administration of long acting HT3RA such as palonosetron or granisetron patch, clinician should consider an agent with different mechanism of action for any breakthrough CINV.
6. Metoclopramide increases gut motility and may be beneficial in the setting of gastroparesis.
7. Cannabinoids may be used to stimulate appetite and manage CINV. However, high doses of cannabinoids may lead to cannabioid hyperemesis.

Useful Tools

NCCN Guidelines on nausea and vomiting, full version: https://www.nccn.org/professionals/physician_gls/pdf/antiemesis.pdf
Quick NCCN Appendix for nausea and vomiting: https://www.nccn.org/docs/default-source/clinical/order-templates/appendix_d.pdf?sfvrsn=d4002e8f_8

References

1. Gupta K, Walton R, Kataria SP. Chemotherapy-induced nausea and vomiting: pathogenesis, recommendations, and new trends. Cancer Treat Res Commun. 2021;26:100278. https://doi.org/10.1016/j.ctarc.2020.100278. Epub 2020 Dec 11
2. Adel N. Overview of chemotherapy-induced nausea and vomiting and evidence-based therapies. Am J Manag Care. 2017;23(14 Suppl):S259–65.
3. Gregory RE, Ettinger DS. 5-HT3 receptor antagonists for the prevention of chemotherapy-induced nausea and vomiting. A comparison of their pharmacology and clinical efficacy. Drugs. 1998;55(2):173–89. https://doi.org/10.2165/00003495-199855020-00002.
4. Hesketh PJ, Kris MG, Grunberg SM, Beck T, Hainsworth JD, Harker G, Aapro MS, Gandara D, Lindley CM. Proposal for classifying the acute emetogenicity of cancer chemotherapy. J Clin Oncol. 1997;15(1):103–9. https://doi.org/10.1200/JCO.1997.15.1.103.
5. James JN. Overview and management of CINV. Am J Manag Care. 2018;24:S0.
6. Navari RM. Managing nausea and vomiting in patients with cancer: what works. Oncology (Williston Park). 2018;32(3):121–5. 131, 136

Chapter 11
Plasma Cell Disorders

Alexis K. Williams and Kimberley Doucette

Case 1 Demonstration

A 59-year-old male with no past medical history presents with increasing low back pain that is worse at night and interfering with his ability to do work in his garden. He is also having increased fatigue. He used to be able to walk around the neighborhood with his family, but now he feels tired after just a block. After physical exam and initial X-ray, he is admitted for compression fractures of L3 and L4. During his initial evaluation, his complete blood count (CBC) shows a hemoglobin of 5.8 mg/dL, and his comprehensive metabolic panel (CMP) shows a calcium level of 13.8 mg/dL, serum albumin of 3.8 mg/dL, and a serum creatinine of 2.3 mg/dL.

Definitions

Multiple myeloma (MM) is part of a spectrum of clonal paraprotein disorders that result in excess immunoglobulins in the blood, called plasma cell dyscrasias. MM is an incurable, uncontrolled growth of monoclonal plasma cells in the bone marrow throughout the body (Fig. 11.1). These cells typically produce monoclonal IgG, IgA, or IgM immunoglobulin (M-protein), which leads to excess nonfunctional immunoglobulin present in the blood. Rarely, these tumors can also produce IgD or

A. K. Williams
Department of Medicine, New York University, New York, NY, USA

K. Doucette (✉)
Medstar Georgetown University Hospital, Washington, DC, USA
e-mail: Kimberley.Doucette@medstar.net

G. Rivero, I. R. Sosa (eds.), *Consulting Hematology and Oncology Handbook*, https://doi.org/10.1007/978-3-031-75810-2_11

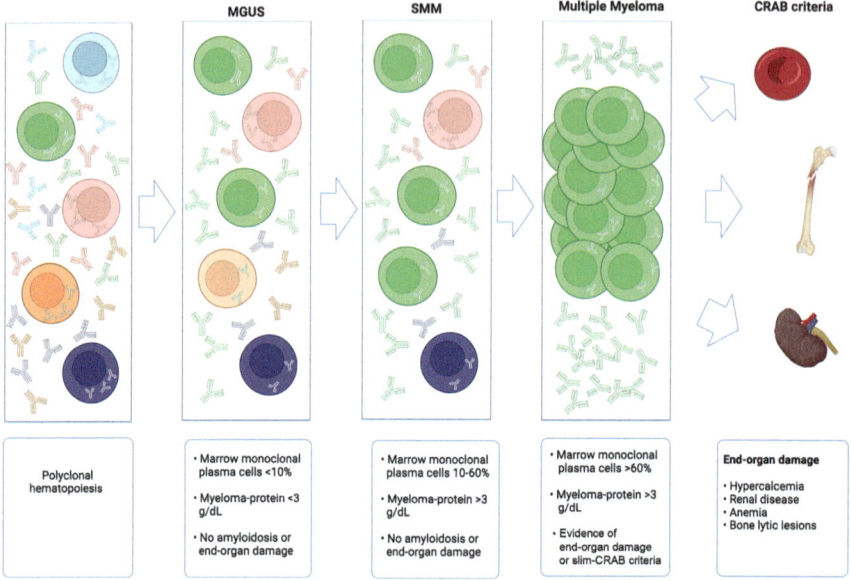

Fig. 11.1 Representation of spectrum of disease of multiple myeloma

IgE, or not produce any immune globulin at all (non-secretory myeloma). Up to 20% of multiple myelomas only produce immunoglobulin light chain without the heavy chain, resulting in excess free light chain (FLC) in the blood and urine [1, 2].

The presence of slim-CRAB criteria indicative of active disease (including lytic bone lesions, anemia, and renal failure) differentiates multiple myeloma from Monoclonal Gammopathy of Uncertain Significance (MGUS) and asymptomatic smoldering myeloma.

Waldenstrom macroglobulinemia is a lymphoplasmacytic lymphoma that produces large amounts of IgM. It is generally characterized by symptoms of hyperviscosity including end-organ damage, particularly ocular damage [3].

Oligo- or non-secretory myeloma is rare, accounting for 1–5% of all myelomas. In oligo- or non-secretory myeloma, a paraproteinemia is not identified although plasma cell tumors are present. Its clinical course does not typically include lytic bone lesions, and incidence of hypogammaglobulinemia is lower [4].

Clinical Context

Multiple myeloma is primarily found in older adults, and it is rarely found in patients younger than 45 years old [1]. The average age of diagnosis is 69 years old. It is twice as common among African Americans as among Caucasians. Multiple myeloma arises from the precursor condition monoclonal gammopathy of undetermined significance (MGUS). Approximately 0.5–1% of MGUS cases transform to MM per year, depending on underlying biologic risk factors. As such, patients diagnosed with MGUS require lifelong screening for MM.

Clinical Manifestations

Multiple myeloma symptoms have classically been defined by the mnemonic "CRAB" as shown in Table 11.1 [5–11]. In 2014, the "SLiM" criteria were added to allow biomarker data to formally contribute to MM diagnosis (Table 11.2) [12]. MM can also present with nonspecific "B" symptoms of malignancy, including fatigue, weakness, and weight loss. If the skull or spine is involved, focal neurological deficits and cranial nerve deficits may occur. Infection is also common, secondary to the lack of diversity of immunoglobulins being produced by the monoclonal plasma cells.

Table 11.1 "CRAB" symptoms of multiple myeloma

Manifestation	Symptoms	Incidence	Most common cytogenetic abnormalities
HyperCalcemia	Constipation, GI disturbances	30%	N/A
Anemia	Fatigue, dizziness, dyspnea on exertion	73%	t(4;14), t(14;16), t(6;14), t(14;20)
Renal failure	Uremia, decreased urine output, electrolyte abnormalities, fatigue	50%	t(14;16), t(6;14), t(14;20)
Bone lytic lesions	Back pain, pathological fractures	90%	N/A

Table 11.2 "SLiM" signs of multiple myeloma

Manifestation	Diagnostic criteria
Sixty percent or higher plasma cells	Seen on bone marrow biopsy
Light chain ratio	Kappa to Lambda free light chain ratio > 100
MRI	Focal lesion >5 mm on MRI

Case 1 (Cont)

A serum protein electrophoresis (SPEP) is obtained, which shows a significant gamma spike. His peripheral blood smear shows a "stacked coin" appearance of the red blood cells. Bone marrow biopsy is done which shows 15% plasma cells with abundant cytoplasm. Urine test is positive for Bence-Jones protein.

Tests to Establish Diagnosis

Initial evaluation includes the following diagnostic tests:

- Comprehensive metabolic panel (CMP): Hypercalcemia, elevated protein, elevated lactate dehydrogenase (LDH) [5].
- Complete blood count (CBC): Anemia (low hemoglobin).
- Serum/urine protein electrophoresis (SPEP/UPEP): Monoclonal spike (see "Useful Tools" section for more information).
- Serum quantitative immunoglobulins (IgA, IgG, IgM, _+/-IgE or IgD in certain circumstances).
- Peripheral blood smear (PBS).
- Bone marrow biopsy (BMB): >10% plasma cells.
- Immunohistochemistry (IHC) of bone marrow: CD138, CD56, anti-Kappa, anti-Lambda [13].

Whole-body CT scan/PET CT scan (or consider whole-body MRI to discern smoldering myeloma from multiple myeloma).
Useful in certain circumstances:

- Congo red stain to assess for AL amyloidosis.
- NT proBNP/BNP if concern for amyloidosis.
- Baseline clone identification and storage of aspirate for future minimal residual disease testing by next-generation sequencing (NGS).
- Hepatitis B, hepatitis C, and HIV testing.
- Echocardiogram.

When a diagnosis of MM has been established, there are several other tests that can help determine prognosis:

- Serum/urine immunofixation assays (SIFE/UIFE): Determine specific type of M-protein produced by tumor [14].
- Serum free light chain (FLC) assay.
- B2-microglobulin: Used for staging and associated with renal function [15].
- 24-h urine studies to assess for paraproteinuria or Bence-Jones protein.
- Viscosity: Test for complications of hyperviscosity; symptomatic hyperviscosity is low prevalence in MM (2–6%).
- Plasma cell fluorescence in situ hybridization (FISH) panel, cytogenetics.

- Consider next-generation sequencing or single nucleotide polymorphism testing.

Identification of Bone Lesions

Traditionally, plain radiographs have been used for the whole skeleton to identify lesions. Recent studies have debated the best imaging method to use for the skeletal survey in MM [16–22]. Whole-body CT and PET/CT have been shown to be more useful than plain radiographs for identifying lesions in the axial skeleton, especially areas that are difficult to visualize on plain radiographs such as the skull. Hinge et al. showed that CT identified lytic lesions in the spine and pelvis in 74% of MM patients whereas plain radiographs showed lesions in only 50% of patients ($p < 0.01$) [17]. However, whole-body CT and PET/CT were not shown to be better than plain films for identifying lesions of the appendicular skeleton. MRI has the highest sensitivity for the axial skeleton but was no better than the plain films for the non-axial skeleton. In one study, MRI found evidence of spinal or pelvic lytic lesions in 69% of patients where plain radiographs found evidence in only 18% of patients [16]. For suspected isolated plasmacytoma or smoldering multiple myeloma, whole-body MRI may be more useful to distinguish these clinical syndromes from active MM.

Risk Stratification

Risk stratification in MM is based on a number of factors, among the most important of which are staging and tumor cytogenetics. Several common cytogenetic abnormalities and their risk stratifications are shown in Table 11.3 [23].

Staging in multiple myeloma is done according to the R2-ISS criteria, established in 2022. First, an ISS score is calculated based on serum B2-microglobulin and albumin at diagnosis (Table 11.4).

Table 11.3 Common cytogenetic abnormalities in multiple myeloma, risk stratification, and average life expectancy

Karyotype	Risk	Mean overall survival
Normal	Standard	7–10 years
Trisomy 3, 5, 7, 9, 11, 15, 17, 19	Standard	7–10 years
t(11;14) (q13;q32)	Standard	7–10 years
t(6;14) (p16;q32)	Standard	7–10 years
t(14;16) (q32;q23)	High	3 years
t(4;14) (p16q32)	Intermediate	5 years
t(14;20) (q32;q11)	High	3 years
Gain 1q21	Intermediate	5 years
Del(17p)	High	3 years

Table 11.4 ISS staging [24]

ISS stage	Serum B2 microglobulin	Serum albumin
I	<3.5 mg/L	≥3.5 g/dL
II	<3.5 mg/L	<3.5 g/dL
II	3.5–5.5 mg/L	N/A
III	*>5.5 mg/L*	*N/A*

Table 11.5 R2-ISS score and risk stratification

R2-ISS Score	Risk/stage	Median progression-free survival (months)
0	Low (I)	NR
0.5–1	Low–intermediate (II)	109 months
1.5–2.5	Intermediate–high (III)	68 months
3–5	High (IV)	38 months

Other factors including mutations and elevated LDH are then assigned point values, which create a point total used to stage MM. The point values for each item are as follows (Table 11.5) [25]:

- 1q+: 0.5 points.
- ISS II: 1 point.
- del(17p): 1 point.
- t(4:14): 1 point.
- LDH high: 1 point.
- ISS III: 1.5 points.

High Risk Disease

- List high risk genetic abnormalities.
- RISS stage III.
- High plasma cell S-phase.
- GEP: High risk signatures.
- Double hit myeloma: Any two high risk genetic abnormalities or triple hit myeloma: three or more high risk genetic abnormalities.

Standard Risk Myeloma

All others including trisomies, t(11;14) and t(6;14).

Case (Cont)

Patient was found to have a t(11;14) translocation, which indicated a standard risk multiple myeloma patient. His projected overall survival is therefore approximately 7–10 years. As a relatively young patient with no past medical history, the goal of treatment for this patient is to achieve early ASCT.

Treatment

Risk stratification of the tumor and eligibility for ASCT are some of the key factors that dictate treatment in multiple myeloma. Some factors in determining eligibility for ASCT include age and renal function, although renal failure does not necessarily exclude an otherwise fit patient from ASCT. In light of this, consultation with a transplant center is always recommended in patients with MM. If a patient is transplant eligible, they will generally receive 4–6 cycles of induction therapy followed by assessment for response via CBC, CMP, SPEP/immunofixation, serum free light chains and ratio, immunoglobulins, and/or repeat whole-body scan especially if oligosecretory or non-secretory disease. If the patient has responded to the induction therapy (ideally > PR), moving onto ASCT is recommended. If not, further experimental therapy such as clinical trial may be necessary. In transplant ineligible patients, intensive induction therapy is usually followed by continuing therapy or transition to maintenance therapy, depending on response. An algorithm for initial treatment of multiple myeloma based on NCCN primary recommendations as well as mSMART guidelines by the Mayo Clinic is shown in Table 11.6 [26–36].

Assessment for response is done following the guidelines set out by the International Myeloma Working Group (IMWG). Table 11.7 shows the clinically relevant response criteria set out by the IMWG [37].

If patients achieve clinical complete response, they should be tested for minimal residual disease (MRD) markers, which are increasingly being recognized as important for understanding the durability of clinical outcomes in MM. MRD markers can be tested either by flow cytometry or next-generation sequencing (NGS) of bone marrow to find clonal plasma cells or tumor mutations, respectively [38].

Supportive Care

One important aspect of MM treatment is supportive care. Bisphosphonates are a cornerstone of MM therapy at all stages to support bone function and prevent fractures. Erythropoietin therapy may be used in patients with significant anemia [10]. In patients with hyperviscosity syndrome, plasmapheresis may be necessary [39, 40]. Finally, for treatment regimens containing immunomodulators, thrombosis prophylaxis is recommended (can use a calculator such as IMPEDE-VTE).

Table 11.6 Treatment algorithm for initial treatment of multiple myeloma based on primary NCCN recommendations and mSMART guidelines

Treatment of multiple myeloma	
Transplant eligible	*Transplant ineligible*
Induction therapy 4–6 cycles of quadruplet regimen with daratumumab, bortezomib, lenalidomide, dexamethasone (now preferred option over triplet)	**Induction therapy** Triplet regimen with daratumumab/lenalidomide/dexamethasone bortezomib/lenalidomide/dexamethasone or quadruplet with antiCD38/lenalidomide/ bortezomib/dexamethasone or certain circumstances: Lenalidomide/low-dose dexamethasone bortezomib/cyclophosphamide/dexamethasone
Collect stem cells Option (1) Autologous stem cell transplant (preferred option) vs Option (2) induction therapy for another 4 cycles *Can consider tandem transplant for high-risk disease*	Continuous myeloma therapy with regimen listed above (for quadruplet, combination of anti CD38 and lenalidomide for continuous therapy after induction)
Maintenance therapy Option (1) Lenalidomide or Daratumumab-Lenalidomide vs Option (2) Lenalidomide until progression, delayed ASCT High-risk disease: Consider proteosome inhibitor for 2 years and lenalidomide	
Progression after ASCT Relapsed refractory standard of care regimens Clinical trial or Second autologous stem cell transplant under certain circumstances (long previous remission) or Rarely, can consider allogeneic stem cell transplant	
Relapse or refractory **Early relapse**	
If non-refractory to lenalidomide *clinical trial* Daratumumab, lenalidomide, dexamethasone Carfilzomib, lenalidomide dexamethasone Elotuzumab, revlimid, dexamethasone	*If refractory to lenalidomide* *clinical trial* Pomalidomide, bortezomib, dexamethasone Daratumumab, carfilzomib, dexamethasone Isatuximab, carfilzomib, dexamethasone Selinexor, bortezomib, dexamethasone Elotuzumab, pomalidomide, dexamethasone Carfilzomib, pomalidomide, dexamethasone Daratumumab, pomalidomide, dexamethasone CAR-T therapy now approved after 1 prior line of therapy

(continued)

Table 11.6 (continued)

Treatment of multiple myeloma
After 1–3 prior lines of therapy
Clinical trials Selinexor combinations Ixazomib combinations Bendamustine monotherapy or in combination with PI Venetoclax/dexamethasone +/ daratumumab if t(11;14) CAR-T cell BCMA and GP6CR bispecific T-cell engagers (after 4 lines of prior therapy)
Treatment-aggressive MM: DCEP VTD PACE KRD PACE

Table 11.7 International Myeloma Working Group (IMWG) response definitions

Complete response (CR)	Negative immunofixation of the serum and urine, disappearance of any soft tissue plasmacytomas, and <5% plasma cells in bone marrow
Strict complete response (sCR)	CR plus normal FLC ratio and absence of clonal cells in bone marrow by immunohistochemistry or immunofluorescence
Very good partial response (VGPR)	Serum and urine M-protein detectable by immunofixation but not by electrophoresis or >90% reduction in serum M-protein plus urine M-protein level <100 mg/24 h
Partial response (PR)	>50% reduction in size of soft tissue plasmacytomas, if present AND > 50% reduction of serum M-protein and reduction in 24 h urinary M-protein by >90% or to <200 mg/24 h OR >50% decrease in difference between involved and uninvolved FLC levels OR >50% reduction in plasma cells in bone marrow, given that initial bone marrow plasma cell percentage was >30%
Progressive disease (PD)	Increase of >25% from lowest response value to in one or more of the following: 1. Serum M-component (absolute increase >0.5 g/dL) 2. Urine M-component (absolute increase >200 mg/24 h) 3. Difference between involved and uninvolved FLC levels (absolute increase >10 mg/dL) 4. Bone marrow plasma cell percentage (must be >10%) 5. Definite increase in number or size of bone lesions or soft tissue plasmacytomas 6. Development of hypercalcemia (>11.5 mg/dL) not otherwise explained
Stable disease	Not meeting criteria for CR, VGPR, PR, or PD
Relapse	Increase in number or size of bone lesions or soft tissue plasmacytomas; hypercalcemia (>11.5 mg/dL), decrease in hemoglobin >2 g/dL, increase in creatinine by 2 mg/dL or more

The majority of patients with MM experience pain at some point during the course of their disease. The most common pain caused by MM is bone pain from lytic lesions which is experienced by up to 90% of patients; it is generally worse with fracture but may be present without fracture. For bone pain due to compressive vertebral fracture, kyphoplasty or vertebroplasty may be considered. Other pain may be treated with a combination of radiotherapy, corticosteroids, non-opioid analgesics such as acetaminophen, and opioids for severe pain. NSAIDs are usually avoided due to nephrotoxicity [41].

MM also carries increased risk of infection both due to the disease itself and in various treatments. Acyclovir prophylaxis for shingles prevention is recommended in patients receiving regimens containing proteasome inhibitors, monoclonal antibody, CAR-T, bispecific antibody, or transplant recipients. Neutropenic patients may also be considered for antifungal prophylaxis with fluconazole if there is prolonged neutropenia. Pneumocystis pneumonia (PJP) prophylaxis is recommended for patients receiving CAR-T or bispecific antibody and should be considered for patients on dexamethasone. Levofloxacin prophylaxis should be considered for new diagnosis (12 weeks duration), CAR-T therapy, or bispecific antibody therapy [42]. The utility of IVIG prophylaxis in MM has mixed evidence in the literature but can be considered if patients are having recurrent infections, and IgG levels are <600 mg/dL. IVIG is recommended currently in patients who have undergone CAR-T or bispecific therapy with IgG levels <400 mg/dL.

For vaccination, patients should follow the CDC guidelines for immunosuppressed patients. This means receiving PCV20 for *Streptococcus pneumoniae* vaccination, yearly influenza shot, and up-to-date COVID-19 vaccinations. After CAR-T therapy or transplant, one may consider repeating these vaccinations 3–6 months after treatment.

Case 1 (Cont)

The patient was determined to be transplant eligible for ASCT based on cardiac, pulmonary, and renal evaluation by a stem cell transplant center. He underwent 4 cycles of daratumumab, bortezomib, lenalidomide, and dexamethasone therapy and had stem cells harvested during induction. He achieved VGPR during induction and was able to undergo successful ASCT, followed by lenalidomide maintenance. He subsequently was found to be MRD negative on repeat bone marrow biopsy following ASCT.

Case 2 Demonstration

An 80-year-old man is undergoing regular medical evaluation. On his yearly comprehensive metabolic panel, he is found to have elevated serum protein. Otherwise, laboratory evaluation including complete blood count (CBC), creatinine, and calcium is normal. He has not had any back pain, and his exercise tolerance is limited somewhat by arthritis but not by shortness of breath or fatigue. He undergoes SPEP which shows an IgA spike of 3.5 mg/dL. MRI survey shows no focal findings.

Definitions

Monoclonal gammopathy of undetermined significance (MGUS) is a clonal expansion of plasma cells resulting in presence of clonal immunoglobulin in the serum without causing symptoms, bone lesions, or sufficiently extensive marrow infiltration to be classified as MM [43]. In order to meet criteria for MGUS, patients must be asymptomatic (no CRAB criteria met) and have an M-spike on SPEP <3 g/dL. If bone marrow biopsy is done, it must show <10% plasma cells. Risk of conversion to active MM for MGUS with various risk factors is shown in Table 11.8.

Smoldering multiple myeloma (SMM) is also an asymptomatic clonal expansion of plasma cells, but it is higher risk for MM than MGUS. M-spike will typically be >3 g/dL and bone marrow biopsy will show plasma cell infiltration of 10–60% [44]. Risk of conversion to MM is 10–20% per year with highest risk in the first 5 years.

Testing

For MGUS, if paraprotein is IgG subtype on immunofixation and is less than 1.5 g/dl, combined with a normal serum free light chain ratio, labs can be repeated at 6 months. If stable, can be repeated yearly to every 2 years for monitoring. Additionally, imaging and bone marrow biopsy are not necessary unless there is concern for progression or new CRAB criteria.

For higher risk MGUS or SMM (elevated free light chain ratio, non-IgG subtype on immunofixation, M-spike >3 g/dL), bone marrow biopsy and whole-body imaging with either CT or MRI should be performed to differentiate SMM from active MM.

Table 11.8 Risk of MGUS conversion to MM

Immunoglobulin class	Risk factors present: Abnormal FLC, M-spike >1.5 g/dL	20-year conversion risk to MM
IgM	Both	55%
IgM	One	41%
IgM	Neither	19%
Non-IgM	Both	30%
Non-IgM	One	20%
Non-IgM	Neither	7%

Table 11.9 Risk
stratification of SMM based
on 2/20/20 criteria

Number of 2/20/20 + cytogenetics risk factors	Risk of progression at 2 years
0	6%
1	22.8%
2	45.5%
3–4	63.1%

SMM can be further risk stratified into several subgroups based on the 2/20/20 criteria: (1) M-spike >2 g/dL, (2) FLC ratio > 20, (3) and bone marrow plasma cells >20% [45]. Of note, there are several smoldering myeloma risk criteria, with 2/20/20 being one of the most utilized. Cytogenetic criteria can also be added to these criteria, with the presence of t(4;14), t(14;16), +1q, del13q, and/or monosomy 13 accounting for an additional risk factor. The risk of progression of SMM is shown in Table 11.9.

Further risk stratification can be done with genetic analysis, with high risk cytogenetics adding additional risk of progression.

Follow-Up

MGUS patients should receive monitoring every 6 months—1 year with SPEP/immunofixation, immunoglobulins, UPEP/UIFE, serum free light chains, and ratio and basic laboratory monitoring to check blood counts, calcium, protein levels, and renal function [46, 47, 48].

SMM patients should undergo more frequent testing every 3–6 months including above serum markers, UPEP/UIFE, and imaging in certain circumstances.

Case 3 Demonstration

A 56-year-old female presents to her primary care doctor with difficulty swallowing. Over the past few months, she has noticed that food seems to "get stuck" in her throat. At first this happened with chewy foods such as meat but recently she has been noticing it even with softer foods and some liquids. She is not having any trouble breathing. She has not noticed any bone pain or any other symptoms. She is sent to ENT clinic, where a pharyngoscopy/laryngoscopy reveals an obstructive mass growing in the oropharynx. On biopsy, plasma cells are demonstrated.

Definitions

Solitary plasmacytomas (SP) are a rare presentation of plasma cell dyscrasia, accounting for approximately 2–5% of all plasma cell dyscrasias. SP is a tumor of plasma cells that is associated with a paraproteinemia and M-spike but is a singular tumor and is not associated with hypercalcemia, anemia, or renal dysfunction [49]. Bone marrow involvement is minimal. Solitary plasmacytomas can occur in the bone (solitary bone plasmacytoma, SBP) or in the soft tissue, most commonly in the head and neck (solitary extramedullary plasmacytoma, SEP).

Diagnostic Testing

The pillars of diagnostic testing for SP include firstly establishing the diagnosis of plasmacytoma and secondly distinguishing from MM. Establishing the presence of a plasmacytoma involves similar testing to MM (see above), but tissue biopsy to determine the character of the tumor is generally necessary. M-spike will be present on SPEP. To distinguish from MM, whole-body MRI should demonstrate no additional plasmacytomas. Bone marrow biopsy should be done as marrow involvement of >10% plasma cells is consistent with active MM as opposed to SP. Any blood testing showing renal dysfunction, anemia, or hypercalcemia in the presence of a plasmacytoma is suggestive of active MM rather than SP. Occasionally, kidney biopsy may be important to distinguish MM from SP and renal disease from alternate cause. Finally, in the case of SP, free light chain analysis and flow cytometry of bone marrow may help further rule out active MM with microscopic bone marrow infiltration.

Treatment

Systemic therapy is generally avoided in true SP when active MM has been ruled out. Patients can be treated with radiation therapy or surgery if required for amelioration of symptoms or prevention of neurologic or airway compromise due to mass effect (i.e., in the spine). Patients should be monitored every 3–6 months similarly to those with SMM with chemistries, CBCs, and more extensive testing as needed to watch for progression to MM.

Useful Tools

How to Read SPEP/UPEP [50]

The SPEP and UPEP separate serum or urine proteins based on size. After electrophoresis, there are five fractions commonly seen, shown as "spikes" on the SPEP/UPEP results: albumin, alpha-1 globulin, alpha-2 globulin, beta globulin, and gamma globulin. Albumin, which makes up the first spike, is the most abundant protein in human serum and therefore is the tallest spike on normal SPEP. Alpha-1 is generally made up of alpha1-antitrypsin, thyroid-binding globulin, and transcortin. Alpha-2 is made up of ceruloplasmin, alpha-2-macroglobulin, and haptoglobin.

As several of these proteins are acute phase reactants, either the alpha-1 or alpha-2 spikes may be increased during inflammation. The beta fraction contains primarily transferrin and beta-lipoprotein. The gamma spike is the final spike on SPEP/UPEP and is the spike that shows the immunoglobulins. This is the spike that is expected to be elevated in multiple myeloma (Fig. 11.2).

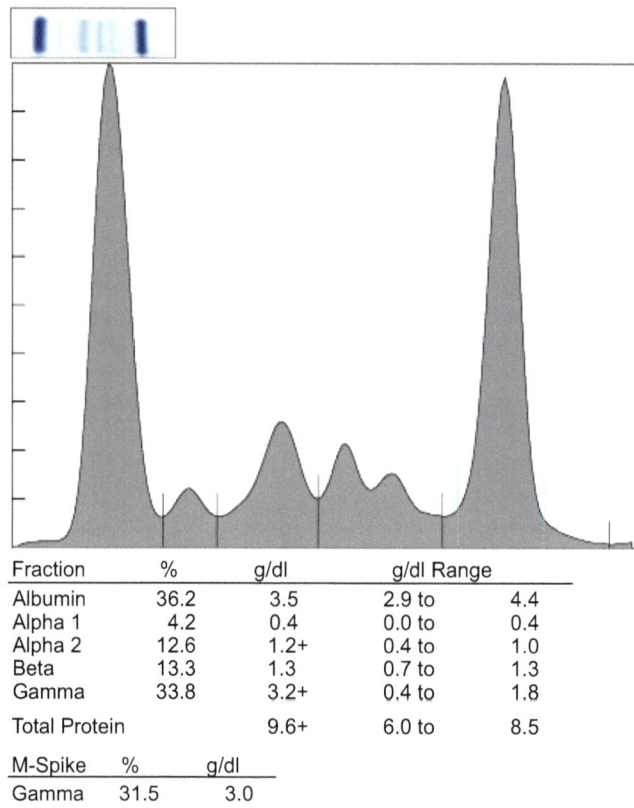

Fraction	%	g/dl	g/dl Range	
Albumin	36.2	3.5	2.9 to	4.4
Alpha 1	4.2	0.4	0.0 to	0.4
Alpha 2	12.6	1.2+	0.4 to	1.0
Beta	13.3	1.3	0.7 to	1.3
Gamma	33.8	3.2+	0.4 to	1.8
Total Protein		9.6+	6.0 to	8.5

M-Spike	%	g/dl
Gamma	31.5	3.0

Fig. 11.2 Serum protein electrophoresis

References

1. Myeloma | CDC. https://www.cdc.gov/cancer/myeloma/index.htm (2021).
2. Kazandjian D. Multiple myeloma epidemiology and survival, a unique malignancy. Semin Oncol. 2016;43:676–81.
3. Owen RG, et al. Clinicopathological definition of Waldenstrom's macroglobulinemia: consensus panel recommendations from the second international workshop on Waldenstrom's Macroglobulinemia. Semin Oncol. 2003;30:110–5.
4. Smith DB, Harris M, Gowland E, Chang J, Scarffe JH. Non-secretory multiple myeloma: a report of 13 cases with a review of the literature. Hematol Oncol. 1986;4:307–13.
5. Brigle K, Rogers B. Pathobiology and diagnosis of multiple myeloma. Semin Oncol Nurs. 2017;33:225–36.
6. Kristinsson SY, Minter AR, Korde N, Tan E, Landgren O. Bone disease in multiple myeloma and precursor disease: novel diagnostic approaches and implications on clinical management. Expert Rev Mol Diagn. 2011;11:593–603.
7. Buege MJ, et al. Corrected calcium versus ionized calcium measurements for identifying hypercalcemia in patients with multiple myeloma. Cancer Treat Res Commun. 2019;21:100159.
8. Yadav P, Cook M, Cockwell P. Current trends of renal impairment in multiple myeloma. Kidney Dis (Basel). 2016;1:241–57.
9. Abdallah N, et al. Cytogenetic abnormalities in multiple myeloma: association with disease characteristics and treatment response. Blood Cancer J. 2020;10:82.
10. Ludwig H, et al. Erythropoietin treatment of anemia associated with multiple myeloma. N Engl J Med. 1990;322:1693–9.
11. Kyle RA, et al. Review of 1027 patients with newly diagnosed multiple myeloma. Mayo Clin Proc. 2003;78:21–33.
12. Ludwig H, Kainz S, Schreder M, Zojer N, Hinke A. SLiM CRAB criteria revisited: temporal trends in prognosis of patients with smoldering multiple myeloma who meet the definition of 'biomarker-defined early multiple myeloma'—a systematic review with meta-analysis. eClinicalMedicine. 2023;58:101910.
13. Dass J, Arava S, Mishra PC, Dinda AK, Pati HP. Role of CD138, CD56, and light chain immunohistochemistry in suspected and diagnosed plasma cell myeloma: a prospective study. South Asian J Cancer. 2019;8:60–4.
14. Kumar SK, et al. Multiple myeloma, version 3.2021, NCCN clinical practice guidelines in oncology. J Natl Compr Cancer Netw. 2020;18:1685–717.
15. Van Dobbenburgh OA, et al. Serum beta2-microglobulin: a real improvement in the management of multiple myeloma? Br J Haematol. 1985;61:611–20.
16. Walker R, et al. Magnetic resonance imaging in multiple myeloma: diagnostic and clinical implications. J Clin Oncol. 2007;25:1121–8.
17. Baseline bone involvement in multiple myeloma—a prospective comparison of conventional X-ray, low-dose computed tomography, and 18flourodeoxyglucose positron emission tomography in previously untreated patients—PubMed. https://pubmed.ncbi.nlm.nih.gov/27390357/.
18. Carlson K, Aström G, Nyman R, Ahlström H, Simonsson B. MR imaging of multiple myeloma in tumour mass measurement at diagnosis and during treatment. Acta Radiol. 1995;36:9–14.
19. Moulopoulos LA, Dimopoulos MA, Alexanian R, Leeds NE, Libshitz HI. Multiple myeloma: MR patterns of response to treatment. Radiology. 1994;193:441–6.
20. Moulopoulos LA, et al. Multiple myeloma: spinal MR imaging in patients with untreated newly diagnosed disease. Radiology. 1992;185:833–40.
21. Lecouvet FE, et al. Skeletal survey in advanced multiple myeloma: radiographic versus MR imaging survey. Br J Haematol. 1999;106:35–9.
22. Tertti R, Alanen A, Remes K. The value of magnetic resonance imaging in screening myeloma lesions of the lumbar spine. Br J Haematol. 1995;91:658–60.
23. Rajkumar SV. Multiple myeloma: 2016 update on diagnosis, risk-stratification, and management. Am J Hematol. 2016;91:719–34.

24. Greipp PR, et al. International staging system for multiple myeloma. JCO. 2005;23:3412–20.
25. D'Agostino M, et al. Second revision of the international staging system (R2-ISS) for over-all survival in multiple myeloma: a European myeloma network (EMN) report within the HARMONY project. JCO. 2022;40:3406–18.
26. Attal M, et al. A prospective, randomized trial of autologous bone marrow transplantation and chemotherapy in multiple myeloma. Intergroupe Français du Myélome. N Engl J Med. 1996;335:91–7.
27. Palumbo A, et al. Autologous transplantation and maintenance therapy in multiple myeloma. N Engl J Med. 2014;371:895–905.
28. Facon T, et al. Daratumumab plus lenalidomide and dexamethasone for untreated myeloma. N Engl J Med. 2019;380:2104–15.
29. Roussel M, et al. Front-line transplantation program with lenalidomide, bortezomib, and dexamethasone combination as induction and consolidation followed by lenalidomide mainte-nance in patients with multiple myeloma: a phase II study by the Intergroupe Francophone du Myélome. J Clin Oncol. 2014;32:2712–7.
30. Attal M, et al. Lenalidomide maintenance after stem-cell transplantation for multiple myeloma. N Engl J Med. 2012;366:1782–91.
31. Rajkumar SV, et al. Lenalidomide plus high-dose dexamethasone versus lenalidomide plus low-dose dexamethasone as initial therapy for newly diagnosed multiple myeloma: an open-label randomised controlled trial. Lancet Oncol. 2010;11:29–37.
32. Richardson PG, et al. Lenalidomide, bortezomib, and dexamethasone combination therapy in patients with newly diagnosed multiple myeloma. Blood. 2010;116:679–86.
33. Berenson JR, et al. Long-term pamidronate treatment of advanced multiple myeloma patients reduces skeletal events. Myeloma Aredia Study Group. J Clin Oncol. 1998;16:593–602.
34. Kumar S, et al. Randomized, multicenter, phase 2 study (EVOLUTION) of combinations of bortezomib, dexamethasone, cyclophosphamide, and lenalidomide in previously untreated multiple myeloma. Blood. 2012;119:4375–82.
35. Sonneveld P, et al. Daratumumab, Bortezomib, Lenalidomide, and Dexamethasone for Multiple Myeloma. N Engl J Med. 2024;390(4):301–313.
36. Treatment of relapsed and refractory multiple myeloma: recommendations from the International Myeloma Working Group—PubMed. https://pubmed.ncbi.nlm.nih.gov/33662288/.
37. Durie BGM, et al. International uniform response criteria for multiple myeloma. Leukemia. 2006;20:1467–73.
38. Kumar S, et al. International Myeloma Working Group consensus criteria for response and minimal residual disease assessment in multiple myeloma. Lancet Oncol. 2016;17:e328–46.
39. Lindsley H, Teller D, Noonan B, Peterson M, Mannik M. Hyperviscosity syndrome in multiple myeloma. A reversible, concentration-dependent aggregation of the myeloma protein. Am J Med. 1973;54:682–8.
40. Mehta J, Singhal S. Hyperviscosity syndrome in plasma cell dyscrasias. Semin Thromb Hemost. 2003;29:467–71.
41. Coluzzi F, Rolke R, Mercadante S. Pain management in patients with multiple myeloma: an update. Cancers (Basel). 2019;11:2037.
42. Drayson MT, et al. Levofloxacin prophylaxis in patients with newly diagnosed myeloma (TEAMM): a multicentre, double-blind, placebo-controlled, randomised, phase 3 trial. Lancet Oncol. 2019;20:1760–72.
43. Rajkumar SV, et al. Serum free light chain ratio is an independent risk factor for progression in monoclonal gammopathy of undetermined significance. Blood. 2005;106:812–7.
44. Kyle RA, et al. Monoclonal gammopathy of undetermined significance (MGUS) and smolder-ing (asymptomatic) multiple myeloma: IMWG consensus perspectives risk factors for pro-gression and guidelines for monitoring and management. Leukemia. 2010;24:1121–7.
45. Mateos M-V, et al. International Myeloma Working Group risk stratification model for smol-dering multiple myeloma (SMM). Blood Cancer J. 2020;10:102.

46. Kyle RA, et al. Long-term follow-up of monoclonal gammopathy of undetermined significance. N Engl J Med. 2018;378:241–9.
47. Bianchi G, et al. Impact of optimal follow-up of monoclonal gammopathy of undetermined significance on early diagnosis and prevention of myeloma-related complications. Blood. 2010;116:2019–25.
48. Landgren O, et al. Association of immune marker changes with progression of monoclonal gammopathy of undetermined significance to multiple myeloma. JAMA Oncol. 2019;5:1293–301.
49. Grammatico S, Scalzulli E, Petrucci MT. Solitary plasmacytoma. Mediterr J Hematol Infect Dis. 2017;9:e2017052.
50. O'Connell T, Horita TJ, Kasravi B. Understanding and interpreting the serum protein electrophoresis. AFP. 2005;71:105–12.

Part II
Benign Hematology

Chapter 12
Primer to Bleeding Disorders

Gregory Hemenway and Iberia Romina Sosa

Case

A 21-year-old female with type O positive blood presents to the emergency room with persistent mucosal bleeding after a dental procedure. She has no personal or family history of bleeding and has undergone a tonsillectomy in the past without complication. Her menses were previously normal but over the past 2 months have become significantly heavier. Initial laboratory testing was significant for a platelet count of 1.5 million/μL, PT 14.0 s, PTT 24.5 s, TT 17.5 s, and fibrinogen 300 mg/dL. The acute bleeding episode is resolved with supportive care. A bone marrow biopsy was performed that showed elevated numbers of megakaryocytes with hyperlobulated nuclei, and genetic testing was positive for a JAK2 mutation. Additional testing for an acquired von Willebrand syndrome was sent and revealed VWF antigen 28%, FVIII activity 45%, VWF function (RCoF) 30%, and decreased high-molecular-weight multimers confirming the diagnosis of acquired von Willebrand syndrome in the setting of newly diagnosed essential thrombocythemia.

G. Hemenway
Department of Internal Medicine, Temple University Hospital, Philadelphia, PA, USA
e-mail: Gregory.hemenway@tuhs.temple.edu

I. R. Sosa (✉)
Department of Hematology/Oncology, Fox Chase Cancer Center, Philadelphia, PA, USA
e-mail: iberia.sosa@fccc.edu

© The Author(s), under exclusive license to Springer Nature
Switzerland AG 2024
G. Rivero, I. R. Sosa (eds.), *Consulting Hematology and Oncology Handbook*,
https://doi.org/10.1007/978-3-031-75810-2_12

143

Clinical Context

A bleeding disorder, also known as a bleeding diathesis or bleeding tendency, is an inherited or acquired disorder affecting primary or secondary hemostasis. The evaluation of a patient with a suspected bleeding disorder can be challenging and the clinical manifestations quite varied: depending on whether the disorder is a primary versus secondary disruption of hemostasis, whether it is inherited or acquired, and consideration of any inciting triggers. Given the complexity of hemostatic physiology, evaluation of each patient should include a detailed family and personal history including ethnicity, consanguinity, and prior medical conditions or surgical procedures (Table 12.1). The diagnostic approach should include an assessment of symptoms and signs, and the approach to testing must be individualized.

The following clinical contexts are associated with specific bleeding diathesis:

Malignancy Associated

Localized bleeding may be a direct result of tumor invasion, while a generalized bleeding diathesis may be due to the malignancy itself.

Table 12.1 Approach to the clinical history and physical exam

Bleeding history	Bleeding during infancy, adolescence, or adulthood
	Any bleeding episode severe enough to require ER visit, surgery, or packing/cautery
	Tolerance of dental procedures
	Prior surgical challenges
	History of poor wound healing
	History of iron deficiency and source of bleeding
	Menstrual history
	Pregnancy history
Family history	Prior history may suggest a congenital etiology
	Transmission pattern can give clues as to the entity (i.e., hemophilia A or B are X-linked
Medication use	Certain medications (SSRI, antibiotics or NSAIDS) as well as herbal supplements can increase bleeding risk
Physical exam	Petechiae, purpura, or ecchymosis
	Telangiectasia around lips, consider hemorrhagic telangiectasia (HHT)
	Perifollicular hemorrhages are seen in scurvy
	Albinism has been described in congenital platelet disorders (Hermansky-Pudlak)
	Splenomegaly (consider liver disease, lymphoma or myeloproliferative neoplasms)
	Macroglossia (consider amyloid)
	Joint laxity (consider Ehlers Danlos)
	Cardiac findings, aortic stenosis (aVWD)
	Skeletal findings (syndromic disorders)

Leukemias, lymphomas, plasma cell disorders, and some solid tumor types (small cell lung cancer, breast cancer, and prostate cancer) can replace normal functioning bone marrow via infiltration and disrupt the microenvironment causing decreased platelet production. Disseminated intravascular coagulopathy (DIC) is often described in the setting of cancer. Gastrointestinal and genitourinary malignancies are particularly susceptible to intraluminal bleeding. Hepatocellular carcinomas are prone to intra-tumoral hemorrhage secondary to spontaneous rupture [1]. Patients with liver metastases experience diminished synthesis of coagulation factors. Acquired inhibitors of coagulation including acquired von Willebrand syndrome (aVWS) and acquired factor VIII inhibitors are described in dysproteinemias [2]. Finally, altered fibrinolysis may contribute to bleeding as some tumor types secrete plasminogen activators to promote tumor cell migration thereby leading to fibrinolysis and bleeding [3].

Radiation therapy may lead to telangiectasia formation and increased risk of gastrointestinal or mucosal hemorrhage [4]. Chemotherapy often results in bone marrow suppression including thrombocytopenia. Platelet destruction occurs due to medications, antibody production, infection, or thrombotic microangiopathy.

Acquired von Willebrand Syndrome

aVWS is a rare, albeit underestimated, bleeding diathesis with laboratory and clinical findings resembling inherited von Willebrand disease but occurring in individuals with no prior personal or family history of bleeding and typically in the context of an underlying systemic disease, such as lymphoproliferative, myeloproliferative, and cardiovascular diseases [2, 5, 6]. Both immune and non-immune mechanisms are responsible for the quantitative or qualitative reduction in von Willebrand factor.

Alcohol Use Disorder

Chronic alcohol use can predispose individuals to bleeding by affecting hemostasis via various mechanisms including decreased platelet count, modulation of clotting factors, fibrinolysis, and platelet function. Alcohol use is a common cause of mild thrombocytopenia independent of liver damage although the mechanism of this is incompletely understood [7]. Experimental models suggest ethanol is directly toxic to mature thrombocytes via mitochondrial damage and apoptosis [7]. The platelets of chronic alcohol users display a relative increase in size and weight suggesting increased production and earlier release into circulation [7]. Alcohol decreases platelet aggregation in response to various activating signals including ADP and collagen. *In vitro* studies show that alcohol inhibits the mobilization of arachidonic acid from phospholipid in platelets, thus inhibiting the formation of TXA_2 [8].

Liver Disease

Liver disease causes a plethora of hemostatic abnormalities, and while it is often considered to increase bleeding risk, it can also increase the risk of thrombosis, ultimately creating a new hemostatic "set point." All aspects of hemostasis can be altered in liver disease including platelet count, platelet function, coagulation factor activity, and changes to fibrinolysis [9].

Thrombocytopenia is a common hematologic sequelae of liver disease, with over 75% of patients experiencing mild thrombocytopenia [10]. The mechanisms responsible for thrombocytopenia include decreased hepatic synthesis of thrombopoietin, platelet sequestration in the spleen due to portal hypertension, and bone marrow suppression from underlying hepatitis C or other infection, alcohol use, or antibiotics [10]. Endothelial changes and disruptions to laminar flow result in reduced platelet function. Additionally, concurrent kidney injury or systemic infection may contribute to platelet dysfunction.

Hepatocytes are responsible for the synthesis of all coagulation factors including fibrinogen, thrombin, and their upstream factors except for factor VIII which is generated in endothelial cells [11]. In addition, posttranslational modifications take place in hepatocytes. Thus, liver disease may impair both factor production and function. In patients with liver disease secondary to alcohol use, concurrent vitamin K deficiency further disrupts the production of factors II, VII, IX, and X [8].

Dissolution of the fibrin clot system, fibrinolysis, is also altered in liver disease. However, like other facets of hemostasis, the fibrinolytic system rebalances in these patients, increasing the risk for both bleeding and clotting [12]. Under certain circumstances, a rare condition known as hyperfibrinolysis may occur, whereby clot dissolution occurs prematurely leading to subsequent consumption of new clotting factors [12]. This condition closely resembles DIC making its identification and diagnosis difficult.

Systemic Lupus Erythematosus

Systemic lupus erythematosus (SLE) manifests clinically with prothrombotic syndromes, notably APLS, as well as bleeding diatheses. Mild to moderate thrombocytopenia is common and is due to bone marrow failure, antiplatelet autoantibodies against GPIIb/IIIa or the thrombopoietin receptor (TPOR), thrombotic microangiopathy, infection, or as a complication of drug therapy [13, 14]. The renal manifestations of lupus may lead to uremia and a subsequent bleeding tendency. In addition to the antiphospholipid antibodies, SLE has been associated with inhibitors to factors II, VIII, IX, XI, XII, and XIII.

Hypothyroidism

Untreated hypothyroidism uncommonly increases bleeding risk due to a type 1 acquired VWS (aVWS). Mechanistically, there is reduced synthesis of factor VIII and VWF in the setting of low thyroid hormone levels [5]. In autoimmune thyroiditis, there may also be autoantibodies against VWF.

Clinical Manifestations

Determining the severity of bleeding or bruising can be difficult due to subjectivity in describing one's experience. Patients without bleeding disorders may report an excess bleeding tendency, while individuals with inherited bleeding disorder may describe minimal bleeding or with symptoms vastly different from peers with the same bleeding disorder. A bleeding assessment tool (BAT) is an objective scoring system used to quantify bleeding by location and severity, predicting the likelihood of a bleeding disorder being present [15, 16].

Importantly, the symptoms described can give a good indication whether the bleeding diathesis is due to primary or secondary hemostasis defect. Primary hemostasis refers to initial steps in clot formation and rely on the integrity of the blood vessel wall and its interaction with platelets and von Willebrand factor. Secondary hemostasis refers to the formation of the fibrin-based clot which relies on coagulation factors. Platelet disorders are more likely to present with petechiae or mucocutaneous bleeding while coagulation factor defects often manifest with deep tissue hematomas [17]. Hence, it is important to pay close attention to a description of the lesions described by the patient, prior history of bleeding challenges, as well performing a good clinical exam for the following:

- *Petechiae* are non-blanching, nonpalpable, flat, red, and small (typically <2 mm), discrete areas on the skin. Typically associated with severe thrombocytopenia, petechiae may also manifest in areas of skin fragility or with the use of certain medications including glucocorticoids.
- *Purpura* refers to a larger area of superficial hemorrhage composed of coalesced petechiae. Both thrombocytopenia and vasculitis elicit purpura. Thrombocytopenia elicits flat, non-blanching skin lesions in dependent areas of the body while vasculitis is most likely to elicit palpable, pruritic skin lesions with a distribution pattern not consistent with dependent areas of the body. Dry purpura describes lesions on the skin, and wet purpura describes lesions in mucocutaneous areas.
- *Bruise/ecchymosis* describes the subcutaneous collection of extravasated blood. The lesions are still flat; however, if the lesion raises the skin profile or occurs in deep tissue, these are called *hematomas* and are most likely to occur in patients with coagulation factor deficiencies. As bruises heal, the color of the skin evolves from purple/blue to red/brown and eventually to green/yellow reflecting the metabolism of hemoglobin to biliverdin and eventually to bilirubin. Several

lesions of the same color suggest a single traumatic event, while multiple lesions of varied colors suggest an evolving process.

- A *bleeding challenge* is an event expected to cause bleeding under normal circumstances, including dental extraction, childbirth, surgery, or trauma. Bleeding in response to one of these inciting events that requires intervention, such as transfusion, surgical correction, and iron repletion, suggests a bleeding diathesis. In a patient presenting with no history of requiring intervention, the likelihood of an inherited bleeding disorder is low. However, if this same patient currently has a bleeding problem, this raises the possibility of an acquired disorder.

Laboratory Investigation

The laboratory investigation of bleeding disorders is essential for precise diagnosis, and the extent and sequence of testing is based on individualized assessment of bleeding risk. It is important to note that most specialized laboratory tests require nuanced sample preparation, handling, and interpretation. It is best to have an experienced hematologist and/or pathologist assisting in the interpretation.

In patients presenting with an undiagnosed bleeding disorder, the following laboratory investigations may help to ascertain primary versus secondary hemostasis.

Tests to Assess Secondary Hemostasis

Coagulation studies, *PT, APTT*

The *prothrombin time (PT)* measures the time, in seconds, for clot formation after the addition of thromboplastin to a patient's plasma. Performing a PT is the first assay to evaluate the extrinsic and common pathways of coagulation (Fig. 12.1). Clot formation is detected via mechanical or optical methods. Thromboplastin contains a mixture of tissue factor, calcium, and phospholipid that is not standardized across laboratories [18]. Therefore, the World Health Organization (WHO) created the international normalized ratio (INR), a dimensionless value, which represents the ratio of a patient's PT divided by a control PT measured using a reference thromboplastin reagent. Calculation of an INR allows for comparison of coagulation across varying time points and centers. A normal INR value for a healthy individual is 1.1 or below, which usually corresponds to a PT range of 10 to 13 s depending on the laboratory.

Common indications for performing a PT include the evaluation of unexplained bleeding, monitoring vitamin K antagonist (VKA) activity such as warfarin, diagnosis of DIC, assessment of the synthetic function of the liver, and establishing a baseline value prior to starting an anticoagulant or performing an invasive procedure. A prolongation of the PT suggests an abnormality involving coagulation factors II, V, VII, X, or fibrinogen. Table 12.2 describes the causes of a prolonged

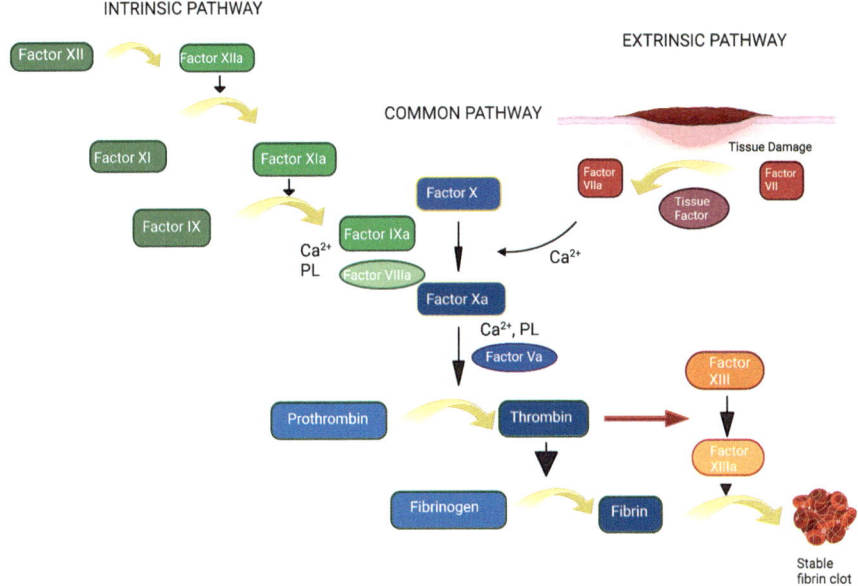

Fig. 12.1 The clotting cascade responsible for secondary hemostasis

Table 12.2 Interpretation of prolonged coagulation studies

PT	aPTT	Underlying disease
Prolonged	Normal	Inherited: Factor VII deficiency Acquired: Liver disease, warfarin, DIC, mild vitamin K deficiency
Normal	Prolonged	Inherited: Deficiency of factor VIII, IX, XI, or XII, vWD (varies) Acquired: Inhibitor of factor VIII, IX, XI, or XII, aVWS, lupus anticoagulant, or anticoagulants[a]
Prolonged	Prolonged	Inherited: Deficiency of fibrinogen, prothrombin, factor V, or factor X Acquired: DIC, liver disease, severe vitamin K deficiency, anticoagulants, acquired inhibitor of fibrinogen, prothrombin, factor V, or factor X (can be in setting of amyloidosis-associated factor X deficiency)

[a]Heparin, dabigatran, argatroban, direct oral factor Xa (DOACs)

PT. Coagulation factors may be deficient due to an inherited disorder or the presence of an acquired autoantibody. Vitamin K deficiency due to malnutrition, antibiotic use, or malabsorption can lead to impaired synthesis of factors II, VII, IX, and X resulting in a prolonged PT. In cases of severe deficiency, the aPTT may also be prolonged. Heparin anticoagulants do not typically prolong the PT due to the addition of heparin-binding agents in the PT reagent. However, high doses of heparin may overcome these chemicals and prolong the PT. Owing to their inhibition of thrombin, all direct oral anticoagulants (DOACs) prolong the PT albeit to varying degrees based on the drug and the reagent used. Thus, measurement of the PT is not clinically useful for monitoring of DOACs.

The *aPTT* is another commonly used assay to evaluate the intrinsic and common pathways of coagulation (Fig. 12.1). This test measures the time it takes plasma to clot after exposure to thromboplastic material (without tissue factor) and a negatively charged molecules such as silica. A source of phospholipid is provided by the thromboplastic material. Unlike the PT, there is no standardization of the aPTT across reagents or instruments, and values from different centers cannot be compared directly. The normal range for the aPTT thus varies but is approximately 25 to 35 s. The clinical uses of the aPTT test are like those for PT, including evaluation of unexplained bleeding, diagnosis of DIC, establishing a baseline prior to start an anticoagulant, and monitoring of therapy with unfractionated heparins and parenteral direct thrombin inhibitor including argatroban. The aPTT cannot be used to monitor low molecular weight heparin (LMW) activity as these agents do not prolong the aPTT. Anti-factor Xa activity is a more accurate means to titrate LWH dosing.

Table 12.2 provides a framework for the causes of prolonged aPTT. The most common reason for a prolonged aPTT while hospitalized is the use of unfractionated heparin. As described above, both liver disease and DIC can cause prolongation of the aPTT with severe disease. Hemophilia A and B, hereditary deficiencies of factor VIII and IX, respectively (Table 12.3), can lead to prolongation of the aPTT. Von Willebrand disease (Fig. 12.2; Table 12.4) can also cause prolongation of the aPTT because factor VIII is carried through the circulation by VWF. Antibodies to factor VIII are the most common factor inhibitors. Factor inhibitors occur due to systemic illness, autoimmune disease, infused factor VIII, or de novo presentation.

Thrombin and Reptilase Time

Both the *thrombin time (TT)* and *reptilase time (RT)* measure the conversion of fibrinogen to fibrin but differ in the reagent that is used. In the TT assay, citrated plasma is incubated in the presence of bovine or human thrombin, and the time to clot formation is measured. The normal range is variable based on lab technique and type of reagent used but typically falls between 14 to 19 s. Conditions that result in low levels of fibrinogen, such as DIC or liver disease, or if an inhibitor of thrombin is present, will prolong the TT. The RT utilizes an enzyme derived from the venom of the *Bothrops* snake, reptilase, which is insensitive to the effects of heparin. RT is also used to detect abnormalities in fibrinogen. Hypofibrinogenemia and dysfibrinogenemia (Table 12.5) with fibrinogen activity levels <100 mg/dL will cause prolongation of the PT, aPTT, TT, and RT [19, 20]. RT's greatest use is detecting the presence of heparin since heparin prolongs the TT but not the RT.

Table 12.3 Types of Hemophilia [22–24]

Type	Deficient clotting factor	Inheritance	Genetic abnormalities	Clinical features[a]	Treatment
A	VIII	X-linked recessive	Inversion of long arm of X chromosome within intron 22 of the FVIII gene in up to 50% of cases[b]	Hemarthrosis, epistaxis, hematuria, GI bleeding, intracranial in infants, musculoskeletal hematomas in children	FVIII replacement product, aminocaproic acid (EACA) or tranexamic acid (TXA) are adjunctive, desmopressin A for mild–moderate disease
B	IX	X-linked recessive	Deletions, point mutations, insertions of the FIX gene	Similar to hemophilia A but often less severe	FIX replacement product, TXA or EACA are adjunctive
C	XI	Autosomal	Many pathogenic variants in FXI gene, in Ashkenazi population missense mutation in exon 9 or premature stop codon in exon 5 are most common	Bleeding in setting of trauma or surgery, slight increase in postpartum hemorrhage, rarely spontaneous	Usually periprocedural TXA or EACA, can use FFP, purified FXI concentrate[c] or rFVIIa in severe cases

[a]Late complications of hemophilia are due to both iatrogenic and non-iatrogenic etiologies including hemophilic arthropathy, cardiovascular disease, inhibitor development and risk of infection from plasma-derived products (screening has greatly reduced the incidence of HIV, Hepatitis B and C viruses)

[b]A rare autosomal recessive, combined deficiency of FVIII and factor V is caused by mutations in the LMAN1 gene

[c]FXI concentrates are not available in the USA

Mixing Studies

In a patient with an unexplained abnormal clotting test, including PT, aPTT, or TT, a mixing study can be performed to determine whether the prolongation is due to factor deficiency versus the presence of an inhibitor. The clotting time is measured via serial dilution of a patient's plasma with normal plasma. In the case of a pure factor deficiency, mixing of patient plasma 1:1 with normal plasma will correct the clotting test as normal plasma will provide at least 50% activity for any deficient factor, enough to normalize the clotting time. Once a pure factor deficiency has been identified, individual factor assays can be used to determine the missing factor. Table 12.6 summarizes various rare coagulation factor deficiencies.

A mixing study that does not correct with the 1:1 addition of normal plasma suggests the presence of an inhibitor. Because some factor inhibitors are time-dependent, the assay is performed immediately after specimen collection as well as after

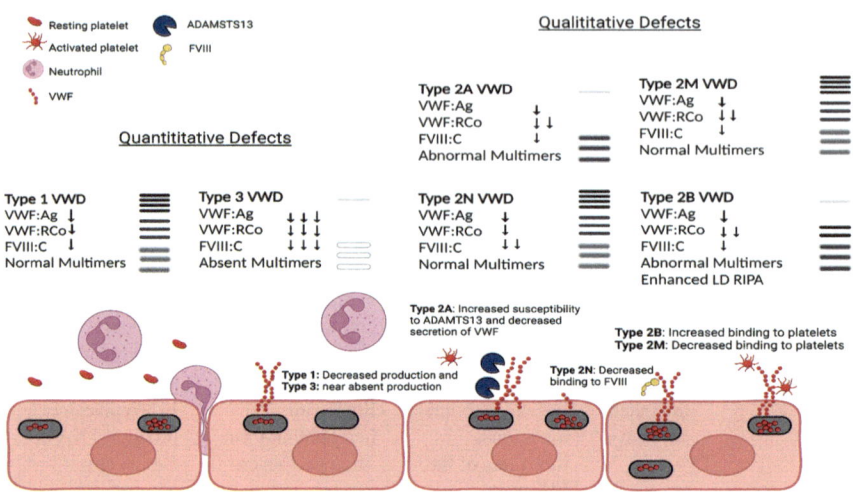

Fig. 12.2 Diagram representation of VWD subtypes and differences in quantitative/qualitative defects

incubation at body temperature for 1 to 2 h. Inhibitors of factor VIII may display delayed onset of action due to slow reaction kinetics. Once it is determined that the mixing study does not correct, subsequent work up will depend on the clinical picture and the most likely underlying etiology. In particular, the presentation and management of alloantibodies in patients with inherited bleeding disorders are quite different from acquired factor inhibitors.

Although rare in the non-hemophilic population, the most described acquired autoantibody leading to a bleeding diathesis is directed against factor VIII, a condition known as acquired hemophilia A (AHA). The reported incidence is approximately one case per million/year and increases with age, with more than 80% of patients aged 65 or older in one prospective study [21]. AHA autoantibodies are predominantly IgG1 and IgG4 and bind similar regions of factor VIII as alloantibodies including A2, A3, and C2 domains [21]. Associated clinical conditions with AHA include malignancy (solid tumor and lymphoproliferative diseases), autoimmune disease (SLE, RA, Sjogren's), Hepatitis B and C, pemphigus, and drug-induced, namely penicillin and interferon. Yet up to 50% of cases remain idiopathic. Bleeding in these patients is severe and often life threatening.

After determining the presence of an inhibitor, characterization can be accomplished by performing additional steps. The addition of phospholipid to a sample of 1:1 mixed plasma with correction suggests the presence of an antiphospholipid antibody.

Table 12.4 Types of von Willebrand disease and their features [25–27]

Type	Pathogenesis	Inheritance	Factor VIII	VWF antigen	Ristocetin cofactor	RIPA	Average ristocetin cofactor: VWF antigen ratio	Multimer analysis
1	Decreased production	AD	Low	Low	Low	Low or normal	1	Normal or all decreased
2A	Defective production and secretion	AD or AR	Low	Low	Very low	Low	0.3	Absent large and intermediate size multimers
2B	Increased turnover	AD	Low or normal	Low or normal	Very low	Increased	0:6	Absent large multimers
2M	Impaired binding to platelets	AD or AR	Low or normal	Low	Very low	Low or normal	<1	Normal
2N	Defective FVIII binding	AD	Very low	Normal	Normal	Normal	1	Normal
3	Defective production	AD	<10%	Undetectable	Undetectable	Very low	Both	All sizes absent
Acquired	Associated with MPN, LPN, valvular disease, drugs	No family history	Low or very low	Low or very low	Low or very low	Low or very low	<1	Type 1 or Type 2 pattern

Table 12.5 Disorders of fibrinogen [19, 20]

Congenital	*Qualitative* Dysfibrinogenemia (autosomal dominant) Hypodysfibrinogenemia (autosomal dominant)
	Quantitative Afibrinogenemia (autosomal recessive) Hypofibrinogenemia (autosomal dominant)
Acquired	*Qualitative* Liver disease Malignancies (renal carcinoma, hepatoma, multiple myeloma) Antifibrinogen antibodies
	Quantitative Hypofibrinogenemia (liver disease, DIC) Hyperfibrinogenemia (pregnancy, malignancy) Medications (fibrinolytic agents, isotretinoin, L-asparaginase, valproic acid)

The Bethesda Assay

The Bethesda Assay is used to characterize FVIII inhibitors. It employs serial dilutions of patient plasma incubated with pooled normal plasma at 37 °C for 2 h, with subsequent measurement of factor VIII activity. The reciprocal dilution of patient plasma that results in 50% factor VIII activity is defined as one Bethesda unit (BU). In general, 1 BU is equivalent to the amount of inhibitor that neutralizes 50% of factor activity. A strong inhibitor is associated with higher dilution to allow for factor VIII activity and subsequently a higher BU titer [29]. Inhibitors with a titer <5 BU despite repeated factor infusions are considered low responding inhibitors, while inhibitors >5BU are considered high-responding [30].

Specific Clotting Factor Assays

If screening assays are abnormal, specific clotting factor assays are performed based on pattern of atypical baseline coagulation: PT/INR and aPTT.

Tests to Assess Primary Hemostasis

- The *platelet function analyzer (PFA)-100* was originally validated to assess the plasma of patients with VWD although it is rarely used for these purposes now. Its main use is for general screening of platelet function when a specific diagnosis is not clear. To perform the test, a small aperture is coated with platelet agonists and the rate of flow is measured as platelets form a hemostatic plug [31]. It is affected by several factors including platelet count, hemoglobin, and vWF levels but can be advantageous because of its ease of use and speed.
- *Platelet aggregometry* is the gold standard for diagnosing platelet function disorders. It measures platelet aggregation in response to various agonists including

Table 12.6 Rare inherited bleeding disorders [28]

Factor deficiency	Laboratory findings	Clinical features	Treatment
I	Prolonged TT, PT, and PTT	Neonatal including umbilical cord bleeding, pregnancy associated hemorrhage, intracerebral	Fibrinogen concentrate or cryoprecipitate
II	Normal TT, prolonged PT and PTT	Hematomas (subcutaneous, muscle), hemarthrosis, mucosal bleeding, post-procedural bleeding	PCC
V	Normal TT, prolonged PT and PTT	Epistaxis, AUB, mucosal bleeding	FFP
VII	Normal TT and PTT, prolonged PT	Epistaxis, AUB	Factor VII, PCC, or recombinant factor VII
X	Normal TT, prolonged PT and PTT	Hematomas (subcutaneous, muscle), hemarthrosis, AUB, umbilical cord bleeding, epistaxis	FFP or PCC
XI	Normal TT and PT, prolonged PTT	Post-procedural bleeding, AUB	FFP or factor XI concentrate
XIII	Normal TT, PT, and PTT Requires specific assays	AUB, neonatal including umbilical cord bleeding and miscarriages, intraperitoneal bleeding	Cryoprecipitate, PCC, or factor XIII concentrate
Combined V and VIII	Normal TT, prolonged PT and PTT	Epistaxis, AUB, postpartum bleeding, post-procedural bleeding	Limited data, FFP
Vitamin K-dependent factors	Normal TT, prolonged PT and PTT	Intracranial, umbilical cord, retroperitoneal bleeding	Vitamin K for prophylaxis; Vitamin K and PCC used for treatment

collagen, adenosine diphosphate (ADP), epinephrine, ristocetin, and arachidonic acid. It is usually performed on platelet-rich plasma stirred in a cuvette at 37 °C. Light transmission through the sample is measured as platelet aggregation occurs in response to the agonists added, thereby improving the transmission with the decreased turbidity of the sample as the clot forms. Interpretation of aggregation depends on the pattern of light transmission to different agonists (Table 12.7). Although aggregometry is a useful tool, it is labor intensive and requires technical expertise for its execution and its interpretation.

- *Electron microscopy* is a useful methodology for the identification of granule subtypes, morphologic changes following platelet activation, and the role of platelet cytoskeleton. It remains the gold standard for identifying various platelet

Table 12.7 Interpretation of aggregometry in platelet disorders

Disorder	Aggregation				Other features
	Primary ADP	Secondary ADP	Collagen	Ristocetin	
VWD	WNL	WNL	WNL	Variable	Platelet morphology is normal VWD panel abnormal
Bernard Soulier	WNL	WNL	WNL	NR	Giant platelets with reduced count
Glanzmann Thrombasthenia	NR	NR	NR	Reduced response	Normal platelet morphology
Storage pool disorder	WNL	NR to reduced response	Reduced response	Reduced response	Electron microscopy is abnormal
Secretion pool defect	WNL	NR to reduced response	Reduced response	Reduced response	Normal platelet morphology an electron microscopy

WNL within normal limits, *NR* no response

abnormalities and storage pool deficiencies (Table 12.8). However, it is important to note it requires technical expertise that are not widely available.

- *Thromboelastography*
- Viscoelastic assays are point of care tests used to determine if hemostasis is preserved. The two main tests available are *thromboelastography (TEG)* and *rotational thromboelastography (ROTEM)* with the former being more widely available. Neither test is capable of distinguishing between thrombocytopenia and specific platelet function defects. To perform the test, a cylindrical cup that holds a sample of whole blood oscillates to and fro at a rotation cycle of 10 s. The physical properties of a forming clot are measured via the torque of the rotating cup which is transmitted to an immersed pin. An electrical signal is generated by the amount of pin rotation and recorded as a tracing which illustrates the different phases of clotting over time. Clot initiation (reaction time R), clot kinetics (clot formation time K and alpha angle), strength (maximal amplitude MA and clot viscoelasticity G), and clot lysis over time (lysis at 30 min LY30) can be ascertained. Platelet function is assessed using the alpha angle and maximal amplitude. TEG and ROTEM cannot distinguish platelet dysfunction from thrombocytopenia. The utility of the TEG remains to be defined. Current clinical applications include transfusion management during surgery, trauma, liver disease, and postpartum hemorrhage.
- *Flow cytometry* is a useful laboratory technique to assess platelet activation and function. It can be performed in whole blood samples as opposed to PRP and it is not adversely affected by thrombocytopenia. In flow cytometry, platelets glycoproteins involved in aggregation are labeled with fluorescent monoclonal antibodies. The cell suspension is passed through a flow chamber equipped by a laser beam that activates the fluorophore. The identification of specific glycoproteins on the platelet surface can provide useful information regarding activation,

Table 12.8 Platelet disorders

Platelet disorder	Underlying etiology	Findings on blood smear and laboratory assessment	Clinical manifestations
Wiskott-Aldrich syndrome [32]	*WAS* mutation, a gene responsible for actin polymerization	Smear: Small platelets with thrombocytopenia Low CD-8T cell count, low memory B cell count, elevated IgA with normal IgG and low IgM	Classic triad of recurrent infections, eczema, and thrombocytopenia usually presenting within the first year of life Petechiae, purpura, prolonged umbilical stump bleeding, hematemesis, melena, epistaxis, hematuria Also associated with autoimmune disease and malignancy including lymphoma
MYH9-related disorders (May-Hegglin anomaly, Sebastian syndrome, Fechtner syndrome, Epstein syndrome) [33]	Autosomal dominant *MYH9* mutation, a gene which encodes non-muscle myosin IIA heavy chain, part of the contractile cytoskeleton of megakaryocytes, platelets, and neutrophils	Smear: Macrothrombocytopenia, neutrophil inclusion bodies (Dohle-like bodies) often seen in cytoplasm Normal platelet aggregation studies	Varies from easy bruising to mucosal bleeding including uterine and spontaneous hemorrhage Kidney disease with associated proteinuria or hematuria that may progress to renal failure, cataracts, sensorineural hearing loss
Quebec syndrome [25]	Autosomal dominant tandem duplication of *PLAU* gene, leading to overexpression and storage of urokinase plasminogen activator by platelets causing increased fibrinolysis	Smear: Thrombocytopenia, usually mild Decreased platelet aggregation in response to epinephrine	Post-surgical bleeding, poor wound healing, heavy menstrual bleeding

(continued)

Table 12.8 (continued)

Platelet disorder	Underlying etiology	Findings on blood smear and laboratory assessment	Clinical manifestations
Bernard-Soulier syndrome [34]	Autosomal recessive mutation in *GP1BA, GP1BB,* and/or *GP9* genes, resulting in a defect in the platelet glycoprotein complex GP1b/IX/V	Smear: Macrothrombocytopenia Platelet aggregation studies are normal except in response to ristocetin	Easy bruising, epistaxis, gingival bleeding, cutaneous bleeding, rarely intracranial hemorrhage
Platelet-type VWD [25, 26]	Gain of function mutation in *GP1BA* gene, causing enhanced VWF and platelet interaction	Smear: Thrombocytopenia with large platelet size and volume, occasional platelet clumping VWF multimer assay shows decreased amount of high-molecular weight VWF multimers	Similar to type 2B VWD with mild to moderate mucocutaneous bleeding
Gray platelet syndrome [25, 35]	Dominant or recessive defect in multiple genes, including *NBEAL2 or HZF*	Smear: Abnormally large, agranular, gray platelets with thrombocytopenia Collagen-induced platelet aggregation is reduced	Associated with bleeding, myelofibrosis, and splenomegaly Epistaxis, easy bruising, uterine bleeding, gastrointestinal bleeding
Glanzmann thrombasthenia [25]	Autosomal recessive defect in the *ITGA2B or ITGB3* gene which encode for platelet integrin $\alpha_{IIb}\beta_3$ (integrin alpha$_{IIb}$beta$_3$)	Smear: Normal platelet count and morphology Prolonged PFA-100 closure time, platelets do not aggregate in response to ADP, collagen, thrombin, and epinephrine but do aggregate in presence of ristocetin	Mucocutaneous bleeding including purpura, epistaxis, heavy menstrual bleeding, gingival hemorrhage, gastrointestinal bleeding
Chediak-Higashi syndrome [25, 36]	Autosomal recessive mutation in *CHS1/ LYST* gene, responsible for regulating size and trafficking of lysosomes	Smear: Large, peroxidase-positive, cytoplasmic granules in platelets and leukocytes Normal platelet count, neutropenia, abnormal bleeding time	Severe immunodeficiency, recurrent bacterial infection, oculocutaneous albinism, progressive neurologic dysfunction, increased risk of HLH and bleeding

(continued)

Table 12.8 (continued)

Platelet disorder	Underlying etiology	Findings on blood smear and laboratory assessment	Clinical manifestations
Hermansky-Pudlak syndrome [25, 37]	Autosomal recessive mutation in 11 different genes that encode for adapter-protein 3 (AP-3) or biogenesis of lysosome-related organelles complex 1, 2, and 3 (BLOC-1, BLOC-2, BLOC-3)	Smear: Usually normal Prolonged bleeding time, reduced delta granule number identified only with electron microscopy	Variable hypopigmentation including oculocutaneous albinism, progressive pulmonary fibrosis, granulomatous colitis, bleeding diathesis Variable degrees of bleeding problems including easy bruising, gingival bleeding, epistaxis, post-surgical bleeding depending on genotype

aggregation, evidence of platelet dysfunction, or congenital deficiency (Table 12.8).

- *Euglobin lysis time* (ECLT) is an assay used to assess the function of the fibrinolytic system. Citrated platelet-poor plasma is mixed with an acid causing the precipitation of clotting factors in a complex called the euglobin fraction. This complex contains fibrinogen, tissue plasminogen activator (tPA), plasminogen, and factor VIII. The euglobin fraction is resuspended in a solution of borate and clotting is activated by the addition of thrombin. Automated methods then measure the time for clot lysis, typically using optical density. A shortened ECLT is indicative of hyperfibrinolysis. The underlying etiologies for hyperfibrinolysis are described in Table 12.9 and include both inherited and acquired defects in the fibrinolytic pathway.

- *D-dimer*

- The D-dimer antigen is a useful, albeit nonspecific, marker of fibrin degradation, indicating active or recent coagulation. D-dimer consists of two D domain moieties from fibrin monomers that have been crosslinked by the activated transglutaminase factor XIII [43]. Commercial assays for measuring D-dimer antigen use a monoclonal antibody to detect a unique and conformationally reactive polypeptide signature that has been modified by factor XIIIa and plasmin (Fig. 12.3). The D-dimer assay importantly distinguishes between fibrin and fibrinogen degradation products. If non-crosslinked fibrinogen was broken down, a D-monomer would be released.

- There are various causes of D-dimer elevation which are described in Table 12.10. Thus, the utility of measuring a D-dimer lies in correlating a positive or negative value with other clinical information to make an informed decision. Current validated scenarios for using a D-dimer antigen include venous thromboembolism

Table 12.9 Disorders of hyperfibrinolysis

Type	Underlying etiology	Clinical features	Diagnostic pearls	Treatment
PAI-1 deficiency [38]	Inherited: Extremely rare, isolated reports on PAI1 gene insertion resulting in nonfunctional enzymatic activity	Post-procedural bleeding, delayed bleeding and wound healing after initial hemostasis, obstetric and gynecologic bleeding, cardiac fibrosis	Shortened or normal ECLT Measurement of PAI-1 antigen and activity[a]	TXA or EACA perioperatively or in women with heavy menstrual bleeding
TAFI deficiency [39]	Inherited: Unreported Acquired: Chronic liver disease	Unknown	Measurement of TAFI antigen and activity	TXA or EACA
Alpha-2-antiplasmin [40, 41]	Inherited: Autosomal co-dominant Acquired: Associated with chronic liver disease, nephrotic syndrome, DIC, APL, amyloidosis, head injury, abdominal aortic aneurysm	Delayed bleeding particularly after dental extraction or surgery, rarely intramedullary hematoma	Shortened ECLT Immunologic or functional alpha-2-antiplasmin assay	TXA, EACA, or FFP transfusion
Quebec platelet disorder [25]	Autosomal dominant tandem duplication of PLAU, the gene that encodes uPA resulting in excess production of uPA in alpha granules of platelets	Moderate to severe bleeding post-procedurally or after trauma	Mild thrombocytopenia, decreased platelet factor V Measurement of uPA, genetic testing	TXA or EACA at time of bleeding or perioperatively

[a]A small proportion of healthy individuals with no history of abnormal bleeding will have PAI-1 levels below the lower limit of detectability [42]

(VTE) exclusion, risk of VTE recurrence in select populations, and the monitoring of DIC.

Management

Treatments for bleeding disorders depend on their etiology and will thus be summarized below by clinical entity.

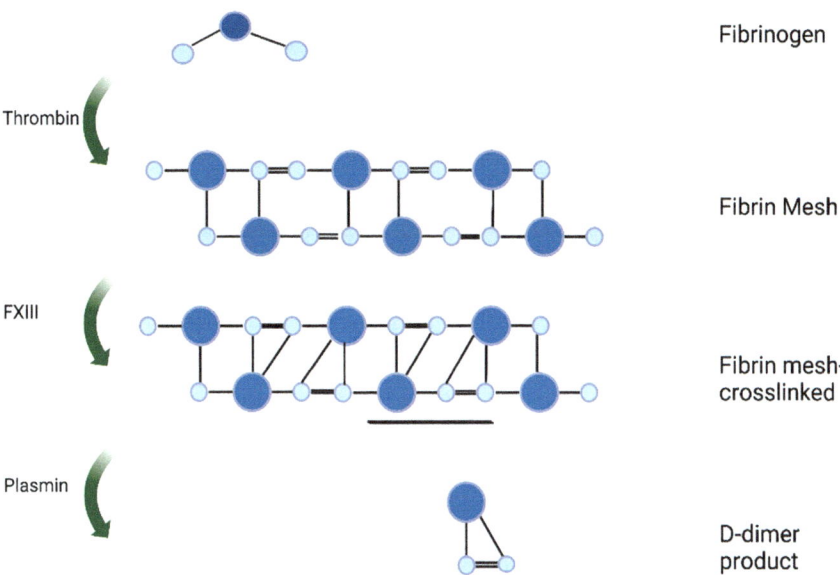

Fig. 12.3   Formation of the fibrin degradation product, D-dimer

Table 12.10 Causes of elevated D-dimer	
	Thromboembolism
	DIC
	Inflammation
	Sepsis
	Surgery/trauma
	Pregnancy
	Sickle cell disease
	Liver disease
	Kidney disease
	Thrombolytic therapy

Management of VWD

The most important tool in the care of patients with VWD is education and counseling of the bleeding risk, importance of planning for surgical procedures and pregnancy, as well as encouraging patients to advocate for themselves in medical emergencies. Treatment options are available based on bleeding risk and severity of disease and include desmopressin (DDAVP), replacement VWF-concentrates, antifibrinolytic agents, or topical therapy (summarized Table 12.11).

Table 12.11 Treatment modalities for VWD and aVWS

Medication	Administration	Notes
DDAVP	Intravenous: 0.3 µg/kg diluted in 50 mL of normal saline given over 20 to 30 min (maximum dose 20 to 30 µg) Intranasal: Weight < 50 kg: 150 µg or one metered spray in one nostril; weight > 50 kg: 300 µg or one metered puff in each nostril	Prophylaxis for minor procedures or acute bleeding episodes Dosing may be repeated every 12-h for two to four doses
VWF concentrate	Minor bleeding or surgery: 30 to 60 ristocetin cofactor units/kg followed by 20 to 40 ristocetin cofactor units/kg every 12 to 48 h to maintain goal VWF level > 30 IU/dL for 3 to 5 days Major bleeding or surgery: 40 to 60 ristocetin cofactor units/kg followed by 20 to 40 ristocetin cofactor units/kg every 12 to 24 h to maintain goal VWF level 50 to 100 IU/dL for 7 to 14 days	Dosing based on clinical picture Can consider continuous intravenous infusion in cases of serious life-threatening bleeding Higher doses may be required in patients with aVWS
Recombinant human VWF	Minor bleeding or surgery: 40 to 50 IU/kg initial dose followed by 40 to 50 IU/kg every 8 to 24 h Major bleeding or surgery: 50 to 80 IU/kg initial dose followed up 40 to 60 IU/kg every 8 to 24 h to keep the VWF level at 50 to 100 IU/kg for 2 to 3 days	Measure factor VIII activity prior to administration and if less than 40%, one dose of recombinant factor VIII is given concurrently with rVWF
Antifibrinolytic agents	*EACA*: 25 to 50 mg/kg per dose orally for up to four doses per day (maximum 5 g dose) *TXA*: 25 mg/kg per dose orally intravenously up to three doses per day	Caution and dose reduction recommended in patients with impaired kidney function Useful for mucosal bleeding

DDAVP

DDAVP is indicated for use prior to minor surgeries or with minor bleeding episodes. Patients with Type I VWD, most of type 2VWD, and some patients with aWVS will respond. However, caution should be exercised in patients with type 2B disease due to the risk for worsening thrombocytopenia. Mechanistically, DDAVP causes indirect release of VWF from endothelial cells. It can be administered intravenously, subcutaneously (Europe only), or intranasally. Side effects include facial flushing, headache, nausea, and paresthesia. Excessive water intake should also be avoided during administration to prevent hyponatremia. Prior to an acute bleeding episode, a DDAVP trial should be performed if possible. Baseline FVIII activity and RCoF blood levels are obtained, and then 0.3 µg/kg of intravenous DDAVP in 50 mL of saline is given over 20 to 30 min. At 1-, 2-, and 4-h post-infusion, FVIII activity and RCoF levels are again checked. A RCoF level of at least 30 IU/dL at 1 h is the threshold for an effective response, with 50 IU/dL indicating an optimal response. The response to DDAVP is transient due to tachyphylaxis and lasts typically from 3 to 5 days.

VWF Concentrates

Several VWF/FVIII replacement therapies exist and are often utilized in severe forms of VWD, in cases of major bleeding or major surgery. Recombinant human VWF products including rVWF, Vonicog Alfa, and Vonvendi contain a range of VWF multimers including the ultra-high-molecular-weight multimers and are highly effective. The clinical application of these agents remains to be defined. Cryoprecipitate contains VWF and can be given but tends to be withheld due to the risk of viral transmission. Intermediate purity FVIII concentrates including Humate P, Alphanate, and Wilate contain both VWF and FVIII and are labeled with RCoF activity. In patients receiving VWF-concentrate, monitoring of VWF activity, FVIII level, and a CBC for platelet count should be monitored daily. Factor VIII level should be maintained at greater than 50% but not over 200% to reduce the risk of thrombosis [27].

Other Agents

Epsilon aminocaproic acid (EACA) and tranexamic acid (TXA) are the two antifibrinolytic agents most used in cases of mild bleeding and work via prevention of fibrin plug degradation. EACA can be administered up to four times daily at doses of 25 to 50 mg/kg, maximum dose of 5 g. TXA is given intravenously up to three times daily at a dose of 10 mg/kg.

Topical Gelfoam or *Surgicel*, agents soaked in topical thrombin, can provide hemostasis in cases of localized bleeding (epistaxis or gingival for example).

In women, *estrogen therapy* has been shown to improve bleeding in patients with type I VWD by partially increasing the synthesis of VWF.

Treatment of Hemophilia

Factor replacement therapy is the mainstay of hemophilia treatment; it has replaced the traditional use of blood products as the standard of care. The use of factor replacement and the delivery of organized care through Hemophilia Treatment Centers has improved quality of life and life expectancy for patients living with hemophilia.

In general, one unit of FVIII concentrate increases FVIII activity by 2%, while one unit of FIX concentrate increases FIX activity by 1%. The available factor replacement products are summarized in Tables 12.12 and 12.13 with the main difference among products being the half-life and source. Overall, the recommendations of replacement are summarized in Table 12.14 with different doses

Table 12.12 Summary of FVIII replacement products for hemophilia A

Factor VIII product	Approximate half-life (h)
Advate (recombinant)	9 to 12
Adynovate (recombinant, pegylated)	13 to 16
Afstyla (recombinant, single chain)	10 to 14
Eloctate (recombinant, Fc fusion)	13 to 20
Esperoct (recombinant, glycol-pegylated)	17–22
Hemofil M (plasma derived, mAb purified)	15
Jivi (recombinant, pegylated)	17–21
Koate (plasma derived, chromatography purified)	16
Kogente FS (recombinant)	11 to 15
Kovaltry (recombinant)	12 to 14
Novoeight (recombinant)	8 to 12
Nuwi (recombinant)	12 to 17
Recombinate (recombinate)	15
Xyntha (recombinant)	8 to 11

Extended half-life products (in italics)

Table 12.13 Summary of FIX replacement products for hemophilia B

Factor IX product	Approximate half-life (h)
Alphanine SD (plasma derived, solvent/detergent treated)[a]	18
Alprolix (recombinant, Fc fusion)	54–90
cBeneFIX (recombinant)	16 to 19
Idelvion (recombinant, albumin fusion)[a]	104
Ixinity (recombinant)	24
Mononine (plasma-derived, monoclonal antibody purified)[a]	23
Rebinyn (recombinant, glyco-pegylated)	103–115
Rixubis (recombinant)	23 to 26

[a]Used only in adults—extended half-life products (in italics)

recommended for prophylaxis/maintenance, bleeding complications, and perioperative management.

The development of autoantibodies against infused factor in patients with hemophilia constitutes a major challenge in delivery of care. The presence of an acquired inhibitor renders the infused factor ineffective. Inhibitors to FVIII concentrates occur in approximately 30% of patients with severe hemophilia A and 3–5% of patients with severe hemophilia B [24]. As previously noted, the Bethesda assay is used to quantitate factor inhibitors and is based on the ability of the patient's plasma to inactivate the factor present in normal plasma.

Table 12.14 Recommendations for factor replacement in hemophilia patients

Type of replacement product		Infusion guidelines
Prophylaxis	Factor VIII concentrate • (standard half-life)	20–40 Units/kg IV 2–4×/week
	• Extended half life	30–50 Units/kg IV twice a week; check specific product information for dosing recommendations
	Factor IX concentrate • (standard half-life)	15–30 Units/kg IV push twice weekly or 25 to 40 Units/kg twice weekly or 40–100 Units/kg 2–3×/week
	• Extended half-life	50 Units/kg once weekly or 100 Units/kg every 10 days; check specific product for dosing recommendations
Major/severe bleeding or Major surgery[a] Goal to raise factor level 80–100%	Factor VIII concentrate	50 Units/kg every 8–12 h
	Factor IX concentrate	100–140 Units/kg every 12–24 h
Hemarthrosis[a] Goal to raise factor level 40–50%	Factor VIII concentrate	25 Units/kg every 8–12 h
	Factor IX concentrate	50–60 Units/kg every 12–24 h
Minor bleeding or minor surgery[a]	Factor VIII concentrate	35 Units/kg every 8–12 h
	Factor IX concentrate	40–70 Units/kg every 12–24 h

[a]See dosing recommendations in product packaging for extended half-life products

Emicizumab-kxwh is a recombinant humanized bispecific monoclonal antibody approved by the FDA for individuals with hemophilia A with and without inhibitors. It works by binding to activated fIX (FIXa) and FX simultaneously, bringing these two molecules together thereby substituting for the scaffold role of factor VIIIa as a cofactor for factor IXa in activating factor X [44]. Emicizumab has been shown to lower bleeding rates in individuals with inhibitors. Therapy is started with a loading dose of 3 mg/kg subcutaneously once weekly for 4 weeks and subsequent maintenance dosing of 1.5 mg/kg subcutaneously once per week, 3 mg/kg subcutaneously once every 2 weeks, or 6 mg/kg subcutaneously once every 4 weeks. Emicizumab is not adequate in patients presenting with acute bleeding. Its use may precipitate rare complications of unusual thrombotic events and thrombotic microangiopathy when activated prothrombin concentrate (aPCC) is co-administered.

Patients with a high responding inhibitor with a titer ≥5 BU and serious bleeding or the need for major surgery require the use of bypassing agents such as recombinant FVIIa (rFVIIa) or aPCC. Bypassing agents (Table 12.15) contain an activated form of a clotting factor in the coagulation cascade. Activated factor VII (FVIIa) can directly activate factor X, bypassing the need for factors VIII and IX, while aPCC

Table 12.15 Bypassing agents and their clinical applications

Type of factor replacement	Active agents	Dosing information	Additional information
4-Factor PCC Kcentra [46]	Contains inactive forms of FII, VII, IX, and X	Initial fixed dose of 1500 to 2000 IU at a rate of 100 units/min. Alternatively, the initial dose may be calculated by body weight and INR [47]	Mostly used for reversal of VKA and DOAC bleeding
3-Factor PCC Profilnine [46]	Contains inactive forms of FII, IX, and X. Contains little to no FVII	1500 to 2000 units IV over 10 min. Check INR 15 min after completion of the infusion. If INR is not ≤1.5, give additional 3F PCC	Used when 4F PCC not available; however, must also give rFVIIa product 20 µg/kg IV OR give FFP 2 units IV by rapid infusion
Activated 4-Factor PCC FEIBA [48]	Contains 4 factors: FII, VII, IX, X with FVII being mostly the activated form	50 to 100 units/kg every 6–12 h, not to exceed 100 units/kg/dose or 200 units/kg/day Check INR 15 min after completion of the infusion. If INR is not ≤1.5, give additional 4F PCC	Bypassing agent for hemophilia patients with inhibitors. Use with caution in hemophilia B patients
Activated FVII NovoSeven [49]	Contains activated FVII	90 to 120 µg/kg every 2–3 h until hemostasis is achieved and at 3–6 h intervals after hemostasis is restored	Bypassing agent for hemophilia patients with inhibitors. Can be used in hemophilia A or B

bypasses FVIII. The rFVIIa products are also appropriate in individuals with hemophilia A who have critical bleeding while receiving emicizumab. For hemophilia B with an inhibitor, rFVIIa products are preferred agent because they do not contain factor IX. This is especially true if the individual experienced an anaphylactic reaction to FIX replacement products. Dosing of bypassing agents is based on clinical response (e.g., cessation of bleeding) rather than laboratory testing [30]. Standard interval dosing is generally continued for at least 48 to 72 h when used for severe bleeding or major surgery, followed by a taper whereby the dosing interval is gradually increased. Although aPCC and/or rFVIIa may be lifesaving in individuals with severe hemophilic bleeding for whom factor replacement is ineffective, these products may be prothrombotic and thus attention to the occurrence of this potential complication should be maintained [45].

Treatment of Acquired and Congenital Platelet Disorders

Treatment for platelet dysfunction is not as straightforward as for coagulation deficiencies. It is recommended that if a patient has clinically significant bleeding suggestive of platelet dysfunction, that appropriate platelet function tests be obtained to properly assess bleeding risk and develop a therapeutic plan that addresses it.

DDAVP is mostly used in mild VWD as previously reviewed. It has also been used in patients with mild platelet defects such as storage pool defects to minimize bleeding with dental procedures and minor surgery [50]. There have been reports that its use reduces bleeding time in patients with cirrhosis [51] or uremia [52], although this correction does not always correlate with a decline in bleeding risk.

As with VWD, the use of *antifibrinolytic agents* such as EACA and TXA may help reduce bleeding in patients with dysfunctional platelets following dental extraction [53].

Hormonal therapies such as conjugated estrogens were previously used in uremic bleeding [54] and can be quite useful in patients with mild to moderate type 1 VWD, especially in patients with gastrointestinal bleeding. Dosing included intravenous estrogen, 0.6 mg/kg daily for 5 days, low dose oral estrogen (2.5–25 mg daily), or transdermal patch 50 to 100 μg weekly. Tamoxifen has had great utility in the treatment of bleeding in hereditary hemorrhagic telangiectasia (HHT); however, a review of this is beyond the scope of this chapter.

Patients with significant platelet dysfunction may ultimately require a *platelet transfusion* to infuse functional platelets. Platelet transfusions are particularly indicated in cases of severe, uncontrolled bleeding who have not responded to other measures (e.g., DDAVP, estrogen) or with anticipated bleeding risk that cannot be empirically treated with available pharmacotherapy.

Patients who cannot receive platelet transfusions because of alloimmunization may benefit from *rFVIIa* infusions. It may act as a local procoagulant at sites of vascular damage or tissue factor-independent thrombin generation induced by the binding of rFVIIa to the surface of activated platelets [55, 56].

Treatment of Acquired and Congenital Fibrinogen Disorders

The goal of management is the prevention and treatment of serious bleeding and thrombosis and the prevention of obstetrical complications. Since many individuals with mild dysfibrinogenemia or mild hypofibrinogenemia are clinically asymptomatic, treatment is not often required. Due to the rarity of these disorders, there is also a lack of evidence-based data to guide best replacement strategy.

For patients with afibrinogenemia, hypofibrinogenemia, or dysfibrinogenemia who have clinically significant bleeding or require emergency surgery, it is recommended fibrinogen be raised to >100 to 150 mg/dL [57]. A higher range is used for more severe bleeding, such as intracerebral hemorrhage, or a particularly challenging surgery with a target of 150 to 200 mg/dL. While cryoprecipitate has been historically utilized, fibrinogen concentrates (Table 12.16) reduce risk of transfusion reactions and volume overload.

Management of bleeding in acquired fibrinogen disorders can be more challenging because often, other coagulation factors (procoagulant and anticoagulant) are likely to be abnormal, for example, DIC. If fibrinogen deficiency is the predominant abnormality, fibrinogen concentrates may be appropriate. If multiple factor

Table 12.16 Fibrinogen replacement therapy [57]

	FFP/24FP	Cryoprecipitate	Fibrinogen concentrate (e.g., RiaStap, Haemocomplettan)
Fibrinogen concentrate per vial or unit	0.5 g	0.3 g	0.9–1.3 g
Volume per vial or unit	250 mL	20 mL	50 mL/vial
Factor concentration	2 g/L Other factors variable amounts: 0.5–1.5 IU/mL	15 g/L FXIII 2.8 IU/mL FVIII 6.3 IU/mL vWF 8.0 IU/mL	Fibrinogen 20 g/L FXIII 1 IU/mL
Pre-transfusion procedure	Thawing; blood type compatibility	Thawing; blood type compatibility	Mix with diluent Blood type compatibility not required
Storage and shelf-life	Frozen 12 months	Frozen 12 months	Store at room temperature 30 months

deficiencies are noted, the individual may benefit from plasma products that contain the deficient coagulation factors.

Routine prophylaxis is not considered necessary unless the patient has previously experienced a life-threatening bleed (secondary prevention) or the individual has a severe family bleeding phenotype (primary prevention) [57]. During pregnancy or if the patient suffered a VTE requiring anticoagulation, a period of prophylactic fibrinogen is considered reasonable, especially for severe deficiency of functional fibrinogen.

Useful Tools

A bleeding assessment tool (BAT) can help quantify extent of bleeding in a patient with a suspected bleeding disorder. BATs are routinely used in hemostasis centers to standardize clinical impression and limit unnecessary testing in patients with a low likelihood of abnormal findings. Unfortunately, BATs are not universally used, and sometimes different tools are used by different institutions making comparisons across establishments less than ideal. The most widely used BATs are those used for standardization of VWD. The International Society on Thrombosis and Hemostasis (ISTH) has made a version of the VWD BAT available online at bleedingscore. certe.nl [15].

References

1. Chearanai O, Plengvanit U, Asavanich C, Damrongsak D, Sindhvananda K, Boonyapisit S. Spontaneous rupture of primary hepatoma: report of 63 cases with particular reference to the pathogenesis and rationale treatment by hepatic artery ligation. Cancer. 1983;51(8):1532–6.
2. Fidalgo T, Ferreira G, Oliveira AC, Silva Pinto C, Martinho P, Mendes MJ, Duarte M, Salvado R, Ribeiro ML. Acquired von Willebrand syndrome in haematologic malignancies—how the clinical-laboratory correlation improves a challenging diagnosis—a case series. Haemophilia. 2017;23(4):e361–5.
3. McMahon B, Kwaan HC. The plasminogen activator system and cancer. Pathophysiol Haemost Thromb. 2008;36(3–4):184–94.
4. Lee JK, Agrawal D, Thosani N, Al-Haddad M, Buxbaum JL, Calderwood AH, Fishman DS, Fujii-Lau LL, Jamil LH, Jue TL, et al. ASGE guideline on the role of endoscopy for bleeding from chronic radiation proctopathy. Gastrointest Endosc. 2019;90(2):171–182e171.
5. Kumar S, Pruthi RK, Nichols WL. Acquired von Willebrand disease. Mayo Clin Proc. 2002;77(2):181–7.
6. Michiels JJ, Budde U, van der Planken M, van Vliet HH, Schroyens W, Berneman Z. Acquired von Willebrand syndromes: clinical features, aetiology, pathophysiology, classification and management. Best Pract Res Clin Haematol. 2001;14(2):401–36.
7. Silczuk A, Habrat B. Alcohol-induced thrombocytopenia: current review. Alcohol. 2020;86:9–16.
8. Mukamal KJ, Jadhav PP, D'Agostino RB, Massaro JM, Mittleman MA, Lipinska I, Sutherland PA, Matheney T, Levy D, Wilson PW, et al. Alcohol consumption and hemostatic factors: analysis of the Framingham offspring cohort. Circulation. 2001;104(12):1367–73.
9. Northup PG, Caldwell SH. Coagulation in liver disease: a guide for the clinician. Clin Gastroenterol Hepatol. 2013;11(9):1064–74.
10. Afdhal N, McHutchison J, Brown R, Jacobson I, Manns M, Poordad F, Weksler B, Esteban R. Thrombocytopenia associated with chronic liver disease. J Hepatol. 2008;48(6):1000–7.
11. Marks PW. Hematologic manifestations of liver disease. Semin Hematol. 2013;50(3):216–21.
12. Lisman T, Porte RJ. Rebalanced hemostasis in patients with liver disease: evidence and clinical consequences. Blood. 2010;116(6):878–85.
13. Cines DB, Liebman H, Stasi R. Pathobiology of secondary immune thrombocytopenia. Semin Hematol. 2009;46(1 Suppl 2):S2–14.
14. Hepburn AL, Narat S, Mason JC. The management of peripheral blood cytopenias in systemic lupus erythematosus. Rheumatology (Oxford). 2010;49(12):2243–54.
15. Rodeghiero F, Tosetto A, Abshire T, Arnold DM, Coller B, James P, Neunert C, Lillicrap D, VWF ISj, Perinatal/Pediatric Hemostasis Subcommittees Working G. ISTH/SSC bleeding assessment tool: a standardized questionnaire and a proposal for a new bleeding score for inherited bleeding disorders. J Thromb Haemost. 2010;8(9):2063–5.
16. Thomas W, Downes K, Desborough MJR. Bleeding of unknown cause and unclassified bleeding disorders; diagnosis, pathophysiology and management. Haemophilia. 2020;26(6):946–57.
17. Girolami A, Luzzatto G, Varvarikis C, Pellati D, Sartori R, Girolami B. Main clinical manifestations of a bleeding diathesis: an often disregarded aspect of medical and surgical history taking. Haemophilia. 2005;11(3):193–202.
18. Levy JH, Szlam F, Wolberg AS, Winkler A. Clinical use of the activated partial thromboplastin time and prothrombin time for screening: a review of the literature and current guidelines for testing. Clin Lab Med. 2014;34(3):453–77.
19. Medved L, Weisel JW, Fibrinogen and Factor XIII Subcommittee of Scientific Standardization Committee of International Society on Thrombosis and Haemostasis. Recommendations for nomenclature on fibrinogen and fibrin. J Thromb Haemost. 2009;7(2):355–9.
20. de Moerloose P, Neerman-Arbez M. Congenital fibrinogen disorders. Semin Thromb Hemost. 2009;35(4):356–66.

21. Franchini M, Mannucci PM. Acquired haemophilia a: a 2013 update. Thromb Haemost. 2013;110(6):1114–20.
22. Blanchette VS, Key NS, Ljung LR, Manco-Johnson MJ, van den Berg HM, Srivastava A, Subcommittee on Factor VIII, Factor IX and Rare Coagulation Disorders of the Scientific and Standardization Committee of the International Society on Thrombosis and Hemostasis. Definitions in hemophilia: communication from the SSC of the ISTH. J Thromb Haemost. 2014;12(11):1935–9.
23. Mauser Bunschoten EP, van Houwelingen JC, Sjamsoedin Visser EJ, van Dijken PJ, Kok AJ, Sixma JJ. Bleeding symptoms in carriers of hemophilia A and B. Thromb Haemost. 1988;59(3):349–52.
24. White GC 2nd, Rosendaal F, Aledort LM, Lusher JM, Rothschild C, Ingerslev J, Factor V, Factor IXS. Definitions in hemophilia. Recommendation of the scientific subcommittee on factor VIII and factor IX of the scientific and standardization committee of the international society on thrombosis and haemostasis. Thromb Haemost. 2001;85(3):560.
25. Carubbi C, Masselli E, Nouvenne A, Russo D, Galli D, Mirandola P, Gobbi G, Vitale M. Laboratory diagnostics of inherited platelet disorders. Clin Chem Lab Med. 2014;52(8):1091–106.
26. Roberts JC, Flood VH. Laboratory diagnosis of von Willebrand disease. Int J Lab Hematol. 2015;37 Suppl 1(Suppl 1):11–7.
27. Nichols WL, Hultin MB, James AH, Manco-Johnson MJ, Montgomery RR, Ortel TL, Rick ME, Sadler JE, Weinstein M, Yawn BP. von Willebrand disease (VWD): evidence-based diagnosis and management guidelines, the National Heart, Lung, and Blood Institute (NHLBI) Expert Panel Report (USA). Haemophilia. 2008;14(2):171–232.
28. Palla R, Peyvandi F, Shapiro AD. Rare bleeding disorders: diagnosis and treatment. Blood. 2015;125(13):2052–61.
29. Duncan E, Collecutt M, Street A. Nijmegen-Bethesda assay to measure factor VIII inhibitors. Methods Mol Biol. 2013;992:321–33.
30. Kempton CL, White GC 2nd. How we treat a hemophilia a patient with a factor VIII inhibitor. Blood. 2009;113(1):11–7.
31. Kundu SK, Heilmann EJ, Sio R, Garcia C, Davidson RM, Ostgaard RA. Description of an in vitro platelet function analyzer—PFA-100. Semin Thromb Hemost. 1995;21(Suppl 2):106–12.
32. Candotti F. Clinical manifestations and pathophysiological mechanisms of the Wiskott-Aldrich syndrome. J Clin Immunol. 2018;38(1):13–27.
33. Balduini CL, Pecci A, Savoia A. Recent advances in the understanding and management of MYH9-related inherited thrombocytopenias. Br J Haematol. 2011;154(2):161–74.
34. Pham A, Wang J. Bernard-Soulier syndrome: an inherited platelet disorder. Arch Pathol Lab Med. 2007;131(12):1834–6.
35. Gunay-Aygun M, Falik-Zaccai TC, Vilboux T, Zivony-Elboum Y, Gumruk F, Cetin M, Khayat M, Boerkoel CF, Kfir N, Huang Y, et al. NBEAL2 is mutated in gray platelet syndrome and is required for biogenesis of platelet alpha-granules. Nat Genet. 2011;43(8):732–4.
36. Kaplan J, De Domenico I, Ward DM. Chediak-Higashi syndrome. Curr Opin Hematol. 2008;15(1):22–9.
37. Huizing M, Helip-Wooley A, Westbroek W, Gunay-Aygun M, Gahl WA. Disorders of lysosome-related organelle biogenesis: clinical and molecular genetics. Annu Rev Genomics Hum Genet. 2008;9:359–86.
38. Minowa H, Takahashi Y, Tanaka T, Naganuma K, Ida S, Maki I, Yoshioka A. Four cases of bleeding diathesis in children due to congenital plasminogen activator inhibitor-1 deficiency. Haemostasis. 1999;29(5):286–91.
39. Colucci M, Binetti BM, Branca MG, Clerici C, Morelli A, Semeraro N, Gresele P. Deficiency of thrombin activatable fibrinolysis inhibitor in cirrhosis is associated with increased plasma fibrinolysis. Hepatology. 2003;38(1):230–7.

40. Carpenter SL, Mathew P. Alpha2-antiplasmin and its deficiency: fibrinolysis out of balance. Haemophilia. 2008;14(6):1250–4.
41. Okajima K, Kohno I, Soe G, Okabe H, Takatsuki K, Binder BR. Direct evidence for systemic fibrinogenolysis in patients with acquired alpha 2-plasmin inhibitor deficiency. Am J Hematol. 1994;45(1):16–24.
42. Agren A, Wiman B, Stiller V, Lindmarker P, Sten-Linder M, Carlsson A, Holmstrom M, Odeberg J, Schulman S. Evaluation of low PAI-1 activity as a risk factor for hemorrhagic diathesis. J Thromb Haemost. 2006;4(1):201–8.
43. Adam SS, Key NS, Greenberg CS. D-dimer antigen: current concepts and future prospects. Blood. 2009;113(13):2878–87.
44. Muto A, Yoshihashi K, Takeda M, Kitazawa T, Soeda T, Igawa T, Sampei Z, Kuramochi T, Sakamoto A, Haraya K, et al. Anti-factor IXa/X bispecific antibody ACE910 prevents joint bleeds in a long-term primate model of acquired hemophilia a. Blood. 2014;124(20):3165–71.
45. Lusher JM. Use of prothrombin complex concentrates in management of bleeding in hemophiliacs with inhibitors--benefits and limitations. Semin Hematol. 1994;31(2 Suppl 4):49–52.
46. Margraf DJ, Brown SJ, Blue HL, Bezdicek TL, Wolfson J, Chapman SA. Comparison of 3-factor versus 4-factor prothrombin complex concentrate for emergent warfarin reversal: a systematic review and meta-analysis. BMC Emerg Med. 2022;22(1):14.
47. Abdoellakhan RA, Khorsand N, Ter Avest E, Lameijer H, Faber LM, Ypma PF, Nieuwenhuizen L, Veeger N, Meijer K. Fixed versus variable dosing of prothrombin complex concentrate for bleeding complications of vitamin K antagonists-the PROPER3 randomized clinical trial. Ann Emerg Med. 2022;79(1):20–30.
48. Hilgartner MW, Knatterud GL. The use of factor eight inhibitor by-passing activity (FEIBA immuno) product for treatment of bleeding episodes in hemophiliacs with inhibitors. Blood. 1983;61(1):36–40.
49. Neufeld EJ, Negrier C, Arkhammar P, Benchikhel Fegoun S, Simonsen MD, Rosholm A, Seremetis S. Safety update on the use of recombinant activated factor VII in approved indications. Blood Rev. 2015;29(Suppl 1):S34–41.
50. Kosch A, Kehrel B, Nowak-Gottl U, Haberle J, Jurgens H. Thrombocytic alpha-delta-storage-pool-disease: shortening of bleeding time after infusion of 1-desamino-8-D-arginine vasopressin. Klin Padiatr. 1999;211(4):198–200.
51. Burroughs AK, Matthews K, Qadiri M, Thomas N, Kernoff P, Tuddenham E, McIntyre N. Desmopressin and bleeding time in patients with cirrhosis. Br Med J (Clin Res Ed). 1985;291(6506):1377–81.
52. Weigert AL, Schafer AI. Uremic bleeding: pathogenesis and therapy. Am J Med Sci. 1998;316(2):94–104.
53. Bolton-Maggs PH, Chalmers EA, Collins PW, Harrison P, Kitchen S, Liesner RJ, Minford A, Mumford AD, Parapia LA, Perry DJ, et al. A review of inherited platelet disorders with guidelines for their management on behalf of the UKHCDO. Br J Haematol. 2006;135(5):603–33.
54. Livio M, Mannucci PM, Vigano G, Mingardi G, Lombardi R, Mecca G, Remuzzi G. Conjugated estrogens for the management of bleeding associated with renal failure. N Engl J Med. 1986;315(12):731–5.
55. Galan AM, Tonda R, Pino M, Reverter JC, Ordinas A, Escolar G. Increased local procoagulant action: a mechanism contributing to the favorable hemostatic effect of recombinant FVIIa in PLT disorders. Transfusion. 2003;43(7):885–92.
56. Wilbourn B, Harrison P, Mackie IJ, Liesner R, Machin SJ. Activation of platelets in whole blood by recombinant factor VIIa by a thrombin-dependent mechanism. Br J Haematol. 2003;122(4):651–61.
57. Levy JH, Goodnough LT. How I use fibrinogen replacement therapy in acquired bleeding. Blood. 2015;125(9):1387–93.

Chapter 13
Interpretation of Blood Clotting Studies

Bittar Gianfranco and Gustavo Rivero

Case Demonstration

A 68-year-old male patient with a past medical history of RA presents to the emergency department with acute right upper quadrant abdominal pain. Physical examination revealed a positive Murphy sign. His abdominal ultrasound findings were consistent with acute calculous cholecystitis. Diffuse skin bruising and hematomas are distributed on his arms and legs. His preoperative evaluation showed a PT, INR, and PTT of 16 s, 1.2, and 78 s.

Definitions

PT or prothrombin time: Coagulation test that assesses the extrinsic and common pathway of the coagulation cascade (Fig. 13.1). It reflects functional integrity for factors I, II, V, VII, and X [1].

    aPTT or activated partial thromboplastin time: Coagulation test that assesses the intrinsic and common pathway of the coagulation cascade. It reflects functional integrity for all clotting factors except VII and XIII.

    TT or Thrombin time: Coagulation test that assesses the conversion of fibrinogen to fibrin using murine or human thrombin [2]. Prolonged times reflect impaired

B. Gianfranco (✉)
Baylor College of Medicine, Baylor St Luke's Medical Center, Houston, TX, USA
e-mail: Gianfranco.bittar@cookcountyhealth.org

G. Rivero
Lombardi Cancer Institute, Georgetown University School of Medicine,
Washington, DC, USA

173

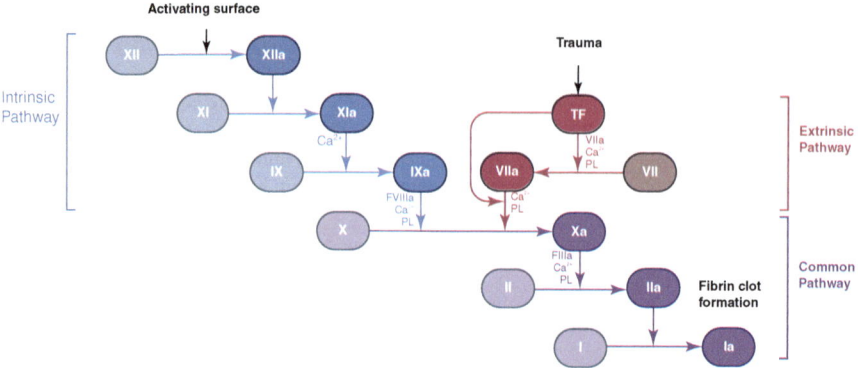

Fig. 13.1 Coagulation pathways. *FVa* activated factor V, *FVIIIa* activated factor VIII, *PL* phospholipid, *TF* tissue factor

fibrinogen conversion due to fibrinogen disorders or inhibition of thrombin activity by heparin or direct thrombin inhibitors.

RT or Reptilase time: Coagulation test that assesses the fibrinogen conversion to fibrin using molecular mimicry of batroxobin (a component of Bothrops snake's venom) with thrombin. It directly activates fibrinogen conversion to fibrin and is resistant to heparin activity and direct thrombin inhibitors such as dabigatran, argatroban, and bivalirudin. It is usually used to distinguish TT prolongation due to fibrinogen abnormalities or specific anticoagulants [3].

Mixing study: The objective of this test is to distinguish the presence of a coagulation inhibitor versus coagulation factor deficiencies as the cause of PT/PTT prolongation. It compares the correction of coagulation times (i.e., PTT) by mixing the patient sample with normal pooled plasma in a 1:1 ratio [4]. This provides 50% of multiple coagulation factors activity, enough to restore the result to normal in patients with coagulation factor deficits. It reports immediate correction and correction after an incubating period [5]. Mixing studies may be performed to assess any coagulation time (PT, PTT, TT, among others).

*Coagulation factor inhibitors***:** These are antibodies directed against coagulation proteins and inhibit their action. Such inhibitors are capable of overcoming intrinsic hemostasis leading to life-threatening infusion-refractory bleeding [6].

Clinical Context

This patient presents with moderate symptomatic elevated PT and aPTT. Initial investigation should include a complete medical and family history. Additionally, we should review medications and perform physical examination to investigate bleeding and thrombosis and to evaluate potential severe infections. Patients should be evaluated for signs of disseminated intravascular coagulation (DIC), severe hepatic failure, and vitamin K deficiency (i.e., prolonged antibiotic use or warfarin use) as potential causes of prolonged PT and PTT. However, most of these scenarios are unlikely in an, otherwise, asymptomatic patient. Potential medications include direct oral anticoagulants (DOACs), vitamin K antagonist (usually after the first week of therapy), and unfractionated heparin. Unfractionated heparin and DOACs (especially argatroban and dabigatran) are usually associated with isolated aPTT elevation, but higher doses may yield PT elevation as well [5]. This patient, however, does not use any anticoagulants.

After considering the above scenarios, elevated coagulation times should be evaluated with mixing studies and thrombin time (TT). TT will evaluate fibrinogen disorders, and its alteration should yield prompt evaluation of fibrinogen antigen levels and fibrinogen activity to distinguish congenital afibrinogenemia, hypofibrinogenemia, hypodysfibrinogenemia, or dysfibrinogenemia, among others.

Complete Correction in a Mixing Study

Correction in mixing studies supports coagulation factor deficiencies. The mixture with normal pooled plasma provides the missing coagulation factors needed to overcome abnormalities. Inherited causes such as hemophilia A or B are unlikely in elderly patients without a history of bleeding. Moderate to severe cases (factor activity levels below 5%) manifest with significant episodes of bleeding in the first 2 years of life in approximately 81% of the patients [7]. Mild hemophilia cases retain a broad spectrum of expression; however, the mean age of diagnosis is 29–36 months [8, 9]. Multiple factor deficiencies are rarer inherited diseases usually involve mutations in transporters or carriers that stabilize multiple factors (LMAN1 and MCFD2 genes) or enzymes responsible for the synthesis of vitamin K-dependent coagulation factors (VKORC1 and GGCX) [10, 11]. Acquired causes of prolonged coagulation times with corrected mixing studies often involve antagonism of vitamin K such as warfarin and rodenticide poisoning.

Further workup should assess coagulation factor activity using one-stage clot-based, chromogenic, or antigenic assays. Clot-based assays evaluate coagulation and correct for activity using specific factor-deficient plasma and are the most commonly used to report coagulation factor activity. Chromogenic assays (usually for factors X and VIII) are reserved for patients with possible interferences with regular coagulation time assessment. Antigenic assays using enzyme-linked immunoassays are preferred to distinguish between functional and absolute deficiencies. Factors to be tested depend on the suspected pathway and frequency of occurrence.

Uncorrected Results

Uncorrected mixing studies suggest interference with the coagulation cascade by anticoagulants (heparin, direct thrombin inhibitors, and DOACs) or antibodies such as lupus anticoagulant or coagulation factor neutralizing antibodies [5, 6]. The addition of phospholipids to an uncorrected mixing study with subsequent correction confirms the presence of lupus anticoagulant based on the three-step procedure (screening with aPTT, mixing study, and phospholipid dependency). This finding should prompt testing for other antiphospholipid antibodies (anticardiolipin and anti-beta-2-glycoprotein I; IgG and IgM) using ELISA.

Investigating anticoagulants use and further testing using thrombin time and reptilase time may help discern remaining etiologies. Prolonged TT with normal RT is characteristic of heparin use, direct thrombin inhibitors use, or heparin contamination [12]. Normal TT and RT suggest upstream inhibition with either direct factor Xa anticoagulants (rivaroxaban, apixaban) or coagulation factor neutralizing antibodies [13].

Factor VIII neutralizing antibodies are the landmark of acquired hemophilia A and are the most common coagulation inhibitors. These may develop in response to recurrent factor infusions in susceptible patients (high-risk HLA alleles DRB1*15 and DQB1*0602) with hemophilia A and due to autoimmunity such as in patients with rheumatologic diseases (i.e., rheumatoid arthritis and lupus exhibiting high-risk HLA alleles DRB1*16 and DQB1*0502). The latter is termed acquired hemophilia A, and could represent a life-threatening emergency. Acquired hemophilia can be observed in women in the postpartum period [14, 15]. They present a characteristic time-dependent pattern in mixing studies with immediate transient correction of aPTT reversing after incubation for 1–2 h with normal pooled plasma [4]. The absence of this pattern does not exclude factor VIII inhibitors but prompts evaluation for factor VII, IX, and XI neutralizing antibodies. Factors to be tested depend on the suspected pathway and, thus, factors affected (Fig. 13.2).

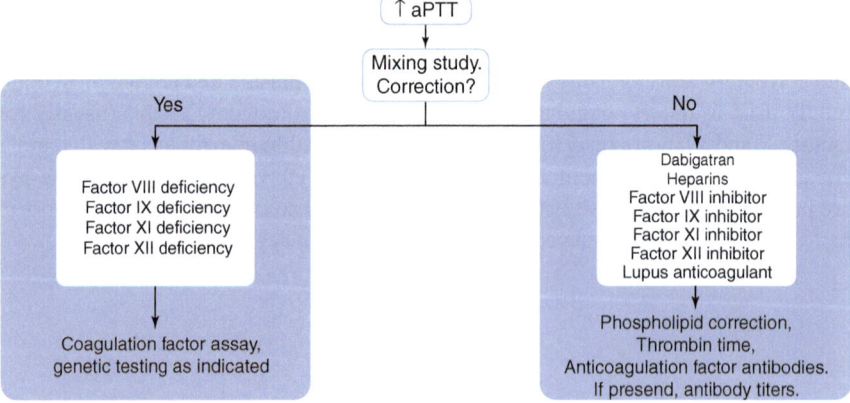

Fig. 13.2 Possible etiologies for an uncorrected mixing study. *DOACs* direct oral anticoagulants, *PT* prothrombin time, *aPTT* activated partial thromboplastin time, *WRR* within reference range [5]

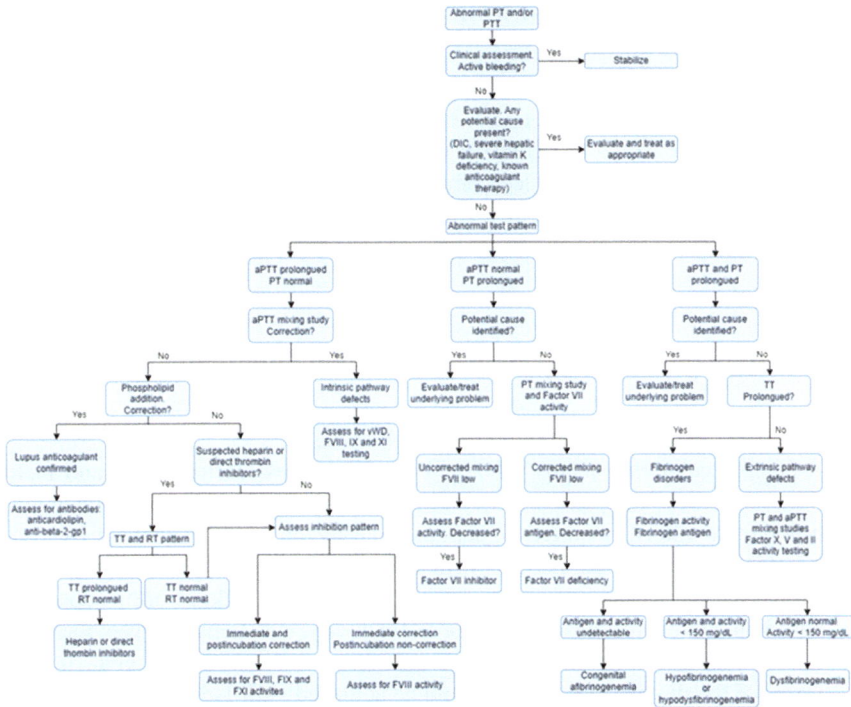

Fig. 13.3 Algorithm for evaluation of abnormal coagulation test and interpretation of mixing studies. *DIC*: disseminated intravascular coagulation; *FII*: factor II; *FV*: factor V; *FVII*: factor VII; *FVIII*: factor VIII; *FIX*: factor IX; *FX*: factor X; *FXI*: factor XI; *PT*: prothrombin time; *aPTT*: activated partial thromboplastin time; *RT*: reptilase time; *TT*: thrombin time; *vWD*: von Willebrand disease [5, 18, 19]

Factor VIII inhibitor is confirmed with the Nijmegen-Bethesda assay or ELISA for anti-factor VIII antibodies. The former test, which consists of serial dilutions, reports Bethesda units as surrogates of antibody titers [16].

Clinically, coagulation factor inhibitors present with mucosal, GI bleeding, GU bleeding, epistaxis, retroperitoneal, and muscular hematomas. Hemarthrosis is uncommon in patients with the acquired disease [17] (Fig. 13.3).

Special Considerations

It is essential to understand that specific conditions may increase false positive and negative results. Mixing studies performed over slightly elevated abnormal coagulation tests (PT greater than 2 s, PTT greater than 5 s) are very likely to correct after the mixture, whereas multiple coagulation factor deficiencies are more prone to remain uncorrected compared to pure factor deficiencies [5].

Case Demonstration, Continued

An aPTT-based mixing study reveals immediate correction that reverses after 2-h incubation, yielding an aPTT of 68 s. Phospholipid addition to the sample does not elicit correction. Factor VIII activity is estimated at 4.7% by clot-based assays. The patient's abdominal pain subsided completely. Nurses report mild oozing bleeding and a 6-cm ecchymosis around the venipuncture site. Patient has suspected diagnosis of acquired hemophilia.

Achieving Hemostasis in Active, Clinically Significant Bleeding

First-line treatment options include the following:
- *Recombinant porcine factor VIII (rpFVIII)*: Low cross-reactivity with anti-factor VIII antibodies. The presence of cross-reacting antibodies and anti-porcine inhibition titers <20 BU required higher doses during the first 24 h with similar clinical efficiency afterward. Patients with anti-rpFVIII titers >20 BU were excluded from the trial. The recommended initial dose is 200 U/kg. Further doses are based on clinical response and factor VIII activity, with activity levels >80% for concerning bleedings and >50% for all others as the treatment goal. In mild forms of the disease, hemostasis could be achieved with 1-deamino-8D-arginine vasopressin (DDAVP). This agent has the ability to increase factor VIII. Doses of 0.3 mg/kg subcutaneously daily for 3 to 5 days could be used in patients without extremely low inhibitor titers (<3 BU) given proven inefficacy to control bleeding [20].
- *Recombinant activated factor VII (rFVIIa)*: Cardiovascular events and thromboembolic phenomena have been reported in up to 5% of patients and 2.9% on average. Administer bolus injections of 90 μg/kg every 2–3 h until hemostasis is achieved. Responses are observed in more than 90% of patients [21].
- *Activated prothrombin concentrate*: Thrombotic events were reported in 4.8% of the patients. Disseminated intravascular coagulation is a potential adverse event seen in supramaximal therapeutic doses. Administer bolus injections of 50–100 U/kg every 8–12 h. Maximum dose: 200 U/kg/day. Responses are observed in more than 80% of patients [22].

No agent has demonstrated superiority over the other. The final decision should rely on their availability, costs, and anti-porcine inhibition titers (required before rpFVIII is considered). In case of first-line treatment failure, switching to alternative first-line option should be considered [23].

Inhibitor Eradication

Immunosuppressive therapy is indicated to achieve elimination of the inhibitor in all patients with acquired hemophilia A. However, patients with WHO performance status >2 require caution since the intervention is associated with four times higher mortality risk. Factor VIII activity <1% was linked with decreased likelihood to achieve partial remission and longer therapy duration. Anti-factor VIII IgA titers >1:80 have correlated with increased relapse [20]. Commonly used agents include the following:

- Prednisone or prednisolone: 1 mg/kg/day PO. Max: 4–6 weeks + tapper.
- Rituximab: 375 mg/m^2/week. Max: 4 cycles.
- Cyclophosphamide: 1.5–2 mg/kg/day PO. Max: 6 weeks.
- Mycophenolate mofetil: 1 g/day for 1 week, followed by 2 g/day.

First-line immunosuppressive regimen depends on factor VIII activity and inhibitor titers. Patients with factor VIII ≥1 IU/dL and inhibitor titers ≤20 BU should be started on corticosteroid therapy for 3–4 weeks. Patients who do not meet these conditions should receive corticosteroids + rituximab or corticosteroid + cytotoxic agents [23].

Second-line therapies include the addition of rituximab or a cytotoxic agent to corticosteroids, whichever was not used as first-line.

Monitoring

In patients not achieving partial remission after 3–4 weeks of corticosteroid treatment but showing continuous improvement, observation is appropriate. Follow-up after complete remission using factor VIII activity is indicated monthly for the first 6 months, every 2–3 months up to 12 months, and every 6 months after [23].

References

1. Onundarson PT, Palsson R, Witt DM, Gudmundsdottir BR. Replacement of traditional prothrombin time monitoring with the new Fiix prothrombin time increases the efficacy of warfarin without increasing bleeding. A review article. Thromb J. 2021;19(1):72.
2. Ignjatovic V. Thrombin clotting time. In: Monagle P, editor. Haemostasis [Internet]. Methods in molecular biology, vol. 992. Totowa, NJ: Humana Press; 2013. p. 131–8. https://doi.org/10.1007/978-1-62703-339-8_10.
3. Karapetian H. Reptilase time (RT). In: Monagle P, editor. Haemostasis [Internet]. Methods in molecular biology, vol. 992. Totowa, NJ: Humana Press; 2013. p. 273–7. https://doi.org/10.1007/978-1-62703-339-8_20.
4. Choi S-H, Rambally S, Shen Y-M. Mixing study for evaluation of abnormal coagulation testing. JAMA. 2016;316(20):2146.

5. Favaloro EJ. Coagulation mixing studies: utility, algorithmic strategies and limitations for lupus anticoagulant testing or follow up of abnormal coagulation tests. Am J Hematol. 2020;95(1):117–28.
6. Hofbauer CJ, Whelan SFJ, Hirschler M, Allacher P, Horling FM, Lawo J-P, et al. Affinity of FVIII-specific antibodies reveals major differences between neutralizing and nonneutralizing antibodies in humans. Blood. 2015;125(7):1180–8.
7. Kulkarni R, Presley RJ, Lusher JM, Shapiro AD, Gill JC, Manco-Johnson M, et al. Complications of haemophilia in babies (first two years of life): a report from the Centers for Disease Control and Prevention Universal Data Collection System. Haemophilia. 2017;23(2):207–14.
8. Benson G, Auerswald G, Dolan G, Duffy A, Hermans C, Ljung R, et al. Diagnosis and care of patients with mild haemophilia: practical recommendations for clinical management. Blood Transfus Trasfus Sangue. 2018;16(6):535–44.
9. CDC. Data & Statistics | Hemophilia | NCBDDD | CDC [Internet]. Centers for Disease Control and Prevention; 2020. https://www.cdc.gov/ncbddd/hemophilia/data.html. Accessed 2 Jan 2022.
10. Hao Z, Jin D-Y, Chen X, Schurgers LJ, Stafford DW, Tie J-K. γ-Glutamyl carboxylase mutations differentially affect the biological function of vitamin K–dependent proteins. Blood. 2021;137(4):533–43.
11. Zheng C, Liu H, Yuan S, Zhou J, Zhang B. Molecular basis of LMAN1 in coordinating LMAN1-MCFD2 cargo receptor formation and ER-to-Golgi transport of FV/FVIII. Blood. 2010;116(25):5698–706.
12. Adcock DM, Gosselin R. Direct oral anticoagulants (DOACs) in the laboratory: 2015 review. Thromb Res. 2015;136(1):7–12.
13. Božič MM. Advances in monitoring anticoagulant therapy. In: Advances in clinical chemistry [Internet]. Amsterdam: Elsevier; 2019. p. 197–213. https://linkinghub.elsevier.com/retrieve/pii/S0065242319300058. Accessed 2 Jan 2022.
14. Pavlova A, Zeitler H, Scharrer I, Brackmann H-H, Oldenburg J. HLA genotype in patients with acquired haemophilia A. Haemophilia. 2010;16(102):107–12.
15. McGill JR, Simhadri VL, Sauna ZE. HLA variants and inhibitor development in hemophilia a: a retrospective case-controlled study using the ATHNdataset. Front Med. 2021;8:663396.
16. Duncan E, Collecutt M, Street A. Nijmegen-Bethesda assay to measure factor VIII inhibitors. In: Monagle P, editor. Haemostasis [Internet]. Methods in molecular biology, vol. 992. Totowa, NJ: Humana Press; 2013. p. 321–33. https://doi.org/10.1007/978-1-62703-339-8_24.
17. Kessler CM, Knöbl P. Acquired haemophilia: an overview for clinical practice. Eur J Haematol. 2015;95:36–44.
18. Fibrinogen disorders algorithm—UpToDate [Internet]. 2022. https://www.uptodate.com/contents/image?imageKey=HEME%2F114258&topicKey=HEME%2F1321&search=mixing%20study&source=outline_link. Accessed 3 Jan 2022.
19. Abnormal PT/aPTT evaluation—UpToDate [Internet]. 2022. https://www.uptodate.com/contents/image?imageKey=HEME%2F103926&topicKey=HEME%2F1368&search=mixing%20study&source=outline_link&selectedTitle=1~29. Accessed 3 Jan 2022.
20. Pai M. Acquired hemophilia A. Hematol Oncol Clin North Am. 2021;35:1131–42.
21. Hay CR, Negrier C, Ludlam CA. The treatment of bleeding in acquired haemophilia with recombinant factor VIIa: a multicentre study. Thromb Haemost. 1997;78(6):1463–7.
22. Sallah S. Treatment of acquired haemophilia with factor eight inhibitor bypassing activity. Haemophilia. 2004;10(2):169–73.
23. Tiede A, Collins P, Knoebl P, Teitel J, Kessler C, Shima M, et al. International recommendations on the diagnosis and treatment of acquired hemophilia A. Haematologica. 2020;105(7):1791–801.

Chapter 14
Venous Thromboembolism

Diana De Oliveira and Gustavo Rivero

Case Demonstration 1

A 32-year-old woman presented to the emergency room with a 4-day history of sudden-onset asymmetric lower right leg pain. Her medications included combined oral contraceptives (OCPs). At examination, her vital signs were normal. The right leg was erythematous, painful, and swollen with a right thigh measurement of 5 cm greater than the left. Doppler ultrasound (US) documented right femoral deep venous thrombosis (DVT).

Definitions

(a) *Venous thromboembolism (VTE)*: Includes deep vein thrombosis (DVT) and pulmonary embolism (PE).
(b) *DVT*: Development of blood clot within a deep vein of the vascular system.

D. De Oliveira (✉)
Baylor College of Medicine, Baylor St Luke's Medical Center, Houston, TX, USA
e-mail: Diana.deoliveiragomes@utsouthwestern.edu

G. Rivero
Lombardi Cancer Institute, Georgetown University School of Medicine, Washington, DC, USA

© The Author(s), under exclusive license to Springer Nature Switzerland AG 2024
G. Rivero, I. R. Sosa (eds.), *Consulting Hematology and Oncology Handbook*, https://doi.org/10.1007/978-3-031-75810-2_14

Clinical Context

~50% of VTE events are associated with a transient risk factor, such as recent surgery, bed rest >3 days, pregnancy, postpartum, trauma, immobility at work, and hormone therapy, among others [1]. These events are frequently described as provoked. Additionally, ~20% of cases are associated with cancer. The incidence of VTE increases with age [2]. In this case, the patient has an increased risk for DVT due to OCPs use. Women who take OCPs have higher risk of VTE, especially those estrogen-containing formulations [3]. Family and personal history of previous DVT was addressed, but both were negative.

Clinical Manifestations

DVT usually presents as leg swelling, pain, erythema, and localized tenderness along the distribution of the deep venous system.

Laboratory and Radiologic Investigation

(a) Complete blood count and differential.
(b) Coagulation profile including PT, PTT, D-dimerc. Doppler ultrasound.

Management of Provoked DVT

Uncomplicated provoked DVT and low-risk PE can be treated as outpatient. Anticoagulation to prevent extension and recurrence are important for management. Prompt anticoagulation initiation even while waiting for confirmatory investigation is important given the high risk of early mortality if untreated. Direct oral anticoagulants (DOACs), which include the direct Xa inhibitors (apixaban, edoxaban, rivaroxaban) and a direct thrombin inhibitor (dabigatran), are preferred over vitamin K antagonists (VKAs). Anticoagulation therapy is achieved in three stages: (1) initial therapy during acute event, (2) primary treatment with a minimal duration of 3 to 6 months, and (3) secondary prevention, which is usually continued indefinitely in patients with chronic risk factors [4]. Our patient was prescribed with rivaroxaban for 6 months. Recommended doses of anticoagulation are shown in Table 14.1.

Table 14.1 Anticoagulants for venous thromboembolism (VTE) [5, 6]

Anticoagulants	Mechanism of action	Usual treatment dose
Unfractionated heparin	Inactivates thrombin and factor Xa through an antithrombin-dependent mechanism	80 IU/kg intravenous bolus, then 18 IU/kg/h IV infusion, target a PTT or antiXa (hospital-specific)
Enoxaparin	Inhibiting factor Xa and factor IIa (thrombin)	1.0 mg/kg subcutaneous twice daily vs. 1.5 mg/kg subcutaneous daily
Apixaban	Selectively inhibits factor Xa	10 mg oral twice daily for 7 days, then 5 mg twice daily
Rivaroxaban	Selectively inhibits factor Xa	15 mg oral twice daily for 21 days, then 20 mg daily
Edoxaban	Inhibits free factor Xa, and prothrombinase activity	60 mg once daily. Decrease to 30 mg once daily for patients with CrCl[a] of 15–50 mL/min, body weight of <60 kg
Dabigatran	Reversible competitive thrombin inhibitor	150 mg oral twice daily. Decrease to 110 mg twice daily if age > 75 years or CrCl 30–49 mL/min
Warfarin	Competitively inhibits the vitamin K epoxide reductase complex 1	Initial dose: 2 to 5 mg orally once a day Maintenance dose: 2 to 10 mg orally once a day Target INR: 2.5 (range: 2 to 3)

[a]*CrCl* creatinine clearance

Caveats

(a) In patients with extensive DVT in whom thrombolysis is considered appropriate, catheter-directed thrombolysis is preferred over systemic thrombolysis.

(b) In patients who have contraindications for anticoagulation (i.e., acute major uncontrollable bleeding), or with repeated episodes of DVT regardless of therapy, and imminent risk of pulmonary embolism, an Inferior Vena Cava Filter (IVC) could be considered [5].

(c) Patients with previous major bleeding (i.e., gastrointestinal or others), who needed blood transfusion or have developed thrombocytopenia, may benefit of antiXa low molecular weight heparin monitoring during lovenox therapy.

(d) For obese patients, especially those with BMI >40 kg/m^2 or >120 kg, the International Society on Thrombosis and Hemostasis (ISTH) is suggested against using DOACs.

(e) The use of low molecular weight heparin in obese patients should be carefully monitored with anti-factor Xa levels if dosing is based on actual body weight.

Case Demonstration 2

A 23-year-old female with previous history of DVT presents with new onset of left lower extremity swelling and pain distributed in her left leg. Her Doppler ultrasound demonstrated acute thrombosis extending from distal left femoral to proximal popliteal vein. Family history was significant for her mother developing first DVT episode at 49 years of age. During her admission, genetic testing demonstrated homozygous factor V gene R506Q mutation. Prior to discharge, rivaroxaban 20 mg orally daily was prescribed for lifelong.

Definitions [7]

Early age thrombosis: Thrombotic events in people younger than 50 years old.

Clinical Context

There are several factors that suggest the presence of hyperthrombotic state including (1) early age at TVE onset, (2) recurrent episodes, and (3) thrombosis in unusual sites (i.e., upper extremities, splanchnic vessels) [7]. Patients developing unprovoked VTE have underlying genetic predisposition in up to 50% of cases. In our case, the patient was diagnosed with factor V Leiden (FVL), which is an autosomal dominant mutation that induces a factor V partially resistant to inactivation by activated protein C (APC) [8]. A diagnostic approach for patients with young patients diagnosed with DVT is depicted in Fig. 14.1.

Laboratory Investigation

In addition to CBC and coagulation studies, thrombophilia screening includes investigation of (1) antithrombin III function, (2) protein C and S deficiency, (3) PCR for factor V Leiden mutation and prothrombin G2021A mutation, and (4) testing for antiphospholipid antibodies and homocysteine level. Table 14.2 summarizes few clinical contexts, in which prothrombotic laboratory testing investigation should be performed.

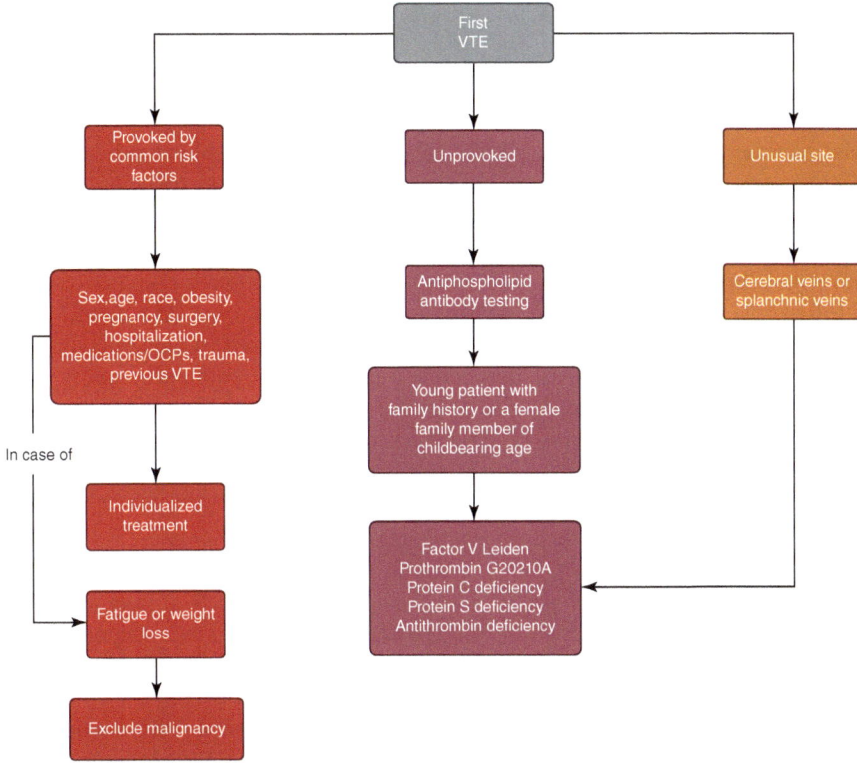

Fig. 14.1 First VTE diagnosis approach. (Adapted from [9])

Table 14.2 Venous thrombophilia screening [10]	
	(a) Age < 50 years
	(b) Young women with previous VTE history before prescribing hormonal replacement
	(c) Women with multiple inexplicable pregnancy losses
	(d) Young women with a positive family history, before prescribing OCPs
	(e) First VTE and a positive family history for VTE
	(f) VTE in unusual sites (cerebral veins or splanchnic veins)
	(g) Young patients with arterial ischemia and right-to-left shunt (paradoxical embolism)

Case Demonstration 2 (Continued)

5 years after diagnosis, the patient returned to the emergency room presenting dyspnea and chest pain. She reported poor adherence to rivaroxaban. At examination, she had tachycardia (120 bpm) and tachypnea (28 bpm); blood pressure was 142/85 mmHg. Her oxygen saturation was 85% on room air. Cardiac auscultation revealed a grade 1/6 holosystolic murmur that increased to grade 2/6 with inspiration at the left lower sternal border. ECG showed sinus tachycardia and T-wave inversions in the anterior leads. Laboratory evaluation showed a D-dimer level of 1380 ng/mL (normal level < 500 ng/mL) and troponin T level of 0.15 ng/mL (normal range, 0–0.1 ng/mL). Contrast-enhanced chest computed tomography demonstrated the presence of a thrombus obliterating the right pulmonary artery. The echocardiogram demonstrated mild tricuspid regurgitation, elevated pulmonary artery systolic pressure (42 mm Hg), right ventricular (RV) enlargement (RV-to-left ventricular [LV] dimension ratio = 1.2), and moderate hypokinesis.

Definitions

(a) *Standard-Risk PE*: Patients with PE who are hemodynamically stable and without evidence of right ventricular dysfunction.
(b) *Intermediate-Risk or Submassive PE*: PE with right ventricular dysfunction evidenced by echocardiography and/or laboratory biomarkers (troponins and brain natriuretic peptide), but without hemodynamic compromise. These patients have worse outcomes than those with those with standard-risk PE [11].
(c) *High-Risk or Massive PE*: For patients with PE and hemodynamic instability, the mortality risk is around 50%.

Clinical Manifestations

PE can remain asymptomatic but most frequently leads to dyspnea, chest pain, hemoptysis, syncope, and palpitations. The clinical signs are tachycardia, tachypnea, elevated jugular pressure, and in severe cases cyanosis and hypotension [12] (Fig. 14.2).

Diagnosis

An algorithm for diagnosis and treatment is proposed below.

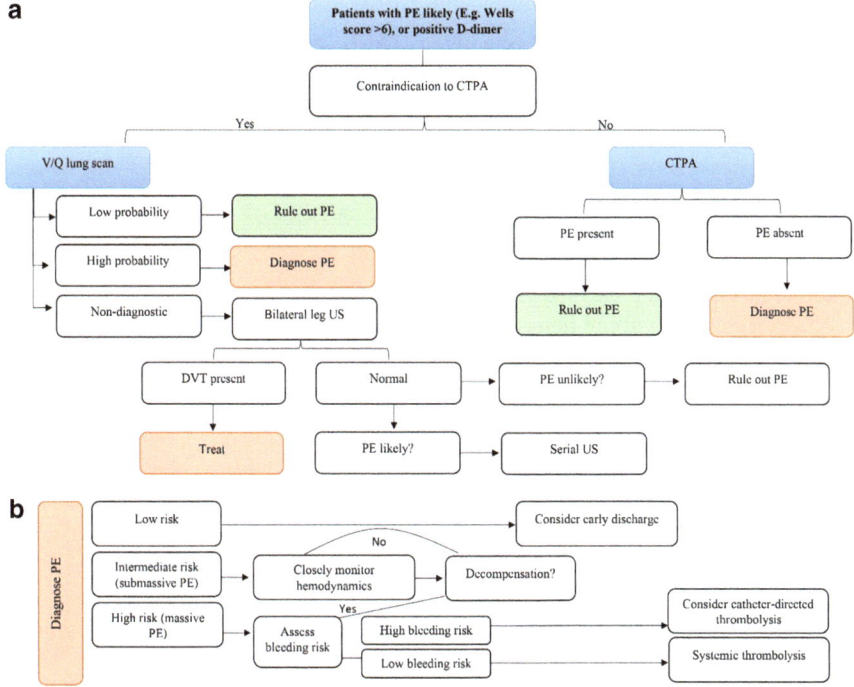

Fig. 14.2 Diagnosis and treatment of PE. (Adapted from [2, 13])

Laboratory Investigation

(a) Electrocardiogram.
(b) Chest computed tomography.
(c) Computed tomography pulmonary angiography (CTPA).
(d) Echocardiography.
(e) Planar ventilation-perfusion lung scan.

Management of PE [4]

In general, treatment approach for acute PE should always consists of three major components:

• Cardiopulmonary support.
• Anticoagulation therapy.
• Reperfusion of the pulmonary artery. Only used in patients with hemodynamic instability. Reperfusion therapies include systemic thrombolysis, catheter-directed thrombolysis, mechanical catheter-based techniques, and surgical embolectomy. Systemic thrombolysis is preferred over catheter-directed throm-

bolysis. Due to the high risk of bleeding associated with this therapy, many relative and absolute contraindications exist, such as blood pressure of ≥180/110 mmHg; recent bleeding, surgery, or invasive procedure; pregnancy; and 75 years old patients, among others [7]. In hemodynamically stable patients, bleeding risk outweighs the benefits.

Submassive PE

Our patient in case 2 presented to the ED with a submassive PE, due to the evidence of RV dysfunction without hemodynamic instability.

(a) In submassive PE, American Society of Hematology (ASH) suggests anticoagulation alone over the routine use of thrombolysis. In younger patients without bleeding risk, or in patients with a cardiopulmonary disease that impose high risk of decompensation, thrombolytic therapy can be considered.
(b) Systemic thrombolysis over catheter-directed thrombolysis is recommended.
(c) ASH *suggests* using DOACs over VKAs (may not include patients with creatinine clearance <30 mL/min, moderate to severe liver disease, or antiphospholipid syndrome).
(d) Patients should be closely monitored for the development of hemodynamic compromise.
(e) Anticoagulation for primary treatment should be extended for 3–6 months. After that, indefinite antithrombotic therapy is recommended:

- In patients on VKAs, maintain a INR between 2.0 and 3.0.
- In patients on DOAC, use a standard dose over a low dose.

During pregnancy, unfractionated heparin and LMWH are the safest options. DOACs and fondaparinux should be avoided because they cross the placenta.

Useful Tools

The Pulmonary Embolism Severity Index (PESI) and simplified PESI are clinical prediction scores widely validated that can be used to predict patient outcomes. Anticoagulation is the cornerstone of therapy in all VTE (Table 14.3).

The PESI and simplified PESI was created to predict the 30-day mortality risk in patients after acute PE diagnosis. It has been shown that patients who are stratified into the higher classes, the mortality rate increases compared to the lower ones. Aujesky et al. [16] demonstrated that 30-day mortality is estimated at 1.1% for those classified into class I, but 24.5% for those in class V. However, in a recent study, with 414 patients, the mortality rates were 13.3% at 30 days, 21.8% at 90 days, 32.6% at 1 year, and 51.0% at 5 years, demonstrating that the long-term mortality in high-risk patients significantly increased up to 5 years of follow-up according to these clinical prediction scores [17].

Table 14.3 The Pulmonary Embolism Severity Index (PESI) and simplified PESI [14, 15]

PESI[a]	
Predictors	Points assigned
Demographic characteristics	
Age > 80 years	Age in years
Male sex	+10
Comorbid conditions	
Cancer	+30
Heart failure	+10
Chronic lung disease	+10
Clinical findings	
Pulse ≥110 beats/min	+20
Systolic blood pressure <100 mmHg	+30
Respiratory rate ≥30 breaths/min	+20
Temperature <36 °C	+20
Altered mental status[b]	+60
Arterial oxygen saturation <90%	+20

[a]≤65 Points = I class; 66–85 = II class; 86–105 = III class; 106–125 = IV class; >125 = V class. Low risk (I–II class), High risk (III–V class)
[b]Defined as disorientation, lethargy, stupor or coma

References

1. Giordano NJ, Jansson PS, Young MN, Hagan KA, Kabrhel C. Epidemiology, pathophysiology, stratification, and natural history of pulmonary embolism. Tech Vasc Interv Radiol. 2017;20(3):135–40.
2. Duffett L, Castellucci LA, Forgie MA. Pulmonary embolism: update on management and controversies. BMJ. 2020;370:m2177.
3. Gialeraki A, Valsami S, Pittaras T, Panayiotakopoulos G, Politou M. Oral contraceptives and HRT risk of thrombosis. Clin Appl Thromb Hemost. 2018;24(2):217–25.
4. Ortel TL, Neumann I, Ageno W, Beyth R, Clark NP, Cuker A, et al. American Society of Hematology 2020 guidelines for management of venous thromboembolism: treatment of deep vein thrombosis and pulmonary embolism. Blood Adv. 2020;4(19):4693–738.
5. Kruger PC, Eikelboom JW, Douketis JD, Hankey GJ. Deep vein thrombosis: update on diagnosis and management. Med J Aust. 2019;210(11):516–24.
6. Shirley M, Dhillon S. Edoxaban: a review in deep vein thrombosis and pulmonary embolism. Drugs. 2015;75(17):2025–34.
7. Senst BTP, Goyal A, et al. Hypercoagulability. In: StatPearls [Internet]. Treasure Island, FL: StatPearls; 2021. https://www.ncbi.nlm.nih.gov/books/NBK538251/.
8. Linnemann B, Hart C. Laboratory diagnostics in thrombophilia. Hamostaseologie. 2019;39(1):49–61.
9. Connors JM. Thrombophilia testing and venous thrombosis. N Engl J Med. 2017;377(12):1177–87.
10. Colucci G, Tsakiris DA. Thrombophilia screening: universal, selected, or neither? Clin Appl Thromb Hemost. 2017;23(8):893–9.
11. Nguyen PC, Stevens H, Peter K, McFadyen JD. Submassive pulmonary embolism: current perspectives and future directions. J Clin Med. 2021;10(15):3383.

12. Huisman MV, Barco S, Cannegieter SC, Le Gal G, Konstantinides SV, Reitsma PH, et al. Pulmonary embolism. Nat Rev Dis Primers. 2018;4:18028.
13. Eberle H, Lyn R, Knight T, Hodge E, Daley M. Clinical update on thrombolytic use in pulmonary embolism: a focus on intermediate-risk patients. Am J Health Syst Pharm. 2018;75(17):1275–85.
14. Chan CM, Woods C, Shorr AF. The validation and reproducibility of the pulmonary embolism severity index. J Thromb Haemost. 2010;8(7):1509–14.
15. Jiménez D, Aujesky D, Moores L, Gómez V, Lobo JL, Uresandi F, et al. Simplification of the pulmonary embolism severity index for prognostication in patients with acute symptomatic pulmonary embolism. Arch Intern Med. 2010;170(15):1383–9.
16. Aujesky D, Obrosky DS, Stone RA, Auble TE, Perrier A, Cornuz J, et al. Derivation and validation of a prognostic model for pulmonary embolism. Am J Respir Crit Care Med. 2005;172(8):1041–6.
17. Sandal A, Korkmaz ET, Aksu F, Köksal D, Toros Selçuk Z, Demir AU, et al. Performance of pulmonary embolism severity index in predicting long-term mortality after acute pulmonary embolism. Anatol J Cardiol. 2021;25(8):544–54.

Chapter 15
Consultation for Thrombocytopenia

Erika Correa and Iberia Romina Sosa

Thrombotic Thrombocytopenic Purpura (TTP)

Case Presentation

A 48-year-old female presented to the emergency room with new confusion, left upper extremity LUE, weakness, and menorrhagia. She had no significant past medical history and did not take any medications. She was a non-smoker and only reported occasional alcohol use. On exam, she was noted to be anxious, with stable vital signs and poor coordination and numbness exhibited in her LUE. EKG and CXR were normal. Labs were consistent with a hemoglobin of 8.6 g/dL and platelet count of 12,000/mL. Hemolysis labs showed reticulocyte of 7%, elevated LDH, and undetectable haptoglobin. Smear evaluation was consistent with >6 schistocytes/high power field.

Definition

Falling under a group of disorders known as thrombotic microangiopathies (TMA), TTP is characterized by microangiopathic hemolytic anemia, thrombocytopenia, and microthrombi that can potentially cause organ injury, leading to a potentially fatal syndrome [1]. It is important to note that not all TMAs will present with

E. Correa (✉)
Fox Chase Cancer Center, Philadelphia, PA, USA

Department of Hematology, Univerity of Miami, Miami, FL, USA

I. R. Sosa
Department of Hematology/Oncology, Fox Chase Cancer Center, Philadelphia, PA, USA
e-mail: iberia.sosa@fccc.edu

© The Author(s), under exclusive license to Springer Nature Switzerland AG 2024
G. Rivero, I. R. Sosa (eds.), *Consulting Hematology and Oncology Handbook*,
https://doi.org/10.1007/978-3-031-75810-2_15

microangiopathic hemolytic anemia (MAHA) and that not all MAHA is caused by a TMA.

TTP is caused by ADAMTS13 deficiency (<10%), in which the acquired form is due to an autoantibody against ADAMTS13 [2]. The inherited form is due to a genetic deficiency of ADAMTS13, known as Upshaw-Shulman syndrome [2]. A normal enzyme in plasma, ADAMTS13 is a protease that cleaves the ultra large multimeric form of von Willebrand factor (ULVWF). Without this enzyme, ULVWF remains uncleaved allowing for tight platelet binding, subsequently causing platelet thrombi in the microvasculature.

Clinical Context

Individuals with TTP usually come to clinical attention due to blood count abnormalities, namely thrombocytopenia and anemia without a clear explanation. The initial evaluation focuses on establishing MAHA and thrombocytopenia and excluding systemic disorders as the cause of these findings. It is important to recognize that MAHA and thrombocytopenia may be caused my multiple clinical entities that are not TTP (Table 15.1).

Pregnancy complications such as preeclampsia with severe features and the HELLP syndrome (hemolysis, elevated liver enzymes, low platelets) are characterized by MAHA and thrombocytopenia and should be considered in the obstetric patient.

A hypertensive crisis, with systolic blood pressure >220 mmHg or diastolic blood pressure >100 mmHg, can cause MAHA and thrombocytopenia, along with kidney injury. If possible, it is important to characterize the temporal relationship between hypertension and hematologic abnormalities.

Systemic infections such as human immunodeficiency virus (HIV), cytomegalovirus (CMV), Rocky Mountain spotted fever (RMSF), red blood cell parasites (e.g., malaria, babesia), and bacterial endocarditis may also mimic TTP. Systemic malignancies may elicit MAHA and thrombocytopenia by microvascular metastases that is not disseminated intravascular coagulation (DIC). Rheumatologic disorders such as systemic lupus erythematosus (SLE), systemic sclerosis, and antiphospholipid syndrome (APS) may also manifest with MAHA and thrombocytopenia by both immune and nonimmune mechanisms. Kidney biopsies in patients with rheumatologic disorders will have evidence of TMA. Patients undergoing acute rejection of a transplanted kidney and patients who have undergone autologous or allogenic bone marrow transplant are also at risk of MAHA and thrombocytopenia. Severe B12 deficiency presents with thrombocytopenia and ineffective erythropoiesis with red blood cell morphology resembling MAHA, although compared with a TTP population, B12 deficient patients are more likely to have teardrops on blood smear and a lower PLASMIC score [3].

Table 15.1 TMA syndromes and systemic disorders

TMA-associated disorder	Clinical and laboratory features
TTP	MAHA and thrombocytopenia with rare renal injury May be inherited or autoimmune. The ADAMTS13 activity and inhibitor can help with differentiation
aHUS	The hallmark is renal failure Inherited disorders have heterozygous mutation of complement pathway (i.e., CFH, CFI, CD46/MCP, C3, CFB, CFHRs) Acquired disorders with antibodies against complement factor H or I
Shiga toxin HUS	Abdominal pain and diarrhea Renal failure is common Positive stool for *E. coli* or *S. dysenteriae* or Shiga toxin
Drug-induced TMA	Exposure to implicated medication. Immune mediated have acute onset, chills, abdominal pain. There is severe kidney injury, drug-dependent antibody to platelets Toxic, dose-related may have gradual or acute onset renal failure and hypertension
Coagulation-mediated TMA	Presents in young children DKGE, thrombomodulin or plasminogen mutation
DIC	Consumption of coagulation factors and platelets which occurs secondary to infection, malignancy, pregnancy complications, or vascular abnormality (i.e., Kasabach-Merritt syndrome)
Infection	Includes bacterial (i.e., rickettsia), viral, or fungal organisms Presentation with high fevers
Malignancy	Breast, prostate, lung, pancreatic, and gastrointestinal tumors are most common
Pregnancy related	Typically seen in third trimester or postpartum HELLP syndrome presents with hypertension, elevated liver enzymes, and low platelets
Hypertensive urgency	Typically presents when systolic BP >200 mmHg May present with neurologic features including PRES
Rheumatoid disease	SLE presents with hypertension, renal insufficiency, and autoimmune cytopenias. Renal biopsy is similar to TMA syndromes Antiphospholipid syndrome can present with arterial and/or venous thrombosis
Transplant	May occur with solid organ, autologous or allogenic transplant Solid tumor can be associated with CMV infection in the setting of immunosuppression Stem cell transplant TMA may be associated to calcineurin inhibitor, radiation, cytotoxic chemotherapy, or infection

Clinical Manifestations

There are no specific clinical features that distinguish TTP. Patients present with nonspecific symptoms, such as weakness, fatigue, purpura, nausea, and diarrhea. Approximately one third of patients will have nonspecific symptoms of confusion and headache, one third will have no neurologic symptoms, and one third will have severe neurologic manifestations such as transient ischemia, aphasia, or stroke.

Patients rarely have purpura or bleeding despite severe thrombocytopenia. The classic pentad of TTP is summarized below, but it is important to note that it is present in only 5% of patients [1]. Fever is classically represented in the pentad but is extremely rare at presentation (Fig. 15.1).

- Fever.
- Hemolytic anemia (schistocytes, elevated LDH, low haptoglobin, low hemoglobin/ hematocrit).
- Thrombocytopenia.
- Renal impairment (elevated creatinine, decreased glomerular filtration rate, elevated blood pressure, abnormal urinalysis).
- Neurological involvement (confusion, seizures, aphasia, numbness).

Due to its variable presentation, clinicians should maintain a high suspicion for diagnosis in patients who present with acute anemia and thrombocytopenia (Fig. 15.2).

Laboratory Investigations

All patients with suspected TTP should have a complete blood count (CBC) to assess degree of anemia and thrombocytopenia. Hemolysis labs including reticulocyte count, lactate dehydrogenase (LDH), haptoglobin, and indirect bilirubin will help support MAHA. Smear review for schistiocytes and serum creatinine elevation

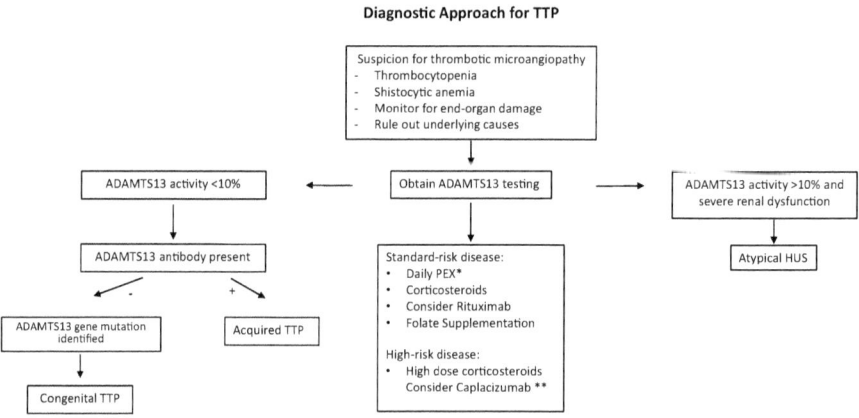

Fig. 15.1 Diagnostic and initial treatment for TTP. *While awaiting ADAMTS13 activity, start plasma exchange. Treatment can be changed once results are obtained. **In settings without reasonable access to ADAMTS13 activity testing, the use of caplacizumab is not recommended, regardless of the pretest probability of TTP

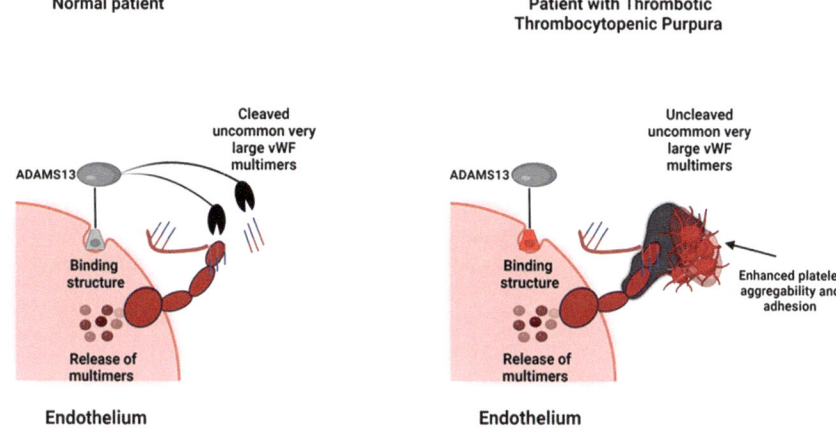

Fig. 15.2 Pathophysiology of acquired TTP. In biologic normal condition, very large vWF multimers are cleaved by ADAMTS13 to avoid pathologic platelet aggregability. ADAMTS13 depletion results in uncleaved large vWF allowing widespread platelet aggregability and adhesion

Table 15.2 Laboratory investigations in TTP	
	CBC with platelet count
	Reticulocyte count
	Lactate dehydrogenase
	Haptoglobin
	Indirect bilirubin
	Creatinine
	Direct antiglobulin test[a]
	PT/aPTT[a]
	Fibrinogen[a]
	D-dimer[a]
	Peripheral smear review
	ADAMTS13 assay (activity/antigen and inhibitor/antibody)

[a]Testing helps rule out other diseases that may look like TMA/ TTP. DAT will rule out autoimmune hemolytic anemia and a smear review will be imperative as well. Coagulation studies, fibrinogen, and D-dimer help to rule out DIC

to establish kidney injury are supportive of MAHA. Coagulation studies, d-dimer, and fibrinogen will help to rule out disseminated intravascular disease (DIC). Once MAHA and thrombocytopenia are established, there should be an urgent request for ADAMST13 activity to confirm acquired TTP that will benefit from plasma exchange, although the treatment should not be delayed if clinical suspicion is high and ADAMTS13 activity is not yet resulted (Tables 15.2 and 15.3).

Table 15.3 TTP treatment paradigm [2, 6]

TTP events	Treatment recommendations
First event, high-risk TTP	PEX + corticosteroids + rituximab ± xaplacizumab Methylprednisolone 1000 mg intravenously per day for 3 days followed by prednisone 1 mg/kg daily orally. Caplacizumab 11 mg IV prior to PEX and 11 mg SC until ADAMTS13 deficiency resolves
First event, standard-risk TTP	PEX + corticosteroids ± rituximab Prednisone 1 mg/kg per day orally Rituximab 375 mg/m² × 4 doses (if no contraindication, conditional recommendation)
Relapsing TTP	PEX + corticosteroids ± rituximab ± caplacizumab
Remission TTP with low ADAMTS13 with no clinical signs	Rituximab maintenance

Table 15.4 Plasmic Diagnostic Score

Parameter	Points
Platelet count <30 × 10⁹/L	1
Combined hemolysis parameter Indirect bilirubin >2 mg/dL, OR Reticulocyte counts >2.5%, OR Haptoglobin undetectable	1
No active cancer	1
No history of solid-organ or stem cell transplant	1
MCV <90 fL	1
INR <1.5	1
Creatinine <2.0 mg/dL	1

Score < 5: low risk for severe ADAMTS13 deficiency. Score 5: intermediate risk. Score > 5: high risk

Management

TTP is a hematological emergency as there is an estimated 50% mortality in the first 24 h [1]. Thrombocytopenia and MAHA in the absence of other identifiable clinical causes are enough to initiate treatment. A PLASMIC score (Table 15.4) in the intermediate to high range (5 to 7 points) also helps make a presumptive diagnosis [4, 5]. Once TTP is suspected, plasma exchange (PEX) should be started promptly. ADAMTS13 testing should be performed prior to the initiation of treatment.

There are relatively limited data from prospective, randomized, and controlled clinical trials to direct the most appropriate use of these treatments. The ISTH provided guidelines intended in helping clinicians make treatment decisions [6].

TTP risk stratification is paramount to initial treatment approach. High-risk disease includes neurological symptoms, decreased level of consciousness, elevated serum troponin, and other signs of critical illness. In general, standard-risk disease is treated with daily PEX, glucocorticoids, and rituximab (unless there is a contraindication). Implications of high-risk disease include the use of high gluco-corticoid dose and initial use of caplacizumab [7]. Daily PEX allows for the removal of autoantibodies and replenishes ADAMTS13. Corticosteroids and rituximab suppress the inappropriate immune response. Caplacizumab hastens platelet recovery and limits microthrombi [8].

In a life-threatening hemorrhage or during invasive procedures, platelet transfusions may be administered.

Assessment of patient should be done daily, with most patients with autoimmune TTP demonstrating improvement in platelet counts within the first week. Moreover, by this time, the results of ADAMTS13 testing should be available. After complete remission, defined as normal platelet count (>150 × 10^9/L), daily PEX should continue for a minimum of 2 days after platelet normalization [2]. A durable treatment response is lasting at least 30 days after discontinuation of PEX.

Relapse TTP is defined as disease recurrence after remission, usually 30 days after the last PEX treatment [1, 9]. Relapse TTP is treated liked a new acute episode, usually mirroring the previous treatment plan.

Refractory TTP is defined by no treatment response by day 30 and/or no durable treatment response by day 6 [1].

In refractory TTP, clinicians can increase the frequency of intensity of PEX ± corticosteroids, or the addition of rituximab or caplacizumab [1]. Furthermore, other immunomodulatory agents such as cyclosporine A, vincristine, cyclophosphamide, mycophenolate mofetil, and bortezomib can be considered. As a salvage option, splenectomy can be considered (Fig. 15.3).

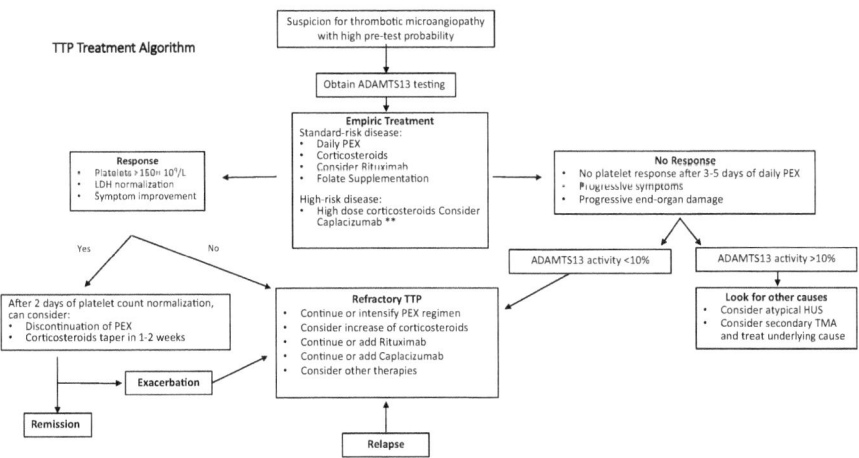

Fig. 15.3 TTP treatment algorithm. *While awaiting ADAMTS13 activity, start plasma exchange. Treatment can be changed once results are obtained. **In settings without reasonable access to ADAMTS13 activity testing, the use of caplacizumab is not recommended, regardless of the pre-test probability of TTP

Monitoring

The highest risk of exacerbation is during the first week. During the first month of remission, CBC and ADAMTS13 activity is monitored weekly.

During the first and second year of remission, ADAMTS13 activity is monitored every 3 months. In subsequent year, ADAMTS13 activity can be monitored annually. The risk of relapse is greatest during the first 2 years, with increased risk for patients with ADAMTS13 < 10%. For patients in clinical remission, but with persistent severe ADAMTS13 deficiency or in whom ADAMTS13 monitored regularly during follow-up becomes less than 10%, maintenance rituximab should be considered [9].

Moreover, in frequent relapses with persistent low ADAMTS12 activity, other immunomodulatory agents or splenectomy can be considered.

Specific Considerations

Long-term follow-up of patients who have recovered from acute episodes of TTP reveals these patients have residual comorbidities following their recovery [10, 11]. They are at increased risk of hypertension, cardiovascular disease, and stroke, presumably resulting from diffuse microvascular thrombi damage. Low ADAMTS13 activity following clinical remission has been noted as a risk factor for stroke [11].

Major depression has been documented in up to 30% of patients who have recovered from an acute episode of TTP, with many of the patients complaining of fatigue and memory problems that are often misdiagnosed [12]. The mechanism for psychiatric sequelae is not well understood but constitutes a real problem in this population as often patients are reluctant to seek out counseling or treatment due to the stigma.

Autoimmune disorders have been reported in approximately 10% of patients who have recovered from TTP, with systemic lupus erythematosus (SLE) being the most common manifestation, but Grave's disease, Addison's disease, and immune thrombocytopenia purpura have also been documented [12].

Pregnancy following recovery from acquired TTP require careful monitoring from a hematologist and maternal fetal medicine specialist with important attention paid to symptoms that may suggest relapse. Clinical relapse is managed with PEX and steroids. We do not typically recommend rituximab in the second or third trimesters unless the patient is refractory to PEX and steroids. There is less concern in the first trimester because rituximab does not significantly cross the placenta before 18 weeks [13]. Importantly, most pregnancies following recovery from acquired TTP are uncomplicated, although the risks of preeclampsia are increased.

Useful Tools

PLASMIC diagnostic score (thrombocytopenia; hemolytic anemia; lack of cancer, macrocytosis, coagulopathy, or renal failure) [4].

Heparin-Induced Thrombocytopenia

Case

A 54-year-old woman was recently discharged from the hospital following hip replacement and was given 2 weeks of unfractionated heparin injections to continue taking at home. She presents to the emergency room 5 days after discharge with left lower extremity swelling and pleuritic chest pain. Physical examination reveals an obese woman in mild distress, with normal blood pressure and heart rate, but decreased oxygen saturation to 93%. Lung fields exhibit decreased air movement bilaterally with right side more affected than left. There is edema and erythema in her left lower limb. Her lower extremity duplex scan showed acute thrombosis of the left common femoral, superficial femoral, and popliteal vein. Complete blood count is significant for hemoglobin 10.5 g/dL and platelet count of 82,000/µL. Hemoglobin at discharge was 10.8 g/dL and platelet count was 168,000/µL.

Definition

Heparin-induced thrombocytopenia (HIT) is a pro-thrombotic life-threatening complication that occurs in a small number of patients following exposure to a heparin product. It is the result of an autoantibody directed against endogenous platelet factor 4 (PF4) complexed to heparin, which results in thrombocytopenia and a hypercoagulable state (Fig. 15.4). It is estimated that 33% to 50% of HIT cases are complicated by thrombosis, which can be limb or life-threatening [14]. Low molecular weight heparin (LMWH) is associated with a fivefold to tenfold lower risk of HIT than unfractionated heparin (UFH) [15]. Untreated HIT has been reported to have a mortality as high as 20%, although these statistics have dramatically improved with early recognition and intervention.

Clinical Context

There are two forms of HIT: type I and type II, with only type II being of clinical significance. The distinction between the two forms of HIT is made based on timing and degree of platelet count drop. HIT type I is a transient drop in platelet count that occurs within 2 days of heparin exposure. The mechanism of platelet drop appears

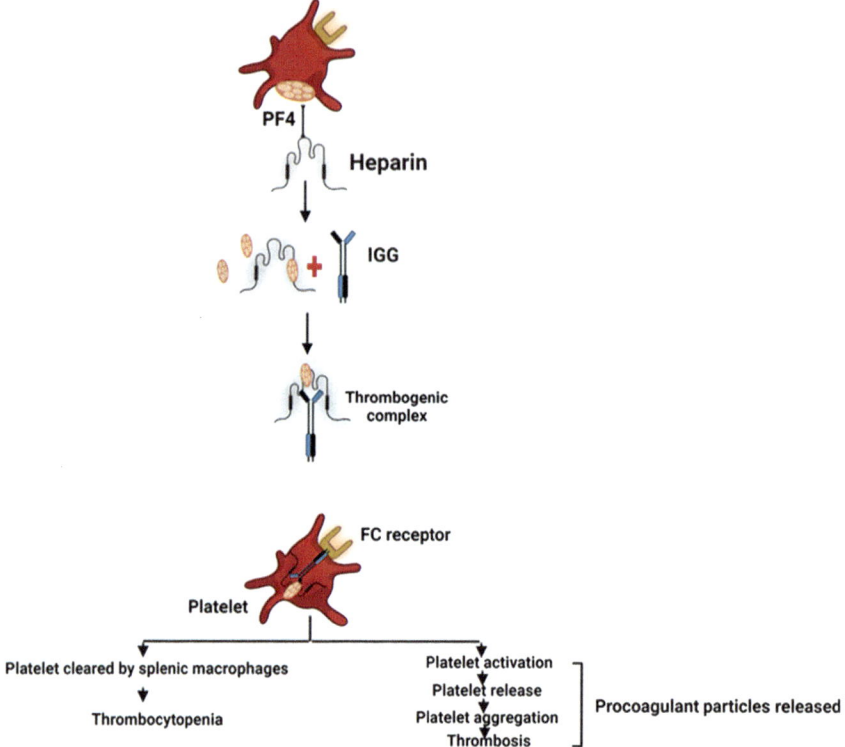

Fig. 15.4 Pathophysiology of HIT. Auto-antibody IGG against platelet factor 4 (PF4)-heparin complex avidly bind platelets and monocytes inducing activation. Platelet aggregability and procoagulant particle release leads to thrombosis

Table 15.5 Characteristics of type I and type II HIT

	HIT type I [14]	HIT type II [14] (antibody-mediated)
Incidence	5–10%	0–3%
Timing of onset	2–3 days after heparin exposure	5–10 days after heparin exposure
Nadir platelet count	100,000/μL	Decreased to >50% decrease in platelets from base value
Complications	None	Thromboembolism, 30–80% Rare hemorrhagic sequalae
Treatment	None	Discontinue heparin products Alternative non-heparin anticoagulation

to be non-immune platelet aggregation. The platelet count often returns to normal with continued heparin administration, and the platelet nadir is typically 100 K/μL without thrombotic or hemorrhagic complications [14] (Table 15.5).

Table 15.6 HIT variants

HIT variants	
Delayed onset HIT [16]	Thrombocytopenia or thrombosis that occurs five or more days after withdrawal of heparin. May be related to high titer antibodies
Refractory (persistent) HIT [17]	Rare presentation of persistent thrombocytopenia and/or thrombosis that lasts weeks after discontinuation of heparin products
Spontaneous HIT [18]	Described in the absence of recent heparin exposure yet there is demonstration of anti-PF4 antibodies of IgG subclass associated with strong in vitro platelet activation in the absence of heparin
Vaccine-induced immune thrombotic thrombocytopenia (VITT) [19]	Described following the ChAdOx1 CoV-19 vaccine. Patients present 5–30 days following vaccination with thrombocytopenia and typical or atypical (cerebral vein, splanchnic vein) thrombosis. No prior heparin exposure, but they have strongly positive heparin/PF4 antibodies on ELISA assay

HIT type II constitutes the clinically significant syndrome triggered by the formation of antibodies against the complex of heparin and PF4 and associated with thrombotic complications; hence the syndrome is more typically referred to as heparin-induced thrombocytopenia and thrombosis (HITT) [14].

There are several variants of HIT that are not typically associated with heparin exposure and are summarized in Table 15.6.

Clinical Manifestations

The most common manifestation of HIT is thrombocytopenia occurring 5–10 days following heparin exposure and experienced by 85% of affected individuals [14]. Nadir is typically 60 K/μL.

with platelet counts <20 K/μL considered rare. Although not all patients will experience thrombocytopenia defined by absolute platelet count, they typically demonstrate 50% reduction in total platelet count, so it is important to see platelet trends to identify this.

Early-onset HIT may be seen following 24 h of heparin exposure in those patients who had a prior exposure to heparin products 1–3 months prior to clinical presentation, presumably due to the presence of circulating HIT antibodies [15].

Patients with HIT may also experience thrombotic sequelae including arterial or venous thrombosis, complication of limb gangrene, or skin necrosis at site of heparin injections [14].

It is important to consider HIT in thrombocytopenia differential when patients are currently receiving heparin or have received it over the preceding 5–10 days and they experience a drop in platelets >50% or absolute thrombocytopenia, new venous or arterial thrombus, necrotic skin lesions, or acute systemic reactions such as anaphylaxis following heparin administration.

A 4T score (Table 15.7) [20] has been established to help the clinician estimate the pretest probability of HIT based on readily available clinical information, prior

Table 15.7 4Ts score for heparin-induced thrombocytopenia

4-T score	Score = 2 points	Score = 1 point	Score = 0 points
Thrombocytopenia	• >50% fall of PLT or PLT nadir of >20 × 10⁹/L with no preceding surgery in the last 3 weeks	• >50% fall but surgery in last 3 days • PLT fall that does not fit score 2 or score 0	• <30% PLT fall • Any PLT fall with nadir <10 × 10⁹/L
Timing	• PLT fall day 5–10 after heparin exposure • PLT fall within 1 day of heparin start and exposure to heparin within past 5–30 days	• PLT fall 5–10 days after heparin exposure but not clear • PLT fall within 1 day of heparin start and exposure to heparin within past 31–100 days • PLT fall after day 10	• PLT fall <day 4 without exposure to heparin in the past 100 days
Thrombosis	• Confirmed new thrombosis • Skin necrosis at injection site • Anaphylactic reaction to heparin • Adrenal hemorrhage	• Recurrent VTE in patient receiving therapeutic anticoagulation • Suspected thrombosis (ultrasound pending) • Erythematous lesions at heparin injection sites	• No thrombosis suspected
Other potential causes of thrombocytopenia	• No alternative explanation for PLT fall evident	Possible other causes evident: • Presumed sepsis • TCP after ventilator support • Other	Possible other causes present: • Surgery within 72 h • Confirmed bacteremia • Chemo/RT within past 20 days • Post transfusion purpura • PLT <20 × 10⁹/L from other drug • Other

Thrombocytopenia, timing of platelet count fall, thrombosis or other sequelae, and other causes of thrombocytopenia enable calculation of pretest clinical score for likelihood of HIT diagnosis:
- <3 points: low probability for HIT, <5%
- 4–5 points: Intermediate probability, ~10%
- 6–8 points: high probability, ~50%

to availability of confirmatory testing. This will be described more thoroughly later in the chapter.

The diagnosis of HIT requires the integration of clinical features and laboratory testing with neither being sufficient to establish a diagnosis. While a presumptive

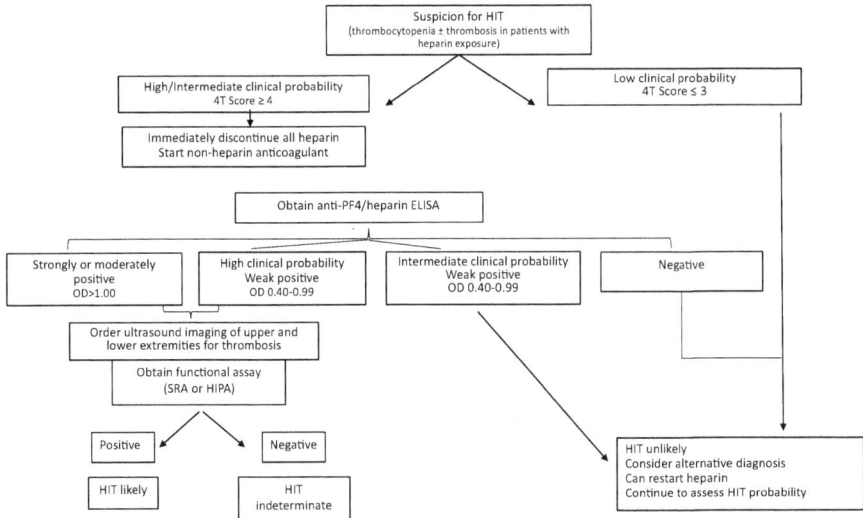

Fig. 15.5 Diagnostic and initial treatment for HIT

diagnostic of HIT is made on clinical presentation, the laboratory evidence is essential for confirmation. We have summarized an algorithm to diagnosis of HIT (Fig. 15.5).

Laboratory Investigations

- CBC.
- PT/ aPTT.
- Fibrinogen.
- D-dimer.
- Anti-PF4/heparin ELISA.
- Serotonin release assay.

Solid phase ELISA is the most used laboratory test to establish the diagnosis of HIT. It detects the presence of anti-PF4/heparin complex in patient serum. It is a quick turnaround assay that requires the addition of patients' serum to a microtiter plate coated with heparin/PF4 complexes. If antibodies are present in serum, they will bind the heparin/PF4 complex and result in colorimetric change whose intensity is measured by optical density (OD) [21]. A higher OD is typically associated with higher antibody titers. Although most assays report positive or negative results based on a predetermined OD cutoff, it is important that the OD of the ELISA is available as it does correlate with the likelihood of HIT [21].

The serotonin release assay (SRA) is considered the gold standard among the diagnostic HIT tests. It measures platelet activation by detecting the release of serotonin from test platelets in the presence of patient serum and heparin [22]. Test platelets are obtained from normal donors and are labeled with ^{14}C-serotonin. A positive test results when the C serotonin is released from platelets following therapeutic concentrations of heparin (0.1 units/mL) but not at higher concentrations (>100 units/mL) since binding of HIT antibodies occurs at certain ratios of heparin to PF4 [22].

Management

Based on strong clinical suspicion, the immediate treatment of HIT starts with the withdrawal of all heparin products. This initial step alone, however, is not sufficient to prevent thrombosis. Consequently, patients should then be started on therapeutic dose of a non-heparin anticoagulant, unless there is a strong contraindication such as high bleeding risk [15]. Anticoagulant choices can be seen on Table 15.8. Figure 15.6 summarizes the best agents based on liver and renal function.

The quantitative result of an immunoassay (ELISA) for PF4 antibodies is helpful in confirming the diagnosis. The magnitude of a positive optical density (OD) result is directly associated with the odds of a positive functional assay [14, 15]. If the results are indeterminate, then a functional assay (serotonin-release assay) is required to confirm or exclude HIT.

All individuals with high suspicion for HIT should be screened for lower extremity deep vein thrombosis, even if asymptomatic [14, 15].

If the diagnosis of HIT is confirmed, then the patient should be continued on a therapeutic dose of a non-heparin anticoagulant. Patients with HIT-associated thromboembolism are maintained on dose-adjusted warfarin for 3 to 6 months [14]. In patient with HIT without thrombosis, the optimal duration of anticoagulation remains unknown. In general, patients are usually maintained on anticoagulation until platelet recovery.

If the diagnosis of HIT is excluded based on pre-test probability and/or HIT testing, the patient may be resumed on heparin therapy, if original indication is present.

Special Considerations

Dosing for direct oral anticoagulants (DOACs) in HIT is not well established based on clinical trials, and their use is based on observational data which suggests the agents may be a good alternative for reducing thrombosis risk in HIT [24]. Case studies have reported their use both as initial therapy and preceded by a parenteral agent [25]. The approach favored by most experts is the path that leads to avoidance of thromboembolism. If a DOAC is started as the initial treatment, the acute treatment dose for VTE should be used for minimum of VTE treatment period or until the platelet count recovers. If DOAC is started after a period of parenteral

Table 15.8 Alternative anticoagulation choices [15]

Agent	Dosing	Monitoring	Dose Adjustments
Argatroban[a] (direct thrombin inhibitor)	No bolus Continuous infusion: 2 µg/kg per minute	Adjust aPTT of 1.5–3.0 times patient baseline	Dose adjustments for hepatic dysfunction, heart failure, post cardiac surgery and anasarca
Lepirudin (direct thrombin inhibitor)	Bolus: 0.2 mg/kg (only for life or limb-threatening thrombosis) Continuous infusion: 0.10 mg/kg/min	Adjust aPTT of 1.5–2.0 times patient baseline	Dose adjustments renal dysfunction
Bivalirudin (direct thrombin inhibitor)	No bolus Continuous infusion: 0.15 mg/kg/h	Adjust aPTT of 1.5–2.5 times patient baseline	Dose adjustment for renal or hepatic dysfunction
Desirudin (direct thrombin inhibitor)	15 mg or 30 mg subcutaneously every 12 h	Not necessary; plasma levels of drug correlate with aPTT	Dose adjustment for renal dysfunction
Danaparanoid (indirect Fxa inhibitor)	Bolus: weight-based Accelerated initial infusion: 400 U/h × 4 h, then 300 U/h × 4 h Maintenance infusion: 200 U/h	Adjust to anti-Fxa of 0.5–0.8 U/mL	Dose adjustment for renal dysfunction
Fondaparinux (indirect FXa inhibitor)	Weigh-based subcutaneous administration	None	Dose adjustment for renal dysfunction
Apixaban (direct FXa inhibitor)	HITT: 10 mg twice per day × 1 week, then 5 mg twice per day Isolated HIT: 5 mg twice per day until platelet count recovery	None	Avoid in moderate to severe hepatic dysfunction
Rivaroxaban (direct FXa inhibitor)	HITT: 15 mg twice per day × 3 weeks, then 20 mg once per day Isolated HIT: 15 mg twice per day until platelet count recovery	None	Avoid in moderate to severe hepatic dysfunction
Dabigatran (direct thrombin inhibitor)	HITT: 150 mg twice per day after ≥5 days of treatment with a parenteral non-heparin anticoagulant Isolated HIT: 150 mg twice per day until platelet count recovery	None	Avoid in moderate to severe hepatic dysfunction

[a]First-line therapy used in the USA [23]

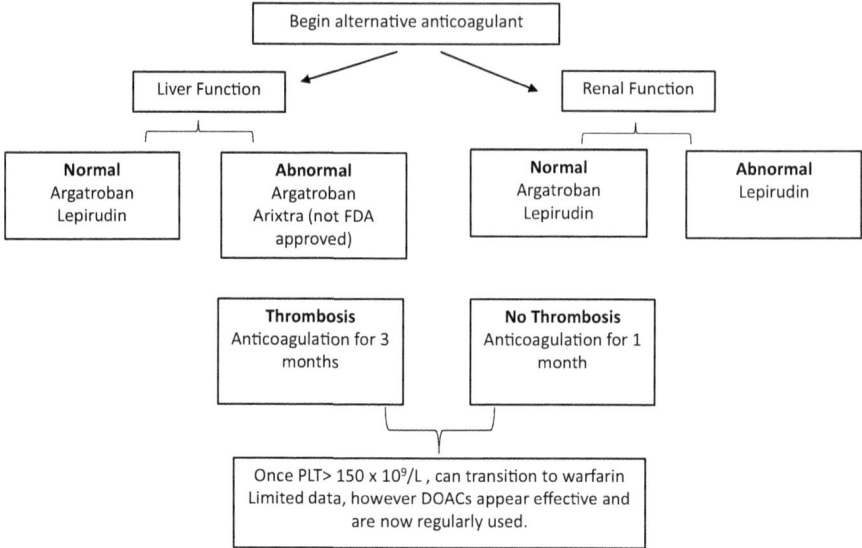

Fig. 15.6 Anticoagulation management

anticoagulation, the usual dose approved for VTE should be used and if the parenteral drug was used for less than 7 days, a loading dose of DOAC should be incorporated into the treatment plan. ASH guidelines recommend a similar approach summarized in Table 15.8 [14].

Other Tools

The 4 T score (Table 15.7) is used to estimate the pretest probability of HIT based on clinical features and makes the presumptive diagnosis of HIT before confirmatory laboratory testing is available [20]. The score assesses the degree of thrombocytopenia, the timing of platelet count drop, and the presence of thrombosis or other sequelae and considers alternative aspects of clinical presentation that may contribute to the observed thrombocytopenia. The sum of the points gives a total of 0 to 8 points and estimates the pretest probability as follows:

- 0 to 3 points—Low probability (<1%)
- 4 to 5 points—Intermediate probability (~10%)
- 6 to 8 points—High probability (~50%).

A meta-analysis of >3000 patients with clinically suspected HIT found that the 4T score had a negative predictive value of 0.998 (CI 0.97–1.0) for those with low-risk probability ultimately having negative functional assay for HIT antibodies. On the other hand, those with intermediate- and high-risk scores had a positive functional assay for HIT antibodies with positive predictive values of 0.14 and 0.64, respectively.

Immune Thrombocytopenia Purpura

Case

A 32-year-old female presents to the emergency room with diffuse petechiae and bruises for 2 days, significant menorrhagia and gum bleeding. She has no known medical issues and does not take any medications. Family history is significant for SLE in her mother. She is otherwise well appearing. There is no blood in the urine or stool. Vital signs are normal; physical exam is notable for diffuse petechiae with scattered bruises and bleeding oral mucosa. Platelet count is 5×10^9/L; hemoglobin, white blood cell count, liver enzymes, and electrolytes (including BUN/creatinine) are within normal range.

Definition

Immune thrombocytopenic purpura (ITP) is an acquired thrombocytopenia caused by autoantibodies against platelet antigens resulting in destruction of circulating platelets and impaired platelet production [26]. Primary ITP is acquired in the auto-immune mechanisms not triggered by another condition. Secondary ITP is an ITP in the setting of an associated condition (Table 15.9; SLE, APS, CLL, immunodeficiency, viral infections, etc.). Drug immune thrombocytopenia can occur due to the presence of drug-dependent platelet antibodies that cause platelet destruction.

Table 15.9 Causes of secondary immune thrombocytopenia

Autoimmune disorders	SLE Evans syndrome Antiphospholipid antibody syndrome Rheumatoid arthritis Inflammatory bowel disease
Immunodeficiency syndromes	HIV Common variable immune deficiency (CVID)
Infections	Cytomegalovirus (CMV) Epstein Barr virus (EBV) Hepatitis C (HCV) HIV Varicella zoster virus (VZV)
Lymphoid malignancies	CLL Lymphoma
Medications	Alemtuzumab Gold Ipilimumab MMR vaccination Nivolumab Pembrolizumab Antibiotics

Based on timing of thrombocytopenia, we further define ITP as follows:

- Acute ITP: Onset of thrombocytopenia up to 3 months.
- Persistent ITP: 3–12 months after diagnosis.
- Chronic ITP: Platelet count <100 × 10⁹/L for longer than 12 months.
- Refractory ITP: ITP that does not respond to, or relapses after, splenectomy.

Clinical Context

The reported incidence of ITP is 3.3/100,000 adults per year with a prevalence of 9.5/100,000 [27]. In younger adults, ITP prevalence is higher in women, but in older patients (age > 65 years), the prevalence is equal in men and women. ITP is a chronic disease in adults but is generally a self-limited process in children.

ITP is challenging to diagnose, as it remains a diagnosis of exclusion. Other causes of thrombocytopenia need to be ruled out, hence the importance of obtaining a detailed history and physical (Table 15.10) [28]. Laboratory investigations are aimed at ruling out etiologies although bone marrow evaluation is no longer recommended [28]. Response to initial treatment is usually the single best diagnostic test [29] although we do not typically do this if the platelet count does not require treatment.

Clinical Manifestations

Due to the wide availability of complete blood counts, patients are often diagnosed due to asymptomatic, chronic thrombocytopenia. The consensus is that a platelet count <100 K/µL, in the absence of anemia, leukopenia, or other apparent cause of thrombocytopenia, is suggestive of ITP. Bleeding manifestations are consistent with the platelet count (Table 15.11).

Laboratory Investigations

CBC and peripheral blood smear are the initial laboratory tests of choice. American Society of Hematology (ASH) evidence-based practice guideline for ITP recommends obtaining additional laboratory tests—HIV, Hepatitis C. In the past, bone marrow examination was recommended for initial evaluation, but ASH evidence-based practice guideline for ITP no longer considers bone marrow examination to be necessary for diagnosis but should be considered in patients who have other cytopenias.

Additional testing is recommended in select patients. Coagulation studies in patients with moderate and severe thrombocytopenia may reveal other causes of thrombocytopenia such as chronic liver disease or disseminated intravascular

Table 15.10 Common causes of thrombocytopenia

Medications	Quinine
	Sulfonamides
	Acetaminophen
	Cimetidine
	Ibuprofen
	Naproxen
	Vancomycin
	Piperacillin
	Glycoprotein IIb/IIIa (abciximab, tirofiban, eptifibatidine)
Food and beverages	Tonic water
	Walnuts
	Certain herbal teas
Infections	HIV
	Hepatitis C
	EBV
	Sepsis
	Helicobacter Pylor
	Intracellular parasites (e.g., malaria, babesia)
Hypersplenism	Due to chronic liver disease
Alcohol	
Nutrient deficiencies	B12
	Folate
	Copper
Pregnancy	Gestational Thromobocytopenia
	Preeclampsia
	HELLP (hemolysis, elevated liver function tests, low platelets)
Autoimmune disorders	SLE
	RA
Bone marrow failure	Myelodysplasia
	Paroxysmal noctural hemoglobinuria
	Aplastic anemia
	Cancer with bone marrow infiltration
Thrombotic Microangiopathy	TTP
	HUS/aHUS
	Drug-induced TMA
Hereditary Thrombocytopenia	Von Willebrand type 2B
	Wiskott-Aldrich syndrome
	Alport syndrome
	May-Hegglin anomaly
	Bernard Soulier syndrome
	Thrombocytopenia absent radius syndrome
	Fanconi anemia

coagulation. *H. pylori* testing is appropriate for patients with gastrointestinal symptoms and thrombocytopenia, especially if they are from countries where *H. pylori* is endemic (e.g., Japan). There are rare reports in patients with thyroid disorders, so testing is appropriate if patients present with clinical signs of hypo- or hyperthyroidism. Testing for antinuclear antibodies (ANA) may be useful in patients who have

Table 15.11 Clinical manifestations of ITP

Petechiae	Flat, red, discrete lesions that do not blanch with pressure as often occur with other types of rash
Purpura	Coalescence of peteciase Nonpalpable and occurs in dependent parts of the body
Epistaxis	Continuous epistaxis may be predictive of greater risk for more serious bleeding
Severe hemorrhage	Less common Includes gastrointestinal or central nervous system bleeding
Fatigue	Common symptoms among ITP patients and may occur even with platelet count mildly reduced
Thrombosis	Rare

symptoms of rheumatologic conditions such as SLE, such as malar rash, arthritis, or myalgias. Mild thrombocytopenia may present with vitamin B12 and folate deficiency in otherwise asymptomatic patients.

Antiplatelet antibody testing has low sensitivity and does not correlate with clinical outcomes; hence we do not recommend these for diagnosis or management of ITP.

Management

Decision to initiate treatment and the type of treatment remains an individualized approach based on a multitude of factors including platelet nadir, bleeding complications, and need for surgical intervention or procedures. We recommend an evidence-based approach summarized in the ASH guidelines based on panel discussion and systematic literature review (Fig. 15.7) [28].

In patient with newly diagnosed ITP and a platelet count of $<30 \times 10^9$/L who are asymptomatic or have minor mucocutaneous bleeding, observation is preferred to medical management [28]. In general, treatment is not required for platelet counts between 20×10^9/L–50×10^9/L in the absence of bleeding. Medical management is best reserved for patients who are bleeding and those with platelet counts $<20 \times 10^9$/L. If newly diagnosed with a platelet count of $<20 \times 10^9$/L, inpatient management is recommended.

If treatment for patient is deemed necessary, a corticosteroid course of less than 6 weeks is favored. Initial glucocorticoid therapy preferences include either prednisone (0.5–2.0 mg/kg per day) or pulse dose dexamethasone (40 mg per day for 4 days). Several studies have suggested a higher complete response (CR) rate using high-dose dexamethasone. However dexamethasone may be poorly tolerated [30]. Prednisone may be preferred due to flexibility in dosing choices to individualize therapy more effectively. It is important to note that the general effectiveness and safety of both prednisone and dexamethasone are similar. Overall, glucocorticoids raise platelet count in approximately two-thirds of patients with ITP, most responses occurring within 5 days, but in some patients requiring up to 2 weeks, primarily if prednisone is utilized. If there is a contraindication to steroids, IVIG can be used

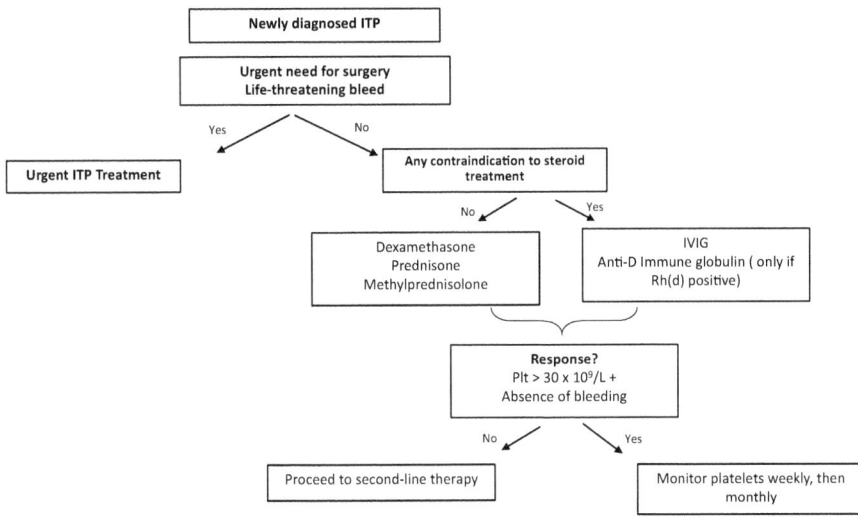

Fig. 15.7   Initial treatment for ITP

Table 15.12   First-line therapies [29, 30]

Treatment	Initial response rate	Time to initial response/peak response time	Duration of response	Toxicity
Corticosteroids	Up to 90%	2–14 days/4–28 days	50–80% remission after 2–5 years follow-up	Hyperglycemia, weight gain, hypertension, edema, cataracts, peptic ulcer disease, avascular necrosis, adrenal insufficiency, immune suppression
• Dexamethasone 40 mg PO daily × 4 days, every 2–3 weeks for 1–4 cycles				
• Prednisone 1 mg/kg/ day × 40 days	70–80%	4–14 days/7–28 days	13–15% estimated remission at 10 years	
• Methylprednisolone 30 mg/kg/ day × 7 days	Up to 95%	4–14 days	23% remission at 20 months	
IVIG	Up to 80%	1–3 days/ 2–7 days	Platelets return to pre-treatment levels within 2–4 weeks	Neutropenia, flu-like illness, aseptic meningitis, thrombosis, anaphylaxis in IgA deficiency
• 1 g/kg/day for 1–2 days				
Anti-D immune globulin	Up to 80%	1–3 days/ 2–7 days	Platelets return to pre-treatment levels within 2–4 weeks	DIC, hemolytic anemia, renal failure
• 50–75 µg/kg				

Fig. 15.8 Urgent
treatment for ITP

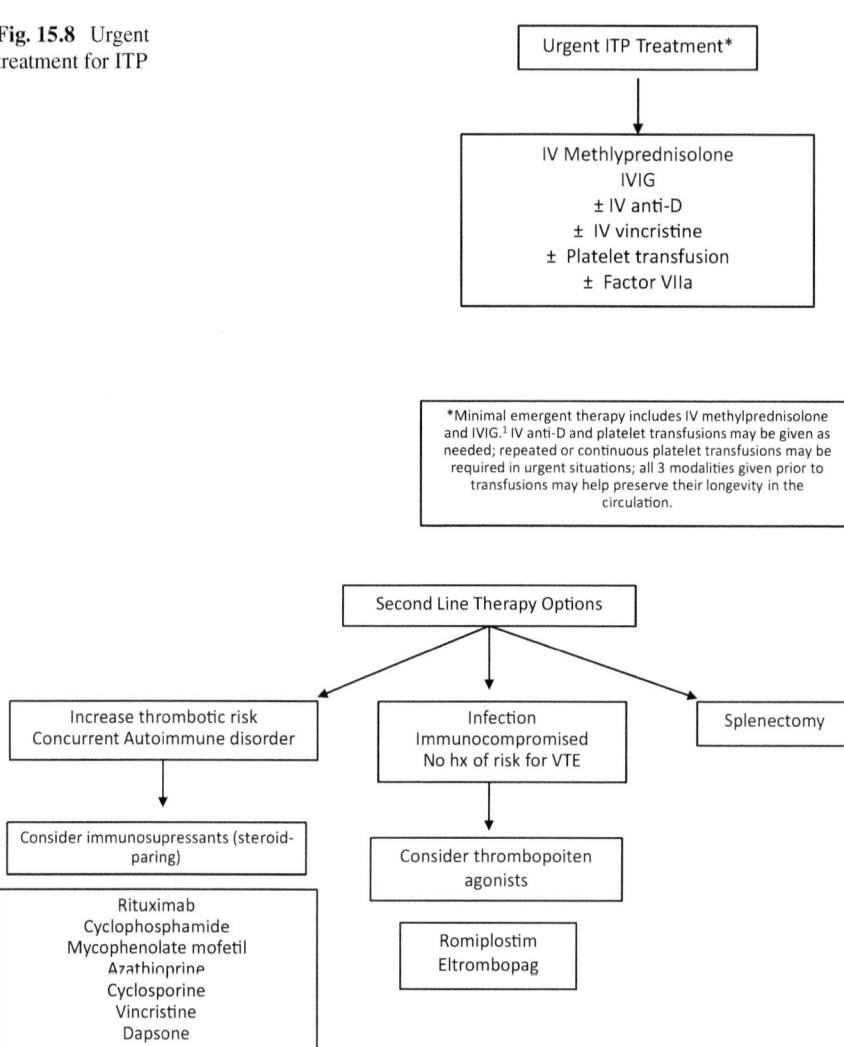

Fig. 15.9 Second line treatment options for ITP

[30]. Complete long-term remissions with glucocorticoids alone have been reported in only 20% of patients (Table 15.12 and Figs. 15.8 and 15.9).

Second-line treatment lacks high-grade evidence. The three agents most commonly used are thrombopoietin receptor agonists (TPO-RAs), rituximab, and mycophenolate mofetil [30]. Additional second-line agents include fostamatinib and immunosuppressive agents (e.g., azathioprine, cyclosporine, and others) [29] (Table 15.13).

Table 15.13 Second-line therapies for ITP [29]

Rituximab	Monoclonal antibody directed against the B-cell surface protein CD20
	Overall efficacy of single-agent rituximab is approximately 40–60%
	Median response of 1 year. Time to response is anywhere from 1 week to 2 months
	Some studies suggest that doses of 100 mg/week × 4 weeks have similar efficacy to higher doses (375 mg/m² weekly × 4 weeks)
	Adverse events include infusion reactions and reactivation of HBV infection. It is recommended patients be tested prior to initiation of therapy. Progressive multifocal encephalopathy has also been described in patients previously immunosuppressed
	Rituximab can interfere with response to immunizations, up to 6 months after administration
TPO-receptor agonists	A good option for those patients who wish to avoid surgery or immunosuppressive therapies
	Does require taking the medication for an extended period; does not induce remission
	Romiplostim is administered as a once-weekly subcutaneous injection
	Eltrombopag and Avatrombopag are once daily oral medication
	Platelet counts may increase in approximately 7–14 days
	Liver enzyme monitoring is recommended for eltrombopag
	There is a small risk of thrombosis
Fostamatinib	Small molecule tyrosine kinase inhibitor approved by FDA in 2018 for patients with chronic ITP who had insufficient response to previous treatment
Mycophenolate mofetil	Often utilized in combination regimens
Danazol	It is an attenuated androgen with efficacy in ITP, better tolerated in men than women due to hirsutism

Splenectomy is a good option for patients who wish to have a single potentially curative surgical procedure, and it does offer a significant opportunity to alter the disease course resulting in sustained remission [31]. However, it is important to note it is also associated with increased risk of thromboembolism and infection with encapsulated organisms. Patients considering splenectomy should receive immunizations for encapsulated organisms at least 2 weeks prior to surgery. Often, optimization of preoperative platelet count is necessary with counts >50 K/μL recommended.

In patients with a life-threatening bleed, minimal emergent therapy includes IV methylprednisolone and IVIG [29]. Platelet transfusions may be given as needed; repeated or continuous platelet transfusions may be required in urgent situations. The use of steroids and IVIG prior to transfusions may help preserve their longevity in the circulation.

Persistent ITP occurs in most patients when steroids are tapered. The goal of therapy is not to achieve a cure, rather to attain a hemostatic platelet count.

Special Considerations

ITP occurs in 1–3/10,000 pregnancies, with platelet counts <50 K/µL in only a small subset [32]. It can occur during any trimester or diagnosis may be known prior to pregnancy. It is expected that the platelet count will decrease during the pregnancy. This is further discussed in Chap. 21.

Disseminated Intravascular Coagulation

Case

A 42-year-old male presented to the emergency department with 2 days of nausea, vomiting, and abdominal pain. He displayed a mottling of irregular purpuric lesions prompting his family to bring him for evaluation. His laboratory studies reveal thrombocytopenia, bandemia, and promyelocyte cells. His coagulation panel shows decreased fibrinogen and elevated PT and aPTT, with elevated fibrin split products. Acute promyelocytic leukemia was confirmed via bone marrow biopsy, flow cytometry, and fluorescent in situ hybridization analysis.

Definition

Disseminated intravascular coagulation (DIC) is a condition characterized by the systemic activation of coagulation and consumption of platelets and coagulation proteins, which leads both to thrombotic and hemorrhagic complications [33]. DIC is due to an underlying condition; therefore, treatment of DIC is the correction of the underlying condition. In DIC, the normal hemostasis is dysregulated with coagulation and fibrinolysis becoming abnormally and massively activated.

DIC is a clinical and laboratory diagnosis; there is no one test that can diagnose DIC. Reliable diagnosis can be obtained by using a simple scoring algorithm. Acute DIC occurs when blood is exposed to large amounts of tissue factor, with significant generation of thrombin leading to rapid consumption of coagulation factors that outpaces their production. It is generally seen in patients with sepsis and hematological malignancy. Chronic DIC occurs when blood is intermittently exposed to small amounts of tissue factor leading to consumption that does not outpace production. It will occur in patients with a history of solid malignancy, especially those with pancreatic, ovarian, gastric, and brain tumors.

Clinical Context

DIC occurs in 1% of admissions to tertiary care hospitals. It is primarily associated with the following medical conditions:

- Malignancy—Often seen in patients with acute promyelocytic leukemia, pancreatic cancer, and other mucin-producing solid tumors such as gastric, prostate, breast, or ovarian cancer [34].
- Infection—Most likely bacterial sepsis.
- Trauma—Occurs in 42% of patients with severe trauma [35].
- Obstetric—Occurs in 20% of patients with HELLP syndrome [36] and 60% of patients with amniotic fluid embolism [37].
- Miscellaneous—Heat stroke, vascular abnormalities, snake bite, acute solid organ transplantation complication.

The differential diagnosis includes other conditions associated with bleeding, hypercoagulability, TMA, and thrombocytopenia such as severe liver disease, HIT, or TTP/aHUS.

Clinical Manifestations

Both acute and chronic DIC patients can be associated with bleeding and/or thrombosis. Acute DIC most often manifests with bleeding. An ill patient in the ICU may experience oozing from intravenous catheter sites and mucocutaneous surfaces. Chronic DIC is more likely to present with thromboembolic complications because procoagulant factors keep pace with ongoing generation of thrombi. DIC can lead to organ dysfunction via thromboembolic mechanisms, hemorrhage, and hypoperfusion. Organ dysfunction is most likely to be seen in acute DIC.

Table 15.14 summarizes clinical manifestations associated with both acute and chronic DIC, although it is important to recognize that none of these are specific to DIC.

Table 15.14   Clinical manifestations of DIC

Acute DIC	Chronic DIC
Bleeding	Thromboembolism, venous or arterial
Renal dysfunction	History of malignancy
Hepatic dysfunction	
Respiratory dysfunction	
Shock	
CNS dysfunction	
Thromboembolism	

Patients with coronavirus disease 2019 (COVID-19) have been reported to manifest clinical and laboratory abnormalities consistent with coagulopathy associated to endothelial cell injury. Typically, the patients most likely exhibit elevated fibrinogen and thromboembolic complications.

Laboratory Investigations

In DIC, the following laboratory abnormalities may be encountered, although none are sensitive or specific for the diagnosis:

- Low platelet count.
- Prolonged PT and aPTT; more likely to occur in acute than chronic DIC.
- Fibrinogen is low especially in acute DIC.
- D-dimer is typically increased in both acute and chronic DIC.
- Smear reveals schistiocytes and helmet cells although these changes are not as pronounced as those encountered in TTP (Table 15.15).

Management

The major principle in the management of DIC is the treatment of the underlying cause. Since DIC occurs due to the dysregulated generation of thrombin, resolution of the stimulus for this process is essential to resolution of DIC.

Supportive measures are the hallmark of therapy and are individualized based on the patient's clinical diagnosis. They include hemodynamic and/or ventilator support, blood product transfusions (Table 15.13) as needed, and aggressive hydration. Best supportive treatment usually results from early patient identification and risk stratification (Table 15.16).

The use of systemic therapies to address bleeding or thrombosis are not used prophylactically. Instead, careful surveillance of the patient for these complications is assumed with complications treated promptly when they develop. Antifibrinolytic therapies such as tranexamic acid (TXA) or epsilon-aminocaproic acid (EACA) are

Table 15.15 Laboratory abnormalities in acute and chronic DIC

	Acute DIC	Chronic DIC
Platelet count	Reduced	Varies
PT/aPTT	Prolonged	Normal
Thrombin time	Prolonged	Normal to slightly prolonged
Fibrinogen	Reduced	Normal
Factor V	Reduced	Normal
FVIII	Reduced	Normal
Fibrin degradation products	Elevated	Elevated
D-dimer	Elevated	Elevated

Table 15.16 Blood products administered as supportive care in DIC

Packed red blood cells (PRBCs)	Anemia 1 unit of PRBC will increase Hgb 1 g/dL and hematocrit 3% points
Fresh frozen plasma	Bleeding in individuals with coagulation factor deficiencies Replacement is 10–20 mg/kg to raise the level of any factor including fibrinogen by 30%
Cryoprecipitate	Bleeding patients with acquired hypofibrinogenemia Increase in plasma fibrinogen 1 unit of cryoprecipitate per 10 kg of body weight will be 50 mg/dL
Platelets	Indicated for bleeding due to severe thrombocytopenia 1 unit of apherised platelets will increase platelet count 30 K/μL in an average sized adult

Table 15.17 Algorithm for diagnosis of DIC

Platelet count
$>100 \times 10^9$/L = 0 $<100 \times 10^9$/L = 1 $<50 \times 10^9$/L = 2
Level of fibrin markers
No increase = 0 Increase but <5× upper limit of normal = 2 Strong increase (≥upper limit of normal) = 3
Prolonged prothrombin time
<3 s = 0 ≥3 to 6 s = 1 ≥6 s = 2
Fibrinogen level
>1.0 g/L = 0 ≤1.0 g/L = 1

contraindicated since blockade of the fibrinolytic system may increase the risk of thrombotic complications. There is no data to support the use of prothrombin complex concentrates in patients with DIC.

Thrombosis is common in patients with infection-related DIC, and they may manifest digital gangrene in digits of hands and feet. Treatment with heparin is appropriate in these cases although the use of prophylactic anticoagulation is not well established. Overall, the use of anticoagulation is generally agreed upon if the patient has acute thrombosis and thrombocytopenia is mild to moderate (>50 K/μL).

The mortality of DIC is highly dependent on the degree of coagulation impairment as well as the treatability of the underlying condition.

Useful Tools

ISTH developed a simple scoring system for the diagnosis of DIC based on laboratory data including platelet count, fibrinogen, coagulation studies, and fibrin degradation products [38]. (Table 15.17).

References

1. Arnold DM, Patriquin CJ, Nazy I. Thrombotic microangiopathies: a general approach to diagnosis and management. CMAJ. 2017;189(4):E153–9.
2. Scully M, Hunt BJ, Benjamin S, Liesner R, Rose P, Peyvandi F, Cheung B, Machin SJ, British Committee for Standards in Haematology. Guidelines on the diagnosis and management of thrombotic thrombocytopenic purpura and other thrombotic microangiopathies. Br J Haematol. 2012;158(3):323–35.
3. Koshy AG, Freed JA. Clinical features of vitamin B12 deficiency mimicking thrombotic microangiopathy. Br J Haematol. 2020;191(5):938–41.
4. Bendapudi PK, Hurwitz S, Fry A, Marques MB, Waldo SW, Li A, Sun L, Upadhyay V, Hamdan A, Brunner AM, et al. Derivation and external validation of the PLASMIC score for rapid assessment of adults with thrombotic microangiopathies: a cohort study. Lancet Haematol. 2017;4(4):e157–64.
5. Bendapudi PK, Upadhyay V, Sun L, Marques MB, Makar RS. Clinical scoring systems in thrombotic microangiopathies. Semin Thromb Hemost. 2017;43(5):540–8.
6. Zheng XL, Vesely SK, Cataland SR, Coppo P, Geldziler B, Iorio A, Matsumoto M, Mustafa RA, Pai M, Rock G, et al. ISTH guidelines for the diagnosis of thrombotic thrombocytopenic purpura. J Thromb Haemost. 2020;18(10):2486–95.
7. Scully M, Cataland SR, Peyvandi F, Coppo P, Knobl P, Kremer Hovinga JA, Metjian A, de la Rubia J, Pavenski K, Callewaert F, et al. Caplacizumab treatment for acquired thrombotic thrombocytopenic purpura. N Engl J Med. 2019;380(4):335–46.
8. Mazepa MA, Masias C, Chaturvedi S. How targeted therapy disrupts the treatment paradigm for acquired TTP: the risks, benefits, and unknowns. Blood. 2019;134(5):415–20.
9. Joly BS, Coppo P, Veyradier A. Thrombotic thrombocytopenic purpura. Blood. 2017;129(21):2836–46.
10. Chaturvedi S, Abbas H, McCrae KR. Increased morbidity during long-term follow-up of survivors of thrombotic thrombocytopenic purpura. Am J Hematol. 2015;90(10):E208.
11. George JN. TTP: long-term outcomes following recovery. Hematology Am Soc Hematol Educ Program. 2018;2018(1):548–52.
12. Han B, Page EE, Stewart LM, Deford CC, Scott JG, Schwartz LH, Perdue JJ, Terrell DR, Vesely SK, George JN. Depression and cognitive impairment following recovery from thrombotic thrombocytopenic purpura. Am J Hematol. 2015;90(8):709–14.
13. Chakravarty EF, Murray ER, Kelman A, Farmer P. Pregnancy outcomes after maternal exposure to rituximab. Blood. 2011;117(5):1499–506.
14. Cuker A, Arepally GM, Chong BH, Cines DB, Greinacher A, Gruel Y, Linkins LA, Rodner SB, Selleng S, Warkentin TE, et al. American Society of Hematology 2018 guidelines for management of venous thromboembolism: heparin-induced thrombocytopenia. Blood Adv. 2018;2(22):3360–92.
15. Cuker A, Cines DB. How I treat heparin-induced thrombocytopenia. Blood. 2012;119(10):2209–18.
16. Warkentin TE, Kelton JG. Delayed-onset heparin-induced thrombocytopenia and thrombosis. Ann Intern Med. 2001;135(7):502–6.
17. Greinacher A, Selleng K, Warkentin TE. Autoimmune heparin-induced thrombocytopenia. J Thromb Haemost. 2017;15(11):2099–114.
18. Warkentin TE, Basciano PA, Knopman J, Bernstein RA. Spontaneous heparin-induced thrombocytopenia syndrome: 2 new cases and a proposal for defining this disorder. Blood. 2014;123(23):3651–4.
19. Schultz NH, Sorvoll IH, Michelsen AE, Munthe LA, Lund-Johansen F, Ahlen MT, Wiedmann M, Aamodt AH, Skattor TH, Tjonnfjord GE, et al. Thrombosis and thrombocytopenia after ChAdOx1 nCoV-19 vaccination. N Engl J Med. 2021;384(22):2124–30.

20. Cuker A, Gimotty PA, Crowther MA, Warkentin TE. Predictive value of the 4Ts scoring system for heparin-induced thrombocytopenia: a systematic review and meta-analysis. Blood. 2012;120(20):4160–7.
21. Warkentin TE, Sheppard JI, Moore JC, Sigouin CS, Kelton JG. Quantitative interpretation of optical density measurements using PF4-dependent enzyme-immunoassays. J Thromb Haemost. 2008;6(8):1304–12.
22. Warkentin TE. Platelet count monitoring and laboratory testing for heparin-induced thrombocytopenia. Arch Pathol Lab Med. 2002;126(11):1415–23.
23. Hook KM, Abrams CS. Treatment options in heparin-induced thrombocytopenia. Curr Opin Hematol. 2010;17(5):424–31.
24. Warkentin TE, Pai M, Linkins LA. Direct oral anticoagulants for treatment of HIT: update of Hamilton experience and literature review. Blood. 2017;130(9):1104–13.
25. Shatzel JJ, Crapster-Pregont M, Deloughery TG. Non-vitamin K antagonist oral anticoagulants for heparin-induced thrombocytopenia. A systematic review of 54 reported cases. Thromb Haemost. 2016;116(2):397–400.
26. Rodeghiero F, Stasi R, Gernsheimer T, Michel M, Provan D, Arnold DM, Bussel JB, Cines DB, Chong BH, Cooper N, et al. Standardization of terminology, definitions and outcome criteria in immune thrombocytopenic purpura of adults and children: report from an international working group. Blood. 2009;113(11):2386–93.
27. Lambert MP, Gernsheimer TB. Clinical updates in adult immune thrombocytopenia. Blood. 2017;129(21):2829–35.
28. Neunert C, Terrell DR, Arnold DM, Buchanan G, Cines DB, Cooper N, Cuker A, Despotovic JM, George JN, Grace RF, et al. American Society of Hematology 2019 guidelines for immune thrombocytopenia. Blood Adv. 2019;3(23):3829–66.
29. Cines DB, Bussel JB. How I treat idiopathic thrombocytopenic purpura (ITP). Blood. 2005;106(7):2244–51.
30. Cooper N. State of the art—how I manage immune thrombocytopenia. Br J Haematol. 2017;177(1):39–54.
31. George JN. Management of immune thrombocytopenia—something old, something new. N Engl J Med. 2010;363(20):1959–61.
32. Care A, Pavord S, Knight M, Alfirevic Z. Severe primary autoimmune thrombocytopenia in pregnancy: a national cohort study. BJOG. 2018;125(5):604–12.
33. Levi M, Scully M. How I treat disseminated intravascular coagulation. Blood. 2018;131(8):845–54.
34. Levi M, Ten Cate H. Disseminated intravascular coagulation. N Engl J Med. 1999;341(8):586–92.
35. Gando S, Nanzaki S, Kemmotsu O. Disseminated intravascular coagulation and sustained systemic inflammatory response syndrome predict organ dysfunctions after trauma: application of clinical decision analysis. Ann Surg. 1999;229(1):121–7.
36. Sibai BM, Ramadan MK, Usta I, Salama M, Mercer BM, Friedman SA. Maternal morbidity and mortality in 442 pregnancies with hemolysis, elevated liver enzymes, and low platelets (HELLP syndrome). Am J Obstet Gynecol. 1993;169(4):1000–6.
37. Gilbert WM, Danielsen B. Amniotic fluid embolism: decreased mortality in a population-based study. Obstet Gynecol. 1999;93(6):973–7.
38. Taylor FB Jr, Toh CH, Hoots WK, Wada H, Levi M, Scientific Subcommittee on Disseminated Intravascular Coagulation (DIC) of the International Society on Thrombosis and Haemostasis (ISTH). Towards definition, clinical and laboratory criteria, and a scoring system for disseminated intravascular coagulation. Thromb Haemost. 2001;86(5):1327–30.

Chapter 16
Erythrocytosis

Diana De Oliveira and Gustavo Rivero

Case Demonstration

A 58-year-old male patient presents to his primary care physician with fatigue, day-time sleepiness, and recurrent headaches for the last 3 months. Past medical history was significant for type 2 diabetes and obesity (body mass index [BMI] of 32 kg/m^2). His wife reports that he snores loudly at night. Laboratory evaluation shows hemoglobin of 21 g/dL, elevated white blood cell count of 12,200/mm^3, and platelets of 320,000/mm^3. Pulse oximetry shows normal saturation. Further evaluation demonstrated increased erythropoietin level of 42 IU/L (normal levels 5–35 IU/L) and normal ferritin (200 ng/mL). Polysomnography showed a markedly increased apnea-hypopnea index of 47.2 (normal level < 5). He was diagnosed with severe obstructive sleep apnea (OSA).

Definitions

- *Erythrocytosis*: Increase in hemoglobin (Hgb) or hematocrit (Hct) greater-than-two-standard-deviation increase adjusted by sex, race, and altitude. It is defined by World Health Organization as a hemoglobin and hematocrit levels of >16.5 g/dL and 49%, respectively, in males and 16 g/dL and 48% in females.
- *Polycythemia*: Increase number of any hematopoietic cell in blood.

D. De Oliveira (✉)
Baylor College of Medicine, Baylor St Luke's Medical Center, Houston, TX, USA
e-mail: Diana.deoliveiragomes@utsouthwestern.edu

G. Rivero
Lombardi Cancer Institute, Georgetown University School of Medicine, Washington, DC, USA

© The Author(s), under exclusive license to Springer Nature Switzerland AG 2024
G. Rivero, I. R. Sosa (eds.), *Consulting Hematology and Oncology Handbook*, https://doi.org/10.1007/978-3-031-75810-2_16

- *Polycythemia Vera (PV)*: myeloproliferative neoplastic disorder caused in 98% of cases by a JAK2 (Janus kinase 2) mutation, which determines a constitutively active protein that drives increased production of RBC, white blood cells, and platelets. The most common are JAK2-V617F (95%) or exon 12 mutations (3%).

Absolute erythrocytosis is present when the red cell mass is greater than 125% of the predicted value for sex and body mass. It is important to distinguish absolute from **relative erythrocytosis**, which is usually caused by contraction of plasma volume, but without a real increase in RBC mass. Relative erythrocytosis is the result of any condition that reduces plasma volume, such as gastrointestinal fluid loss or diuretic use. Furthermore, it has been associated with obesity, alcohol excess, smoking, and hypertension [1].

Erythropoiesis involves the proliferation, differentiation, and maturation of hematopoietic stem cells into RBC. It is regulated in the bone marrow mostly by erythropoietin (EPO), a peptide hormone produced in specialized peritubular fibroblast cells of the kidney under the regulation of Hypoxia Inducible Factor (HIF) transcription family. Binding of Epo to its receptor (EpoR) produces autophosphorylation of the receptor-associated tyrosine kinase JAK2, which activates the signal transducer and activator of transcription protein 5 (STAT5). STAT5 homodimerizes and translocates to the nucleus to affect gene transcription, enhancing proliferation and reducing apoptosis of erythroid progenitors [2]. Other cytokines, such as interleukin (IL)-1, IL-3, IL-6, granulocyte-macrophage colony-stimulating factor (GM-CSF), and stem cell factor (SCF), also regulate the process, where multipotent hematopoietic stem cells differentiate into unipotent erythroid progenitor called proerythroblast. Further differentiation involves the maturation of the cell into different stages: erythroblasts, normoblasts, and reticulocytes. Finally, the reticulocytes are released into bloodstream where they become mature RBC in up to 2 days (Fig. 16.1) [3].

According to the pathogenic mechanism, the increase in RBC is categorized as primary (clonal) or secondary (non-clonal). Primary erythrocytosis is due to a mutational defect in the erythroid progenitor cell lineage (usually JAK2 mutation) and associated with suppressed endogenous EPO level. Secondary erythrocytosis results

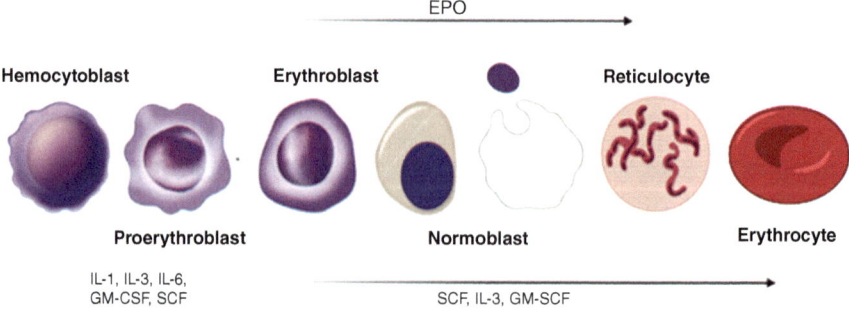

Fig. 16.1 The regulation pathway of erythropoiesis

from medullary response to increased EPO or other growth factors, caused by an acquired (hypoxia from respiratory or cardiac disease, renal disorders, among others) or hereditary conditions (high-oxygen affinity hemoglobins, erythropoietin receptor mutations, and alterations in oxygen-sensing molecular pathways). A less common cause of erythrocytosis is Chuvash polycythemia, which is a hereditary condition characterized by an increased level of HIF-1 and HIF-2 and upregulation of the hypoxic response even when oxygen levels are normal. When no etiology is identified, erythrocytosis is termed idiopathic (Fig. 16.2). In our previously described case, the patient has an increase in RBC due to hypoxia caused by OSA. His polysomnography showed a markedly increased apnea-hypopnea index of 47.2 (normal level < 5). Respiratory hypoxia is the most common cause of secondary erythrocytosis. It is observed in 2–8% of patients with OSA.

Clinical Context and Manifestations

Many patients with erythrocytosis are asymptomatic, or they may complain of non-specific symptoms associated with an increase in blood viscosity. Symptoms of hyperviscosity include chest and abdominal pain, myalgia and weakness, fatigue, headache, blurred vision or symptoms to suggest amaurosis fugax, and paresthesia, among others. Patients with PV or other myeloproliferative neoplasms can present

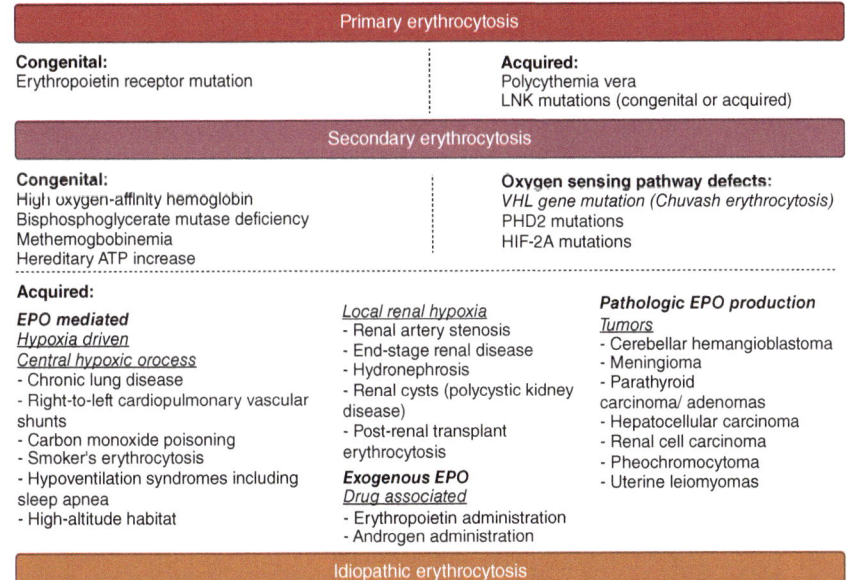

Fig. 16.2 Classification of erythrocytosis. (Adapted from [1, 4] "Created with BioRender.com")

with two specific symptoms: pruritus and erythromelalgia. Diagnosis criteria of PV are depicted in Table 16.1.

In a patient presenting with high RBC, a history and physical examination should be completed to rule out relative erythrocytosis. A detailed medical and drug history includes smoking status, alcohol consumption, and use of medication such as diuretics, testosterone, and anabolic drugs. Additionally, possible causes of hypoxia such as residing in a place with high altitude, symptoms of OSA, COPD, and cardiac or renal disease should be investigated.

Physical examination can give clues to detect possible causes of secondary polycythemia. In cases of chronic hypoxia, cyanosis and clubbing can be seen. Abdominal examination can detect the presence of organomegaly or erythropoietin-producing intraabdominal tumors as paraneoplastic manifestation (e.g., hepatocellular or renal cell carcinoma). In cases of renal artery stenosis, a bruit may be heard on auscultation [5].

A diagnosis approach for erythrocytosis is proposed in Fig. 16.3. In cases of persistent asymptomatic erythrocytosis with low serum EPO levels, and without PV mutations, an EPOR germline mutation evaluation is recommended. This condition is characterized by evidence of an autosomal dominant condition where family members exhibit history of erythrocytosis and are usually asymptomatic. Moreover, if the EPO level is normal or elevated, other group of diseases such as high-affinity hemoglobin or germline mutations in genes as HIF or VHL can be considered [7].

Laboratory Investigation

Initial

- Complete blood count, repeated at least 1 week after the first assessment, to determine if the rise in RBC is transient. PV may be associated with expansion of all myeloid elements of the bone marrow, so leukocytosis and thrombocytosis may be observed.
- Serum EPO levels.
- Blood smear.

Table 16.1 2016 World Health Organization criteria for Polycythemia vera [6]

Diagnosis criteria
1. All 3 major criteria
2. First 2 major criteria + 1 minor criteria
Major criteria
1. Hemoglobin >16.5 g/dL(men)/>16.0 g/dL (women) or hematocrit >49% (men)/48% (women)
2. BM biopsy showing trilineage myeloproliferation with pleomorphic megakaryocytes
3. Presence of JAK2 or JAK2 exon 12 mutation
Minor criteria
1. Subnormal serum erythropoietin level

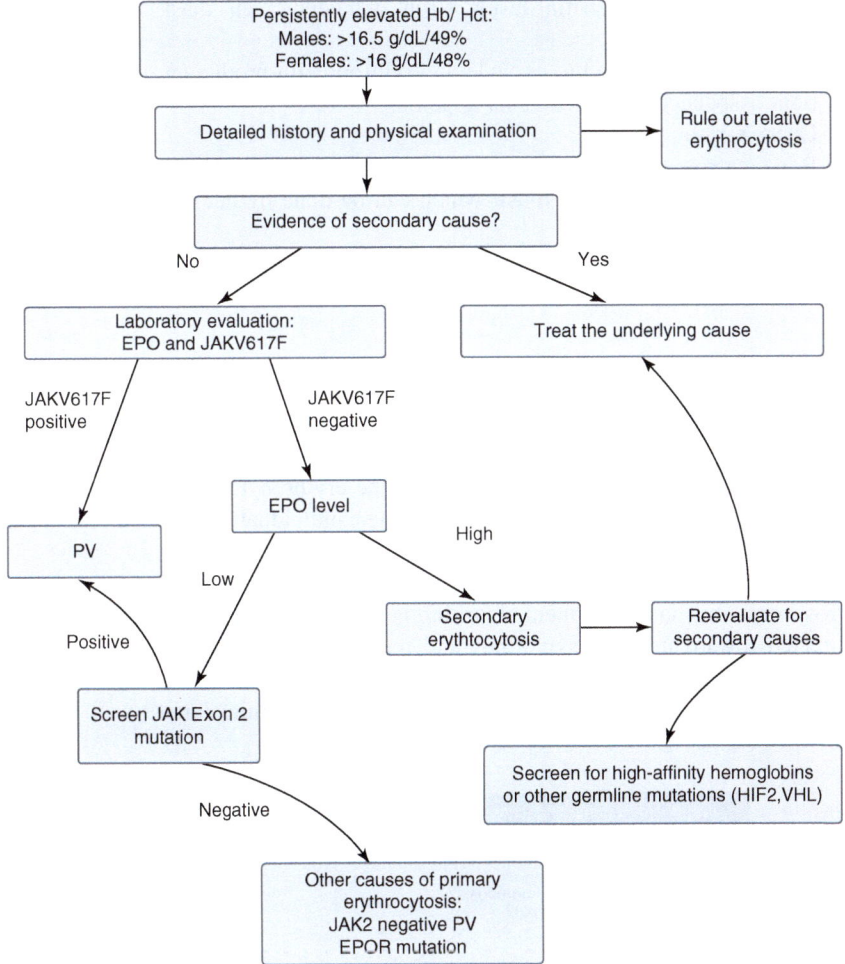

Fig. 16.3 Diagnosis approach of erythrocytosis. (Adapted from [1, 8] "Created with BioRender.com")

- JAK2 assessment in patients with no secondary cause of erythrocytosis or in whom PV is suspected.
- Oxygen saturation: <92% on room air by pulse oximetry suggest a secondary cause. Some causes of secondary hypoxia present with normal oxygen saturation (OSA, high-oxygen-affinity hemoglobins, or carboxyhemoglobinemia in smokers).

Depending on the assessment, further tests are needed to confirm the specific cause:

- Renal and liver function test.

- Iron studies and ferritin levels (iron deficiency can mask the degree of erythrocytosis).
- Abdominal ultrasound to exclude an erythropoietin-producing tumor or conditions associated with local renal hypoxia.
- Chest X-ray.
- Bone marrow aspirate.
- Measurement of red cell mass, which can be done by nuclear isotope dilution (not widely available).
- Other tests including polysomnography, EPO receptor gene analysis, and VHL analysis, among others.

Management

First, it is important to assess the cause of the erythrocytosis. Intervention is not always indicated; the decision to treat is often individualized after a risk-benefit assessment.

Patients with PV have increased risk of thrombosis and progression to myelofibrosis or leukemia. A treatment algorithm is depicted in Fig. 16.4. The treatment is directed toward mitigate symptoms and reduces the risk of arterial and venous thromboembolism. In patients with PV, the risk of arterial thrombus is higher than venous suggesting that low-dose aspirin should be administered to all patients.

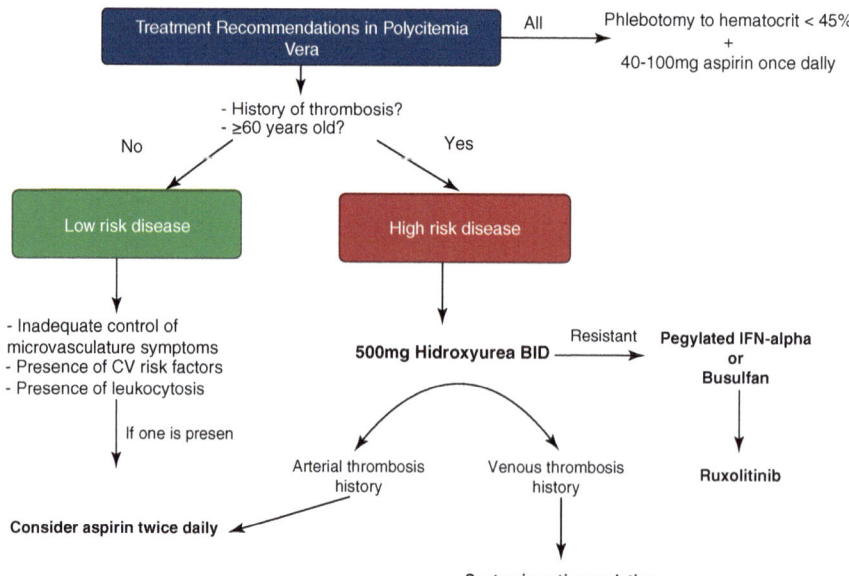

Fig. 16.4 Treatment PV. (Adapted from [10] "Created with BioRender.com")

Additionally, the hematocrit should be maintained below 45%, which is achieved pharmacologically or by phlebotomy. The CYTO-PV trial demonstrated significant lower rate of cardiovascular death and major thrombosis in patients achieving Hct <45% [9]. PV patients require long-term follow-up to monitor signs of disease progression to the myelofibrotic stage. When the risk for thrombosis is high, cytoreduction is considered, most commonly with hydroxyurea or interferon alpha, (Fig. 16.4). In patients who are resistant to this treatment, the JAK inhibitor ruxolitinib can be used [8].

In cases of secondary polycythemia, the most important step is the correction of the precipitating factor. There is no definitive evidence that there is an increased risk of thromboembolism in patients with secondary erythrocytosis; therefore, the treatment is evaluated according to the presence of symptoms attributable to high hematocrit and/or the history of thrombosis; as shown in Fig. 16.5, phlebotomy is not routinely recommended.

In patients diagnosed with OSA, a pulmonary disease specialist should evaluate the need for continuous positive airway pressure (CPAP) or BiPAP. Additionally, in patients with hypoxic lung disease, long-term oxygen therapy should be considered, including nocturnal oxygenation with noninvasive ventilation. The development of erythrocytosis in patients with hypoxic lung disease is related with an increased risk of cor pulmonale and poor median survival. Smoking cessation should be strongly advised [4].

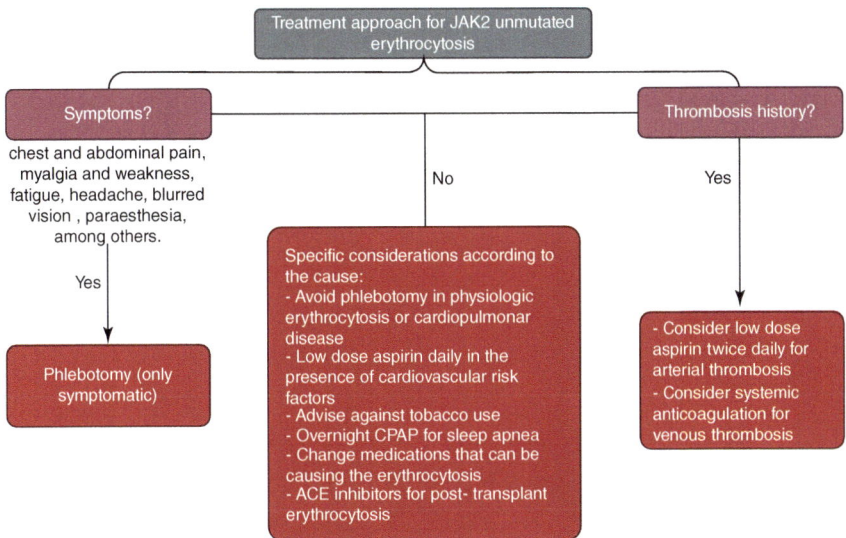

Fig. 16.5 Treatment approach for JAK2 unmutated erythrocytosis. (Adapted from [11] "Created with BioRender.com")

Specific Considerations

In cases of hereditary erythrocytosis with normal or elevated EPO, venous p50 measurement (oxygen tension at which Hgb is 50% saturated) could be performed. A venous p50 < 24 mmHg suggests a diagnosis of high-oxygen affinity Hgb and defective 2,3 BPG mutase causing 2,3 BPG deficiency or methemoglobinemia. Meanwhile, a normal venous p50 should raise suspicion of mutations in the oxygen-sensing pathway (VHL, PHD2, HIF2A) [11].

References

1. Mithoowani S, Laureano M, Crowther MA, Hillis CM. Investigation and management of erythrocytosis. Can Med Assoc J. 2020;192(32):E913–e8.
2. Patnaik MM, Tefferi A. The complete evaluation of erythrocytosis: congenital and acquired. Leukemia. 2009;23(5):834–44.
3. Gašperšič J, Kristan A, Kunej T, Zupan IP, Debeljak N. Erythrocytosis: genes and pathways involved in disease development. Blood Transfus. 2021;19(6):518–32.
4. McMullin MF. Investigation and management of erythrocytosis. Curr Hematol Malig Rep. 2016;11(5):342–7.
5. Haider MZAF. Secondary polycythemia. In: StatPearls [Internet]. Treasure Island, FL: StatPearls; 2021. https://www.ncbi.nlm.nih.gov/books/NBK562233/?report=classic.
6. Barbui T, Thiele J, Gisslinger H, Kvasnicka HM, Vannucchi AM, Guglielmelli P. The 2016 WHO classification and diagnostic criteria for myeloproliferative neoplasms: document summary and in-depth discussion. Blood Cancer J. 2018;8(2):15.
7. Pozdnyakova O. Erythrocytosis. In: Wang SA, Hasserjian RP, editors. Diagnosis of blood and bone marrow disorders. Cham: Springer International; 2018. p. 243–56.
8. Lee G, Arcasoy MO. The clinical and laboratory evaluation of the patient with erythrocytosis. Eur J Intern Med. 2015;26(5):297–302.
9. Assi TB, Baz E. Current applications of therapeutic phlebotomy. Blood Transfus. 2014;12 Suppl 1(Suppl 1):s75–83.
10. Tefferi A, Barbui T. Polycythemia vera and essential thrombocythemia: 2021 update on diagnosis, risk-stratification and management. Am J Hematol. 2020;95(12):1599–613.
11. Gangat N, Szuber N, Pardanani A, Tefferi A. JAK2 unmutated erythrocytosis: current diagnostic approach and therapeutic views. Leukemia. 2021;35(8):2166–81.

Chapter 17
Anemia

Ishara Lareef and Iberia Romina Sosa

Case

A 52-year-old man with a history of untreated diabetes and hypertension presents to clinic for evaluation of worsening fatigue over the past several months. His labs are pertinent for a hemoglobin of 8.2 g/dL, an MCV of 90 fL, and a GFR of 20 mL/min/1.73 m². Iron studies are suggestive of iron deficiency anemia. It is discussed with him that his fatigue is likely due to anemia related to his renal disease. Treatment is initiated for his chronic conditions, nephrotoxins are removed from his medication list, and he is started on parenteral iron infusions and epoetin alfa. He returns to the clinic in 3 months with an increased hemoglobin to 11.5 g/dL and his fatigue is significantly improved.

Clinical Context

Anemia is defined functionally as insufficient red blood cell (RBC) mass to adequately deliver oxygen to peripheral tissues. This may be due to a reduced number of RBCs circulating in the blood or to a reduced amount of hemoglobin. Anemia is typically quantified as a hemoglobin less than 14 g/dL for men or 12 g/dL for women [1].

I. Lareef
Temple University, Philadelphia, PA, USA
e-mail: ishara.lareef@tuhs.temple.edu

I. R. Sosa (✉)
Department of Hematology/Oncology, Fox Chase Cancer Center, Philadelphia, PA, USA
e-mail: iberia.sosa@fccc.edu

© The Author(s), under exclusive license to Springer Nature
Switzerland AG 2024
G. Rivero, I. R. Sosa (eds.), *Consulting Hematology and Oncology Handbook*,
https://doi.org/10.1007/978-3-031-75810-2_17

About 27% of the world population, or about two billion people, suffer from anemia [2]. Anemia has various etiologies, from nutritional deficiency to congenital and acquired enzyme deficiency or membranopathy. The clinical context of common disorders causing anemia will be discussed here and will be delineated by mean corpuscular volume (MCV), a useful laboratory marker that is discussed in further detail in the section "Laboratory Evaluation."

Low MCV < 80 fL

Iron deficiency anemia results from low dietary iron intake, iron malabsorption (e.g., celiac disease), or chronic blood loss. The development of iron deficiency is largely dependent on the baseline iron stores. Normal body iron content in an adult is approximately 3–4 g with the bulk of that found in the circulating RBCs (Fig. 17.1). Additional iron can be found in myoglobin, enzymes, and proteins responsible for iron storage (ferritin) and transport (transferrin).

Iron deficiency typically occurs in different stages, defined by rapidity of depletion of iron storage and subsequently of iron available for hemoglobin synthesis. Often, iron stores can be completely depleted without evidence of anemia. Individuals can feel fatigued despite absence of anemia if iron stores are low. Further loss of iron from a "labile" pool derived from hemoglobin turnover will ultimately

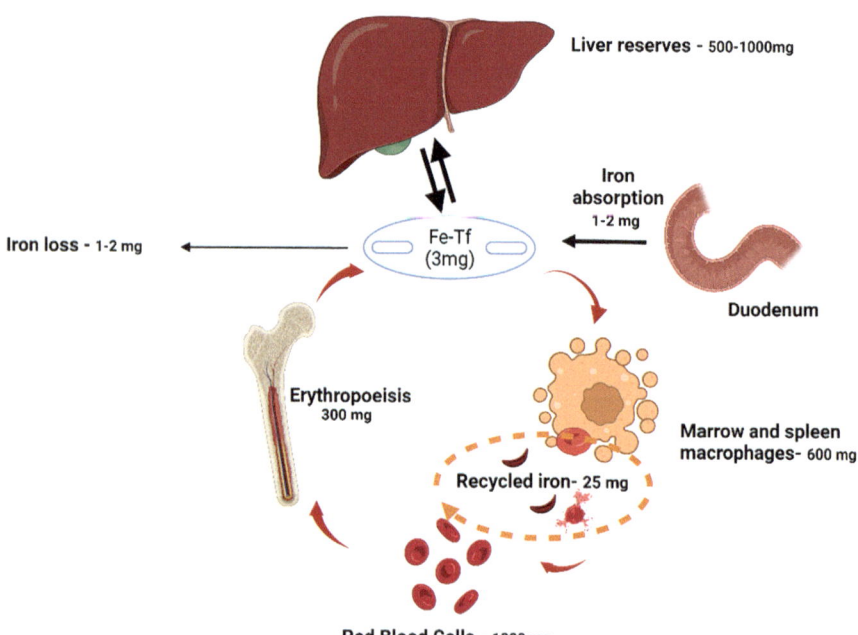

Fig. 17.1 Iron content in the body

lead to anemia and eventually microcytosis [3]. Useful laboratory tests include the serum iron level; total iron binding capacity (TIBC) which measures the total amount of iron bound by proteins in the blood; and ferritin, which reflects total body iron storage (Tables 17.1 and 17.2) [3, 4]. It is important to note that both transferrin and ferritin are synthesized by the liver, but the former is a negative acute phase reaction (levels fall in inflammation) and the latter is a positive acute phase reactant (levels rise in inflammation).

Thalassemias are inherited conditions due to defective synthesis in one or more of the polypeptide chains comprising hemoglobin. Thalassemias are further divided into alpha and beta thalassemia, depending on which of the chains is defective. Alpha and beta thalassemia are then further defined by the number of missing alleles or genotype, respectively. Alpha thalassemias are due to mutated alleles in the genes HBA1 and HBA2 which are inherited in an autosomal recessive fashion [5] (Table 17.3). Reduced production of alpha globin is compensated for by excess beta globin chains which then form unstable tetramers which cannot bind oxygen appropriately. Beta thalassemias are due to mutated alleles in the HBB gene and are similarly inherited in an autosomal recessive fashion. These alleles are characterized as B^+ if partially functional or B^0 if non-functional [5] (Table 17.4). There are additionally rare combination hemoglobinopathies involving the delta chains, hemoglobin

Table 17.1 Laboratory parameters in iron deficiency

	Normal	Iron deficiency without anemia	Iron deficiency with anemia
Hemoglobin	Men:14–17.5 g/dL Women: 12.0 to 15.0 g/dL	Men:14–17.5 g/dL Women: 12.0 to 15.0 g/dL	Low; Hgb <12 g/dL
MCV	Normal	Normal	Low
Serum iron	Normal	Normal	Low
TIBC	Normal	Normal to high	High
Ferritin	40 to 200 ng/mL	<40 ng/mL	<20 ng/mL
Transferrin saturation	20–50%	20%	<15%

Table 17.2 Expected iron studies in microcytic anemia [3]

Etiology	Serum iron	TIBC	Ferritin	Transferrin saturation
Iron deficiency	↓	↑	↓	↓
Thalassemia	↑	↓	↑	↑
Anemia of chronic disease[a]	↓	↓	Normal/↑	Normal/↓

[a]MCV may be low or in the normal range

Table 17.3 Alpha thalassemia subtypes [5]

Type of alpha thalassemia	Number of missing alleles	Phenotype
Silent carrier	1	Asymptomatic (no anemia)
Alpha thalassemia trait	2	Mild anemia
Hemoglobin H disease	3	Mild–moderate anemia
Hydrops fetalis	4	Intrauterine fetal demise or shortly after birth

Table 17.4 Beta thalassemia subtypes [5]

Type of beta thalassemia	Genotypes	Phenotype
Beta thalassemia trait Thalassemia minor	B/B^0 B/B^+	Mild anemia
Beta thalassemia intermedia	B^+/B^+ B^+/B^0	Mild–moderate anemia Can have extramedullary hematopoiesis Iron overload May need occasional transfusions
Thalassemia major	B^0/B^0	Severe anemia Transfusion dependence Splenomegaly Iron overload Extramedullary hematopoiesis

S, and hemoglobin C. Due to the ineffective erythropoiesis in thalassemia, these individuals may exhibit hemolytic anemia [5] and iron overload [6].

Normal MCV (80–100) fL

Anemia of chronic disease (ACD), or anemia of inflammation, can occur in individuals with infectious, inflammatory, autoimmune, or neoplastic diseases that persist for an extended duration. This type of anemia will characteristically show low transferrin saturation and normal to elevated ferritin levels. ACD is a cytokine-mediated process, in which inflammation triggers the release of TNF, IL-1, IL-6, and interferons. These cytokines drive iron metabolism disturbances due to increase in the acute phase reactant hepcidin, shortened lifespan of erythrocytes, and reduced erythropoietin release resulting in impaired marrow response [7]. ACD is characterized by functional iron deficiency, where iron storage is not available for RBC production. Treatment of anemia is directed at the underlying chronic disease [7].

Anemia is associated with chronic kidney disease, which is defined as when creatinine clearance falls below 60 mL/min/1.73 m^2 BSA for 3 months or more [8]. The degree of anemia tends to correlate with the degree of renal failure. This anemia is driven by reduced renal secretion of erythropoietin, shortened lifespan of erythrocytes, and further suppression of marrow response due to buildup of uremic toxins and secondary hyperparathyroidism. Uremia can also contribute to anemia through hemolysis. Iron deficiency is common in patients with renal insufficiency and is a result of increased hepcidin which blocks intestinal absorption of iron and release of stored iron [9]. Treatment is with epoetin alpha and with iron supplementation [9].

Hemolytic anemia occurs when RBC is unable to maintain an intact structure, leading to reduced lifespan and increased turnover culminating in a compensatory increase in RBC by the bone marrow [10]. An inability of the marrow to compensate for the diminished RBC lifespan leads to anemia, which can be intravascular and/or extravascular based on site of RBC demise. Symptoms of hemolytic anemia include fatigue and dyspnea as in other anemias but is also characterized by pigmented gallstones and/or jaundice due to the accumulation of bilirubin. Both non-congenital hemolytic anemias and congenital hemolytic anemias are further described below.

Acquired Hemolytic Anemia

Autoimmune hemolytic anemias (AIHA) are characterized by the presence of auto-antibodies which bind the erythrocyte and facilitate RBC destruction. They are classified by the temperature at which the antibodies are active, as either cold, warm, or mixed activity antibodies. Cold active antibodies typically are IgM, fix complement, and lead to intravascular hemolysis at below normal cold body temperature. Cold agglutinin disease (CAD) can be primary or idiopathic, or secondary to mycoplasma pneumoniae infection, infectious mononucleosis, autoimmune disorders, or B-cell lymphoproliferative disorders [11].

Warm active antibodies are more often IgG, may or may not fix complement, and cause anemia by splenic clearance of erythrocytes. Like CAD, warm autoimmune hemolytic anemia can be primary or idiopathic, or due to secondary causes including lymphoproliferative disorders (e.g., lymphoma or CLL), rheumatoid disorders (e.g., systemic lupus erythematosus (SLE)), non-lymphoid neoplasms (e.g., ovarian tumors), chronic inflammatory disorders (e.g., ulcerative colitis), and drugs (e.g., a-methyldopa) [12]. Diagnosis of both cold and warm AIHA is facilitated by the Coomb's test [13].

Paroxysmal nocturnal hemoglobinuria (PNH) is a rare, acquired disorder of hematopoietic stem cells and their cellular progeny, exhibiting reduced or absent glycosylphosphatidylinositol (GPI) resulting from an acquired defect of the PIG-A gene (Fig. 17.2a). Loss of GPI-linked complement inhibitors CD55 and CD59 leads to reduced protection from complement-mediated destruction [14] (Fig. 17.2b). This disease entity may present with general signs of hemolysis as listed above, with systemic vasoconstriction, venous thromboembolism (VTE), and pancytopenia. Laboratory workup will be consistent with evidence of hemolysis with reticulocytosis, elevated LDH and low haptoglobin but negative for direct Coombs test. It can be seen as an isolated etiology but may also occur in aplastic anemia or

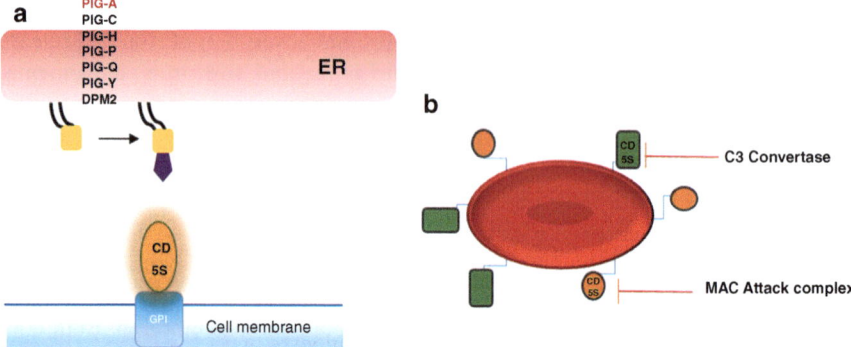

Fig. 17.2 Pathophysiology of PNH. (**a**) PNH is the result of expansion of hematopoietic stem cell with severe deficiency or absence of GPI as a result of a somatic mutation in the PIG-A gene, which is responsible for the first step in the synthesis of GPI anchor that attaches a subset of proteins to the cell surface [14]. (**b**) An inability to anchor complement inhibitory proteins, CD55 and CD59, two GPI-linked proteins result in chronic complement-mediated hemolysis in GPI-deficient RBCs

myelodysplastic syndrome. Complications of PNH can include Budd-Chiari syndrome, acute leukemia, and infections [14].

Congenital Hemolytic Anemias

Hereditary spherocytosis (HS) is the result of mutation(s) in the genes coding for the spectrin (alpha and beta), ankyrin, band-3, or protein 4.2 proteins [15]. These proteins play a role in the erythrocyte membrane. The pathogenic membrane protein variants reduce the level of one or more RBC membrane proteins that link the cytoskeleton to the overlying plasma membrane thereby reducing vertical associations between the cytoskeleton and membrane, leading to microvesiculation and progressive membrane loss [16]. The implications of this are that the erythrocytes are less flexible and do not travel as well in the capillaries due to their shape. They become more susceptible to osmotic and mechanical stressors leading to their destruction. These abnormal erythrocytes are broken down by the spleen and the result is hemolytic anemia. HS is typically inherited in autosomal dominant fashion (75% of cases) and is estimated to affect between 1 in 2000 to 1 in 5000 individuals from Northern Europe and Northern America [17]. Gold standard of diagnosis is the eosin 5′ maleimide test [18], which is described in further detail under the section "Laboratory Testing."

Hereditary elliptocytosis (HE) is similarly a result of mutations in cytoskeletal proteins alpha spectrin (65%), beta spectrin (30%), and protein 4.1 (5%) that result in reduced horizontal associations, in this case leading to elliptoid or oval-shaped erythrocytes [19]. It is typically asymptomatic but can result in a mild or moderate hemolytic anemia with splenomegaly. The true incidence of elliptocytosis is poorly understood, as it is likely that many individuals with this trait are undiagnosed, but estimates range from 1/2000 to 1/4000 individuals worldwide [20].

Glucose-6-phosphate dehydrogenase (G6PD) deficiency is an X-linked recessive disorder that causes hemolytic anemia due to a defective G6PD enzyme and is estimated to affect 400 million individuals globally [21]. G6PD is an enzyme in the pentose phosphate pathway that reduces NADP to NADPH while oxidizing glucose-6-phosphate. The result of this deficiency is a reduced amount of NADPH in the erythrocyte, which results in reduced regeneration of glutathione which then results in a buildup of reactive oxygen species. This impacts erythrocyte membrane integrity and results in hemolysis. Intracellular hemoglobin precipitates, forming "Heinz bodies," the oxidized insoluble hemoglobin, which can be appreciated on evaluation of peripheral blood smear. It can present in the newborn as jaundice in the setting of chronic hemolytic anemia but can also present episodically in those with the deficiency after exposure to an oxidative stressor such as medications, food (e.g., fava beans), or infection [22]. Resolution of symptoms typically occurs 4–7 days after exposure to the stressor, when reticulocyte count increases and newer erythrocytes with higher G6PD activity are present [22]. Several common drugs can precipitate a hemolytic attack in individuals with G6PD deficiency and are summarized in Table 17.5 [21, 23].

Pyruvate kinase deficiency is caused by a mutation of the PKLR gene. Pyruvate kinase (PK) is involved in glycolysis and functions to transfer a phosphate group from phosphenol pyruvate to ADP thereby creating ATP and pyruvate. A deficiency in pyruvate kinase thus results in the inability to create ATP. This is especially relevant for mature erythrocytes, which lack a nucleus and mitochondria and thus rely

Table 17.5 Common drugs implicated in G6PD deficiency exacerbation

Drugs to avoid in G6PD deficiency	Drugs to be used with caution in G6PD deficiency
Dapsone	Acetaminophen
Methylene blye	Aspirin
Flutamide	Antazolinc
Isobutyl nitrite	Chloramphenicol
Niridazole	Chloroquine
Nitrofurantoin	Colchicine
Phenazopyridine	Diphenhydramine
Primaquine	Isoniazid
Rasburicase	Glyburide
Sulfonamides	Benzhexol
	IV vitamin C
	Quinine
	L-Dopa
	Streptomycin
	Sulfacytine
	Sulfadiazine
	Trimethoprim
	Vitamin K
	Tripelennamine

Adapted from Luzatto et al. [23]

on anaerobic glycolysis to generate ATP. A resultant lack in ATP results in cessation of function of sodium potassium ATPase, causing potassium to leak out of the cell, followed by water and ultimately leading to erythrocyte dehydration and hemolysis [24]. Most commonly, the treatment is with blood transfusions.

Aldolase A deficiency is an autosomal recessive disorder of metabolism caused by the deficiency of the aldolase A enzyme which is found in muscle tissue and erythrocytes. This deficiency results in hemolytic anemia and exercise intolerance and may even result in rhabdomyolysis. Similar to that which is described above with pyruvate kinase deficiency, aldolase A deficiency results in hemolysis as it is the enzyme which catabolizes the fourth step of glycolysis; a deficiency in this enzyme thus results in lack of ATP and hemolysis [25].

Sickle cell disease is discussed in depth in Chap. 7. This disease is characterized by the formation of defective hemoglobin S, leading to sickle formation of RBC during episodes of hypoxia and chronic hemolysis [26].

Thalassemia, discussed above in microcytic anemia, has elements of hemolysis and may have laboratory evidence suggestive of this (see Table 17.6).

Hemolytic anemia can be subcategorized by the etiology of hemolysis, that is, whether the hemolysis is "intrinsic", i.e., that the hemolysis is due to a defect in the erythrocyte, or "extrinsic", i.e., that the hemolysis is due to the inappropriate breakdown of normal erythrocytes (Tables 17.7 and 17.8).

High MCV > 100 fL

Macrocytic anemia can be characterized as *megaloblastic* or *nonmegaloblastic*. If megaloblastic, consider impaired DNA synthesis in the erythrocyte, which may be due to B12 or folate deficiency. Both can be caused by poor diet. B12 deficiency can be related to pernicious anemia, where autoantibodies are present against intrinsic

Table 17.6 Laboratory signs of hemolysis (not including peripheral blood smear)

Marker	Description
Haptoglobin	A protein produced by the liver which binds free hemoglobin to reduce its oxidative ability Low level, <25 mg/dL is both sensitive and specific for hemolysis
Lactate dehydrogenase	Nonspecific, implies cellular breakdown, will be increased in hemolysis
Unconjugated (indirect) bilirubin	Heme breakdown product, will be increased in hemolysis
Hemoglobinuria	Urine dipstick positive for heme but no RBCs seen on urine microscopy Typically seen in early intravascular hemolysis
Hemosiderinuria	Hemosiderin is the storage form of hemic iron. It can be found in the urine in the context of proximal tubule cells, which filter hemoglobin Typically seen in late intravascular hemolysis
Urobilinogen	Byproduct of indirect bilirubin breakdown in the gut resulting in excess urobilinogen in the systemic circulation Typically seen in extravascular hemolysis

Table 17.7 Causes of hemolysis

Intrinsic hemolysis	Extrinsic hemolysis
Hemolysis due to a defect within the erythrocyte (by location) – RBC membrane defects: Hereditary spherocytosis, paroxysmal nocturnal hemoglobinuria – Enzyme defects: G6PD deficiency, pyruvate kinase deficiency – Hemoglobinopathies: Sickle cell disease, thalassemia, hemoglobin C disease, hemoglobin Zurich	Inappropriate breakdown of normal erythrocytes: – Mechanical destruction: microangiopathic and macroangiopathic hemolytic anemias – Autoimmune mediated hemolysis – Alloimmune-mediated hemolysis – Immune reaction to an infection (mycoplasma) or tumor (e.g., CLL) – Infections themselves causing destruction (Babesiosis, malaria, bartonella) – Hypersplenism

Table 17.8 Mechanisms of hemolysis [24]

Intravascular hemolysis	Extravascular hemolysis
Erythrocyte contents are released into the vascular system, causing hyperbilirubinemia Etiologies: Complement-mediated hemolysis (e.g., PNH), alloimmune-mediated hemolysis (transfusion reaction, cold agglutinin disease, hemolytic anemia of the newborn), enzyme deficiency (G6PD), macroangiopathic hemolytic anemia (artificial valves), microangiopathic hemolytic anemia (DIC, HUS/TTP, HELLP), toxins (some rattlesnake bites), and oxidative (copper poisoning)	Occurs in the reticuloendothelial system (spleen, liver, marrow, and lymph nodes). Macrophages destroy RBC contents which are therefore not released into the vascular system If extensive, hemosiderin can be deposited into the above organs Etiologies: Antibody mediated (warm and cold agglutinin disease, defects in the RBC (hereditary spherocytosis, elliptocytosis, sickle cell disease, pyruvate kinase deficiency)

Adapted from Noronha et al. [27]

factor; due to altered GI anatomy as can occur in gastric or ileal resection; or due to malabsorption as may occur in small intestinal bowel overgrowth or drug-induced malabsorption [1, 28]. The Schilling test was previously used to diagnose pernicious anemia. Folate deficiency can be related to tropical sprue and jejunal disease and can be in the setting of increased needs during pregnancy [28].

Nonmegaloblastic anemia can be associated with alcohol toxicity, hypothyroidism, liver disease, myelodysplastic syndrome, red cell aplasia, acquired sideroblastic anemia, or hereditary dyserythropoietic anemias. In these cases, reticulocyte count will be normal or decreased. If there is an increased reticulocyte count in a nonmegaloblastic anemia, consider hemorrhagic anemias [5]. Anemia in individuals with hypothyroidism occurs with an estimated prevalence of ~40% [29]. The etiology of anemia is poorly understood, but is thought to involve reduced erythropoietin production, marrow suppression, comorbid autoimmune anemias, or comorbid iron, B12, or folate deficiencies [30].

Clinical Manifestations

Clinical manifestations vary based on the chronicity of the anemia, with sudden, acute drops in hemoglobin causing more severe symptoms, while chronic drops in hemoglobin result in subtle symptoms. General symptoms include the following:

- Shortness of breath, especially with exertion.
- Fatigue and reduced exercise tolerance.
- Palpitations.
- Lightheadedness.

   Exam findings of anemia may include the following:

- Severe anemia can appreciate a loud systolic murmur in the precordium and apical regions thought to be related to relative tricuspid and mitral stenosis due to dilatation of the ventricles greater than the A-V ostia.
- Tachycardia.
- Pallor (best observed in mucous membranes of oropharynx, nail beds, lips, conjunctivae).

   Findings in specific types of anemia may include the following:

- Pernicious anemia: glossitis, early graying of the hair, concavity of the nails, paresthesias, limb pain, and difficulty walking.
- Hemolytic anemias: scleral icterus, jaundice and splenomegaly.

Laboratory Investigation

The initial workup of anemia requires close attention to the complete blood count (CBC), RBC indices, reticulocyte count, and peripheral smear.

   The reticulocyte count is used to assess if there is appropriate marrow response to the anemia. Calculate the absolute reticulocyte count: ARC = % reticulocytes x RBC count

- If the reticulocyte count is increased appropriately, then the marrow is functioning properly, if not, then consider disorders of hypoproliferation or marrow failure.
- If the anemia is associated with reticulocytosis, evaluate for hemolysis (see Table 17.9).
- In patients with low reticulocyte count, evaluate for etiology based on mean corpuscular volume (MCV). MCV normal ranges for adults provided below, but ranges vary based on age for the pediatric population. Additionally, MCV are mean values and as such may represent a combination of etiologies. Differential based on MCV is discussed in detail in the section "Clinical Context."

Table 17.9 Mean corpuscular volume

Definition	MCV range	Etiologies
Microcytic anemia	MCV < 80	Iron deficiency, thalassemia
Normocytic anemia	80 < MCV < 100),	Chronic disease, hemolysis
Macrocytic anemia	MCV >100	Megaloblastic anemia, nonmegaloblastic anemia

Table 17.10 Peripheral blood smear and anemia

Peripheral blood smear findings	Clinical correlation
Schistocyte, helmet cells	Hemolytic disease
Teardrop cells, nucleated RBCs, early WBC precursors, abnormal platelet size/shape	Marrow infiltrative disease
Rouleaux, agglutination	Multiple myeloma Cold agglutinin disease
Dimorphic erythrocytes	Sideroblastic anemia
Oval macrocytes, hypersegmented neutrophils	Macrocytic anemia

- MCHC is helpful in late-stage iron deficiency evaluation, when severe hypochromia may occur.
- RDW, red cell distribution width, assesses the degree of heterogeneity of RBC size. Increased RDW is an early finding of iron deficiency and most megaloblastic anemias.

The peripheral blood smear can be helpful for qualitative assessment, with various shapes and features of erythrocytes providing diagnostic clues (Table 17.10). It can also be useful in assessing variation in RBC diameter (micro/macro/normocytic) and pigmentation (chromia) and can be especially helpful in the case of combined etiologies.

- Normal size of an RBC is the size of a lymphocyte's nucleus; normal area of central pallor is 1/3–1/2 the diameter of an RBC.

Bone marrow biopsy is useful as an adjunct to the peripheral smear. It can be helpful in which marrow failure is suspected: aplastic anemia, myelofibrosis, granulomas (myelophthisic anemias), leukemic, or tumor invasion. Furthermore, a bone marrow biopsy showing ringed sideroblasts can confirm the diagnosis of sideroblastic anemia. Additional laboratory tests (Table 17.11) can assist with identifying the etiology of hemolytic anemia.

Table 17.11 Special laboratory tests may help to identify anemia subtypes

Test name	Utility	Details	Special considerations
Direct Coomb's test/direct antiglobulin test (DAT) (Fig. 17.3) [13]	Determine if anemia is autoimmune mediated (warm vs. cold)	Warm autoimmune hemolytic anemia (IgG+ and C3 +/−) cold agglutinin disease (C3+)	Will be negative in the case of anemias which involve IgA, IgG4, and about 1–10% of AIHA
Osmotic fragility test, acidified glycerol test	Hereditary spherocytosis and elliptocytosis	Spherocytes and elliptocytes rupture in salt and water or glycerol due to increased membrane permeability	Historic test
Eosin 5' maleimide test [18]	Hereditary spherocytosis	Reduced fluorescence in the presence of spherocytes secondary to reduced ability of the eosin 5'maleimide (EMA) dye to bind to the sulfhydryl groups found on band 3 and Rh complex (CD47, RhAG, and Rh polypeptide) on the erythrocyte plasma membrane	Gold standard test for HS may also detect other membranopathies such as hereditary elliptocytosis and hereditary ovalocytosis
Pyruvate kinase enzyme activity [31] PKLR gene sequencing	Pyruvate kinase deficiency	Reduced enzyme activity in deficient state	Gold standard test
G6PD enzyme activity	G6PD deficiency	Reduced enzyme activity in deficient state measured with reduced NADPH generation to screen Confirm with quantitative G6PD assays which measure enzymatic activity [29]	Do not test in the midst of a hemolytic episode since the RBCs with the most severely reduced G6PD will have hemolyzed and new RBC (reticulocytes) typically have normal G6PD activity
Hemoglobin electrophoresis	Sickle cell disease, sickle cell trait, and beta thalassemia	Discern between normal hemoglobin variants and the structurally different variants	Does not assess for alpha thalassemia (must use an alpha gene mutation panel)

Management

Treatment of anemia is targeted at the underlying etiology. For example, nutritional deficiencies are treated with replacement and correction of the underlying etiology (Table 17.12).

For those with iron deficiency due to chronic blood loss, a referral to gynecology or gastroenterology for correction of bleeding source is imperative. In individuals with non-dialysis anemia of CKD, the choice is to treat iron deficiency anemia with IV iron in those with severe iron deficiency (transferrin saturation < 12%), severe

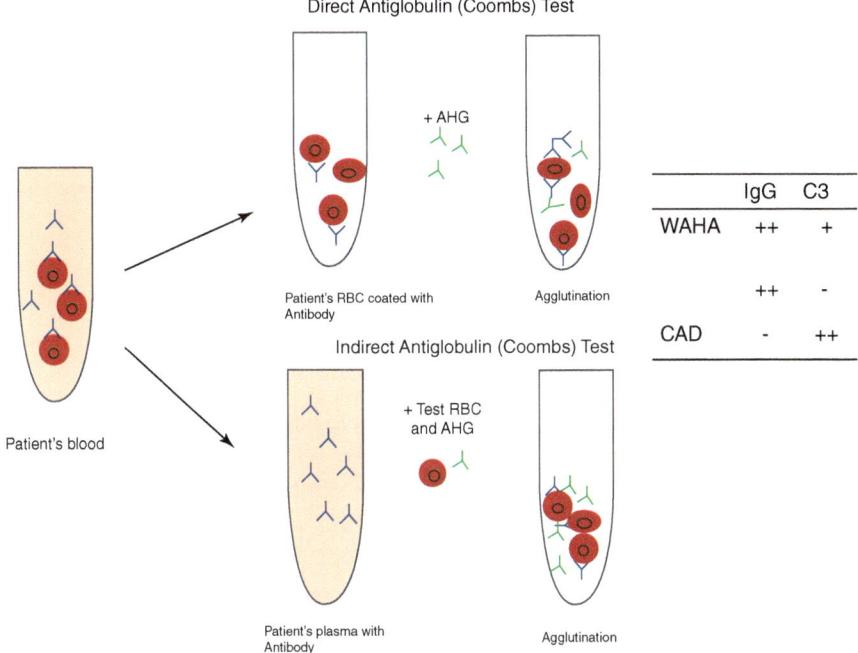

Fig. 17.3 Antiglobulin (Coombs) test [13]

Table 17.12 Treatment of B12 and folate deficiencies [30]

Deficiency	Treatment
B12 deficiency	1000 μg IM once per week until deficiency is corrected, then 1000 μg once per month, or oral 1000–2000 μg per day
Folate deficiency[a]	Oral folic acid 1–5 mg daily

[a]Doses for supplementation will vary in those who are pregnant (see Chap. 21)

anemia (hemoglobin <7 g/dL), ongoing bleeding, significant side effects, or poor response to oral iron [32]. A meta-analysis comparing oral vs. IV iron in those with CKD showed greater hemoglobin response to parenteral iron rather than oral iron but could not determine a mortality benefit, infectious risk difference, or quality of life difference [33]. In iron deficiency anemia, treatment can be with oral or parenteral iron. The choice between which to use depends on individual patient's side effect tolerability, access to centers which can provide the IV infusions, and whether the patient has a malabsorptive syndrome which prevents adequate absorption of oral iron. Several preparations of oral iron tablets (Table 17.13) and liquid formulations exist. Studies have shown that they are equivalent in effectiveness. These formulations may be taken with alternate day dosing and can be titrated to reduce side effects [34]. Oral iron preparations are thought to have improved absorption with ascorbic acid tablets or orange juice; however, the data around this remains

Table 17.13 Oral iron preparations

Drug	Concentration of elemental iron	Available strengths
Ferrous sulfate	65 mg	325 mg
Ferrous gluconate	28–36 mg	240, 324, 325 mg
Ferrous fumarate	106 mg	324 or 325 mg
Ferrous sulfate elixir	44–60 mg/5 mL	220–300 mg

Adapted from Bohm (2021) [34]

Table 17.14 Parental iron preparations

Drug	Concentration of elemental iron	Recommended infusion dose	Test dose	Side effects
Ferric derisomaltose	100 mg/mL	>50 kg, single dose of 1000 mg	Not recommended	Flushing, headaches, chills, BP variations
Ferric carboxymaltose (FCM)	50 mg/mL	>50 kg, 1–2 doses of 750 mg at least 7 d apart	Not recommended	Flushing, headaches, chills, fatigue, hypophosphatemia, BP variations
Ferumoxytol	30 mg/mL	2 doses of 510 mg given 3–8 d apart	Not recommended	Flushing, headaches, chills, BP variations
Sodium ferric gluconate	12.5 mg/mL	Multiple doses of 125 mg	Not recommended	Flushing, headaches, chills, BP variations
Iron sucrose	20 mg/mL	Multiple doses of 100–200 mg	Not recommended	
Low molecular weight iron dextran	50 mg/mL	Based on formula: Single 1000 mg dose or multiple doses of 100 mg	Highly recommended: 25 mg prior to first dose	Anaphylactic and allergic reactions

inconclusive. It is recommended to avoid taking oral iron with antacids, H2 blockers, and PPIs as these reduce the pH of the stomach and may impair iron absorption. Side effects of oral iron include constipation, diarrhea, nausea, and black or green tarry stools [35].

Parenteral iron is also available in different formulations with equal effectiveness. These products vary by cost and frequency of visits required to obtain the full dosage. In the United States, low molecular weight iron tends to be the most inexpensive formulation but requires longer transfusion time [34]. The dose of IV iron required to replete iron stores is based on the patient's hemoglobin deficit, body weight, and the amount of elemental iron available in the product (Ganzoni equation, see "special considerations"). Current recommendations, however, are to provide a fixed dose of ~1000 mg total as either a single dose or in several infusions depending on the product. Choice of product will depend on patient comorbidities, total dose of repletion, and availability (Table 17.14) [36, 37].

Most congenital hemolytic anemias are treated with supportive care, such as RBC transfusions as needed. Avoidance of specific toxins and triggers is also recommended (see section "G6PD Deficiency"). Splenectomy is indicated in some hereditary hemolytic anemias such as HS, HE, and PK deficiency, if the patients are transfusion dependent and have poor quality of life [16, 31].

Warm autoimmune hemolytic anemia can be treated by treating the underlying disorder and with the immunologic medications listed below (Table 17.15) [12].

Table 17.15 Treatment of warm autoimmune hemolytic anemia

Treatment	Dose	Response rate/time to response	Comments
1st line treatments			
Glucocorticoids	Oral prednisone 1–2 mg/kg/day IV methylprednisolone 500–1000 mg/day Taper slowly 4–6 months if Hgb > 10 g/dL after 1–3 weeks	75–80%/TTR 7–25 days	Monitor for: Glucose, osteoporosis, risk of infections, hypertension, cushingoid syndrome, mood swings Remission rate 20–30%
2nd line treatments			
Rituximab	IV 375 mg/m² of BSA weekly × 4 doses May be effective even at low doses (100 mg weekly)	80–90%/TTR 3–6 weeks	Monitor for reactivation of hepatitis B infection, progressive multifocal leukoencephalopathy Retreatment usually effective Relapse free survival: 70% when combined with steroids, vs. 45% with monotherapy alone
Splenectomy	Surgical consult	80%/TTR 7–10 days	Thrombosis 10–15% Complications of bacterial infections due to encapsulated organisms Vaccination against H. influenza, meningococcus and pneumococcus recommended 8–10 weeks prior to treatment Potentially curative 20–50%
IVIG	0.4 g/kg/day × 5 days or 1 g/kg × 2 days	30–40%/TTR 1–5 days	Monitor for septic meningitis, renal insufficiency and hemolytic anemia Responses are transient

(continued)

Table 17.15 (continued)

Treatment	Dose	Response rate/time to response	Comments
3rd and fourth line treatment			
Mycophenolate mofetil	500–1000 mg every 12 h	Highly variable, 25–100%/TTR 1–3 months	Monitor for pancytopenia, lymphoma, infections, nausea, headache, diarrhea
Sirolimus	2 mg/m^2/day; trough goal 5–15 ng/mL		Monitor for complications of lymphoma, lung disease opportunistic infections Hypertension, mucositis Consider this option for patients with autoimmune lymphoproliferative syndrome
Azathioprine	1–2 mg/kg/day Max dose is 150 mg/kg/day	40–60%/1–3 months	Monitor for pancytopenia, infection, liver function abnormalities Particularly useful in autoimmune conditions, Evans
Cyclophosphamide	500–1000 mg/m^2; 1–3 doses every 2–3 weeks		Monitor for pancytopenia, infection, secondary cancer, infertility
Cyclosporine A	5 mg/kg/day divided every 12 h Target trough level between 150–300 ng/mL	40–60%/1–3 months	Monitor for renal and hepatic dysfunction, lymphoma, hypertension and excessive hair growth Steroid sparing agent, especially useful in systemic autoimmune conditions
Danazol	200 mg orally/day; increased to 600–800 mg/day based on response	40%/1–3 months	Complications of hepatotoxicity. and androgenic effects Do not use in men with prostatic adenoma or carcinoma

Adapted from Brodsky [12]

Second-line therapy may include splenectomy. In contrast, steroids and splenectomy are not effective in the treatment of cold hemolytic anemia. Treatment for cold hemolytic anemia will include rituximab alone or with adjunctive bendamustine, interferon alpha, or fludarabine (Table 17.16). Sutimlimab is a recently FDA-approved IgG4 monoclonal antibody which inhibits complement C1 and has shown to be effective in reducing hemolysis, anemia, and fatigue in patients with CAD requiring frequent transfusion [38].

Table 17.16 Treatment of cold agglutinin disease

	Bendamustine + rituximab	Fludarabine + rituximab	Rituximab [39]	Sutimlimab
Regimen	Day 1: Rituximab 375 mg/m² and bendamustine 90 mg/m² Day 2: Bendamustine 90 mg/m²	Day 1: Rituximab 375 mg/m² and Fludarabine (PO) 40 mg/m² Days 2–5: Fludarabine (PO) 40 mg/m²	Day 1: Rituximab 375 mg/m²	39–75 kg: 6.5 g IV once per week for 2 weeks, then 6.5 g IV once every 2 weeks thereafter 75 kg+: 7.5 g IV once weekly for 2 weeks, then 7.5 g IV once every 2 weeks thereafter
Cycle interval	28 day	28 day	1 week	Weekly, then every 2 weeks
Number of cycles	4	4	4	As tolerated

Adapted from Hill and Hill, 2018 [10]

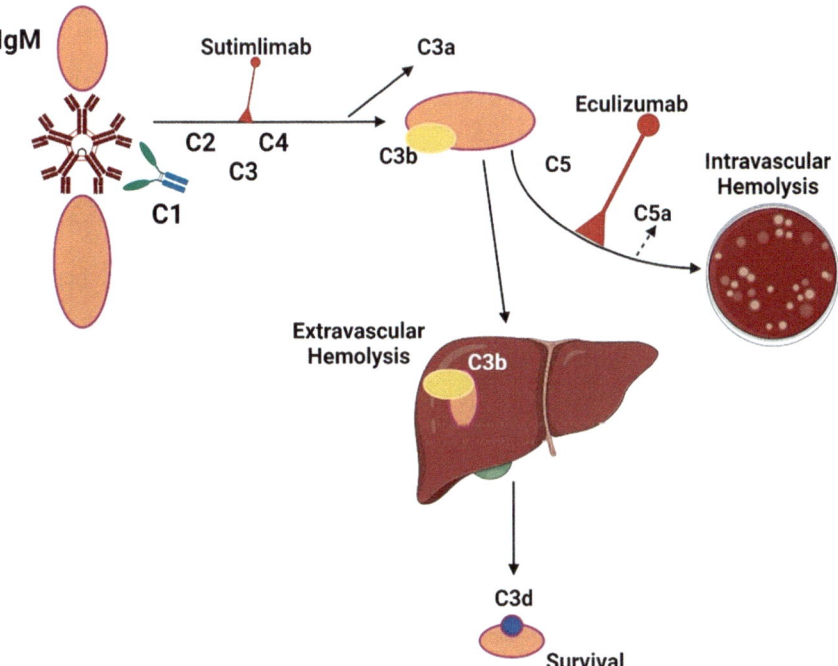

Fig. 17.4 Treatment options for PNH

Anticomplement directed therapies, such as eculizumab and ravulizumab, are approved in PNH (Fig. 17.4) [39]. Treatment is indicated for PNH when the patient is experiencing symptoms of chronic hemolysis with fatigue, frequent pain paroxysms, and reduced quality of life. Thrombosis is also an indication for initiation of anticomplement therapy.

Special Considerations

- Consider marrow failure when anemia occurs with other cytopenias (Chap. 10). In these cases, consider aplastic anemia, leukemia, or other disease of the marrow. It can also be secondary to peripheral destruction or splenic sequestration. Anemia in liver disease is multifactorial in etiology, stemming from hemolysis, intravascular dilution in the setting of hypervolemia, and poor marrow response. Spur cells, or acanthocytes, are abnormal erythrocytes that are characterized by their spike-like projections. Spur cells are characteristic of liver disease which is associated with hemolysis and arise due to defective membrane lipids and proteins. One can also see target cells in liver-disease associated anemia. Anemia is often noted in individuals with HIV and is notably associated with the development of AIDS [40]. This anemia is also multifactorial related to decreased erythropoietin levels, changes in the production of cytokines that are linked to hematopoiesis, concurrent opportunistic infection (e.g., MAC), and frequently used medications (trimethoprim-sulfamethoxazole, ganciclovir, zidovudine). Parvovirus B19 infection in those with hemolytic anemia can additionally cause aplastic anemia [41].

Useful Tools

- Ganzoni formula is used to calculate the total iron dose for repletion:
  - Total iron deficit = [body weight x (target hemoglobin-actual hemoglobin)] × 2.4 + iron stores.
- Absolute reticulocyte count: ARC = % reticulocytes × RBC count.

References

1. Means RT. General hematology of anemia. In: Nutritional anemia: scientific principles, clinical practice, and public health; 2019. p. 1–9.
2. Kassebaum NJ, Collaborators GBDA. The global burden of anemia. Hematol Oncol Clin North Am. 2016;30(2):247–308.
3. DeLoughery TG. Iron deficiency anemia. Med Clin North Am. 2017;101(2):319–32.
4. Faruqi A, Mukkamalla SKR. Iron binding capacity. In: StatPearls. Treasure Island, FL: StatPearls; 2022.
5. Martin A, Thompson AA. Thalassemias. Pediatr Clin North Am. 2013;60(6):1383–91.
6. Taher AT, Saliba AN. Iron overload in thalassemia: different organs at different rates. Hematology Am Soc Hematol Educ Program. 2017;2017(1):265–71.
7. Weiss DJ, Krehbiel JD, Lund JE. Studies of the pathogenesis of anemia of inflammation: mechanism of impaired erythropoiesis. Am J Vet Res. 1983;44(10):1832–5.
8. Levey AS, Eckardt KU, Tsukamoto Y, Levin A, Coresh J, Rossert J, De Zeeuw D, Hostetter TH, Lameire N, Eknoyan G. Definition and classification of chronic kidney disease: a posi-

tion statement from kidney disease: improving global outcomes (KDIGO). Kidney Int. 2005;67(6):2089–100.

9. Gutierrez OM. Treatment of iron deficiency anemia in CKD and end-stage kidney disease. Kidney Int Rep. 2021;6(9):2261–9.

10. Hill A, Hill QA. Autoimmune hemolytic anemia. Hematology Am Soc Hematol Educ Program. 2018;2018(1):382–9.

11. Berentsen S, Roth A, Randen U, Jilma B, Tjonnfjord GE. Cold agglutinin disease: current challenges and future prospects. J Blood Med. 2019;10:93–103.

12. Brodsky RA. Warm autoimmune hemolytic anemia. N Engl J Med. 2019;381(7):647–54.

13. Zantek ND, Koepsell SA, Tharp DR Jr, Cohn CS. The direct antiglobulin test: a critical step in the evaluation of hemolysis. Am J Hematol. 2012;87(7):707–9.

14. Hill A, DeZern AE, Kinoshita T, Brodsky RA. Paroxysmal nocturnal haemoglobinuria. Nat Rev Dis Primers. 2017;3:17028.

15. Gallagher PG, Forget BG. Hematologically important mutations: spectrin and ankyrin variants in hereditary spherocytosis. Blood Cells Mol Dis. 1998;24(4):539–43.

16. Perrotta S, Gallagher PG, Mohandas N. Hereditary spherocytosis. Lancet. 2008;372(9647):1411–26.

17. Wang C, Cui Y, Li Y, Liu X, Han J. A systematic review of hereditary spherocytosis reported in Chinese biomedical journals from 1978 to 2013 and estimation of the prevalence of the disease using a disease model. Intractable Rare Dis Res. 2015;4(2):76–81.

18. Wu Y, Liao L, Lin F. The diagnostic protocol for hereditary spherocytosis—2021 update. J Clin Lab Anal. 2021;35(12):e24034.

19. Gallagher PG, Ferriera JD. Molecular basis of erythrocyte membrane disorders. Curr Opin Hematol. 1997;4(2):128–35.

20. Gallagher PG. Abnormalities of the erythrocyte membrane. Pediatr Clin North Am. 2013;60(6):1349–62.

21. Cappellini MD, Fiorelli G. Glucose-6-phosphate dehydrogenase deficiency. Lancet. 2008;371(9606):64–74.

22. Luzzatto L, Ally M, Notaro R. Glucose-6-phosphate dehydrogenase deficiency. Blood. 2020;136(11):1225–40.

23. Luzzatto L, Nannelli C, Notaro R. Glucose-6-phosphate dehydrogenase deficiency. Hematol Oncol Clin North Am. 2016;30(2):373–93.

24. Risinger M, Kalfa TA. Red cell membrane disorders: structure meets function. Blood. 2020;136(11):1250–61.

25. Yao DC, Tolan DR, Murray MF, Harris DJ, Darras BT, Geva A, Neufeld EJ. Hemolytic anemia and severe rhabdomyolysis caused by compound heterozygous mutations of the gene for erythrocyte/muscle isozyme of aldolase, ALDOA(Arg303X/Cys338Tyr). Blood. 2004;103(6):2401–3.

26. Kato GJ, Steinberg MH, Gladwin MT. Intravascular hemolysis and the pathophysiology of sickle cell disease. J Clin Invest. 2017;127(3):750–60.

27. Noronha SA. Acquired and congenital hemolytic anemia. Pediatr Rev. 2016;37(6):235–46.

28. Green R, Datta Mitra A. Megaloblastic anemias: nutritional and other causes. Med Clin North Am. 2017;101(2):297–317.

29. Soliman AT, De Sanctis V, Yassin M, Wagdy M, Soliman N. Chronic anemia and thyroid function. Acta Biomed. 2017;88(1):119–27.

30. Szczepanek-Parulska E, Hernik A, Ruchala M. Anemia in thyroid diseases. Pol Arch Intern Med. 2017;127(5):352–60.

31. Grace RF, Barcellini W. Management of pyruvate kinase deficiency in children and adults. Blood. 2020;136(11):1241–9.

32. Batchelor EK, Kapitsinou P, Pergola PE, Kovesdy CP, Jalal DI. Iron deficiency in chronic kidney disease: updates on pathophysiology, diagnosis, and treatment. J Am Soc Nephrol. 2020;31(3):456–68.

33. O'Lone EL, Hodson EM, Nistor I, Bolignano D, Webster AC, Craig JC. Parenteral versus oral iron therapy for adults and children with chronic kidney disease. Cochrane Database Syst Rev. 2019;2:CD007857.
34. Bohm N. Diagnosis and management of iron deficiency anemia in inflammatory bowel disease. Am J Manag Care. 2021;27(11 Suppl):S211–8.
35. DeLoughery TG. Safety of oral and intravenous iron. Acta Haematol. 2019;142(1):8–12.
36. Auerbach M, Achebe MM, Thomsen LL, Derman RJ. Efficacy and safety of ferric derisomaltose (FDI) compared with iron sucrose (IS) in patients with iron deficiency anemia after bariatric surgery. Obes Surg. 2022;32(3):810–8.
37. Auerbach M, Henry D, DeLoughery TG. Intravenous ferric derisomaltose for the treatment of iron deficiency anemia. Am J Hematol. 2021;96(6):727–34.
38. Röth A, Barcellini W, D'Sa S, Miyakawa Y, Broome CM, Michel M, Kuter DJ, Jilma B, Tvedt THA, Fruebis J, et al. Sutimlimab in cold agglutinin disease. N Engl J Med. 2021;384(14):1323–34.
39. Kulasekararaj AG, Hill A, Rottinghaus ST, Langemeijer S, Wells R, Gonzalez-Fernandez FA, Gaya A, Lee JW, Gutierrez EO, Piatek CI, et al. Ravulizumab (ALXN1210) vs eculizumab in C5-inhibitor-experienced adult patients with PNH: the 302 study. Blood. 2019;133(6):540–9.
40. Sullivan PS, Hanson DL, Chu SY, Jones JL, Ward JW. Epidemiology of anemia in human immunodeficiency virus (HIV)-infected persons: results from the multistate adult and adolescent spectrum of HIV disease surveillance project. Blood. 1998;91(1):301–8.
41. Qian X, Zheng Y, Zhang G, Jiao X, Li Z. Relationship between human parvovirus B19 infection and aplastic anemia. Chin Med Sci J. 2001;16(3):172–4.

Chapter 18
Bone Marrow Failure Syndromes

Paul Sackstein and Gustavo Rivero

Case 1 (Hypercellular MDS)

A 63-year-old female presents to hematology clinic for worsening fatigue. Labs are notable for WBC 4.0×10^9/L with ANC 2100/μL, hemoglobin 7.8 g/dL, MCV 102 fL, and platelet count 180×10^9/L with no evidence of circulating blasts. Reticulocyte count is 0.2% and serum erythropoietin (EPO) level is 60 mIU/mL. Bone marrow biopsy with aspirate is performed and demonstrates hypercellularity (80%) with dyserythropoiesis and 30% ring sideroblasts. Cytogenetics were normal; however, NGS reveals *SF3B1* gene mutation with VAF 30%. She is diagnosed with myelodysplastic syndrome (MDS) with ring sideroblasts (Fig. 18.1).

Definition of Bone Marrow Failure

Bone marrow failure refers to intrinsic bone marrow disorders that arise from damage to the hematopoietic stem cell (HSC) compartment, leading to impaired white blood cell (WBC), red blood cell (RBC), and/or platelet production [1]. HSC injury can occur through immune-mediated destruction, apoptosis, or ineffective hematopoiesis caused by HSC gene mutations [2]. Bone marrow failure is always an

P. Sackstein
Georgetown University School of Medicine, Washington, DC, USA

Georgetown University School of Medicine, MedStar Georgetown University Hospital, Washington, USA
e-mail: paul.e.sackstein@medstar.net

G. Rivero (✉)
Lombardi Cancer Institute, Georgetown University School of Medicine, Washington, DC, USA

© The Author(s), under exclusive license to Springer Nature Switzerland AG 2024
G. Rivero, I. R. Sosa (eds.), *Consulting Hematology and Oncology Handbook*,
https://doi.org/10.1007/978-3-031-75810-2_18

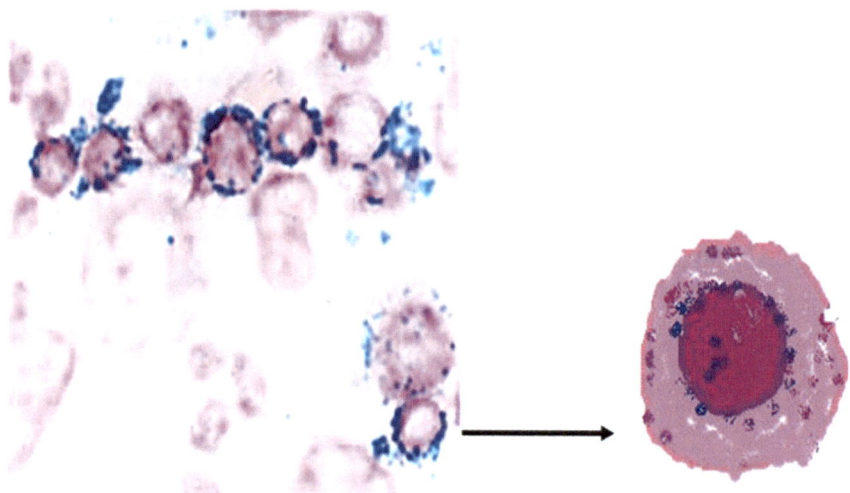

Fig. 18.1 Myelodysplastic syndrome with ring sideroblasts and single lineage dysplasi

important consideration in the differential diagnosis of pancytopenia. Bone marrow failure syndromes can be inherited due to germline mutations (Fanconi anemia, Dyskeratosis congenita, Shwachman-Diamond syndrome, Diamond-Blackfan anemia, etc.) or acquired due to somatic HSC mutations, most commonly aplastic anemia (AA), myelodysplastic syndrome (MDS), or paroxysmal nocturnal hemoglobinuria (PNH). The management of bone marrow failure syndromes varies widely based on the underlying etiology.

Clinical Evaluation of Bone Marrow Failure

If bone marrow failure is suspected, a careful medical history should be obtained to evaluate for infections, offending medications and prior toxin exposure including solvents, benzene, and pesticides (Table 18.1). Laboratory evaluation includes CBC with differential and peripheral smear review, basic metabolic panel, liver function tests, direct antiglobulin test (DAT), PT and aPTT, and fetal hemoglobin % (HbF %). Additional laboratory studies including HIV, hepatitis B and C serologies, parvovirus, EBV, CMV and serum folate, vitamin B12, and copper and zinc levels should be obtained to rule out viral infection or metabolic deficiencies. Testing for paroxysmal nocturnal hemoglobinuria (PNH) using flow cytometry and fluorescent-labeled aerolysin (FLAER) should also be considered. Bone marrow aspirate and biopsy should be performed to assess cellularity, dyspoiesis, and megakaryocyte morphology with immunohistochemistry. Cytogenetics and next-generation sequencing (NGS) should also be conducted as this has prognostic and treatment implications.

Table 18.1 Diagnostic evaluation of suspected bone marrow failure

Rule out reversible causes
• Medications
Valproic acid
Immunosuppressants
Mycophenolate, tacrolimus
Ganciclovir
Chemotherapy
• Toxins
Heavy metals (arsenic, lead)
Alcohol
• Viral infections
HIV
HBV
HCV
Parvovirus
EBV
CMV
• Vitamin or mineral deficiency
Folate
Vitamin B12
Copper
Zinc
Laboratory evaluation
• CBC with differential
• Peripheral blood smear
• Basic metabolic panel
• Liver function tests
• Direct antiglobulin test (DAT)
• PT and aPTT
• Hemoglobin F%
• HLA typing
Molecular evaluation
• Bone marrow biopsy with aspirate
• Cytogenetics
• Next generation sequencing (NGS)
Additional testing to consider:
• PNH FLAER
• Testing for inherited bone marrow failure syndromes

aPTT activated partial thromboplastin time, *FLAER* fluorescent aerolysin, *PNH* paroxysmal nocturnal hemoglobinuria

Acquired Causes of Bone Marrow Failure

Myelodysplastic Syndrome

Definition

MDS is a clonal hematopoietic disorder characterized by ineffective hematopoiesis resulting in cytopenias and dysplastic cellular morphology [3]. The median age of diagnosis is 76 years [3]. The World Health Organization (WHO) fifth edition classification differentiates MDS based on defining genetic abnormalities or morphologically for those without genetic abnormalities (Table 18.2) [4]. Historically, the prognosis of MDS was determined through risk stratification using the revised international prognostic symptom score (IPSS-R). The IPSS-R score classifies patients as having very low-, low-, intermediate-, high-, or very high-risk disease based on blast percentage, cytogenetic abnormalities, hemoglobin, platelet count, and ANC. However, the molecular IPSS (IPSS-M) risk calculator now incorporates molecular data in addition to clinical data and cytogenetics. Figure 18.2 depicts incidence of M-IPSS subtypes [5]. In the era of genetic-based MDS classification, the IPSS-M score should be used for more accurate risk stratification and prognostication.

Table 18.2 World Health Organization MDS 2022 classification

	Subtypes	Blasts
MDS with defining genetic abnormalities	MDS with low blasts and isolated 5q deletion	<5% BM and <2% PB
	MDS with low blasts and *SF3B1* gene mutation	
	MDS with biallelic *TP53* gene mutation	<20% BM and PB
MDS defined by morphology	MDS with low blasts	<5% BM and <2% PB
	MDS, hypoplastic	≤25% age-adjusted bone marrow cellularity
	MDS with increased blasts	
	MDS-IB1	5–9% BM
	MDS-IB2	10–19% BM

BM bone marrow, *IB* increased blasts, *MDS* myelodysplastic syndrome, *PB* peripheral blood, *SF3B1* splicing factor 3b subunit 1, *TP53* Tumor protein p53

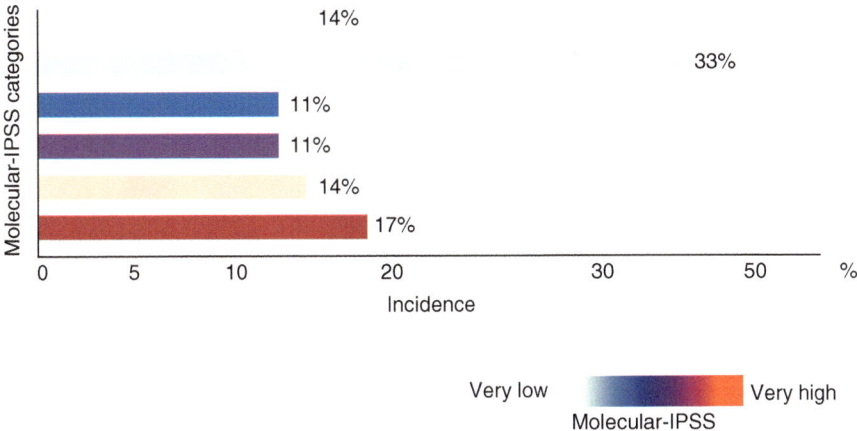

Fig. 18.2 Incidence of myelodysplastic syndrome subtypes according to Molecular-International Prognostic Score System (IPSS)

Diagnosis

MDS should be considered in patients with unexplained cytopenias, bone marrow failure, or bone marrow dysplasia. The diagnostic criteria for MDS include the following:

- At least one cytopenia which cannot be attributed to vitamin deficiency, toxin, or medication effect.

  - Hemoglobin <10 g/dL.
  - Absolute neutrophil count (ANC) <1800/μL.
  - Platelet count <100 × 10⁹/L.

- Dysplasia in ≥10% of at least one hematopoietic lineage.
- Defining cytogenetic or molecular abnormalities.
- <20% blasts in bone marrow or peripheral blood.

Importantly, a blast percentage ≥20% or the presence of t(8;21) *RUNX1::RUNX1T1*, inv(16) or t(15;17) *PML::RARA* are suggestive of acute myelogenous leukemia (AML) and would exclude the diagnosis of MDS [4].

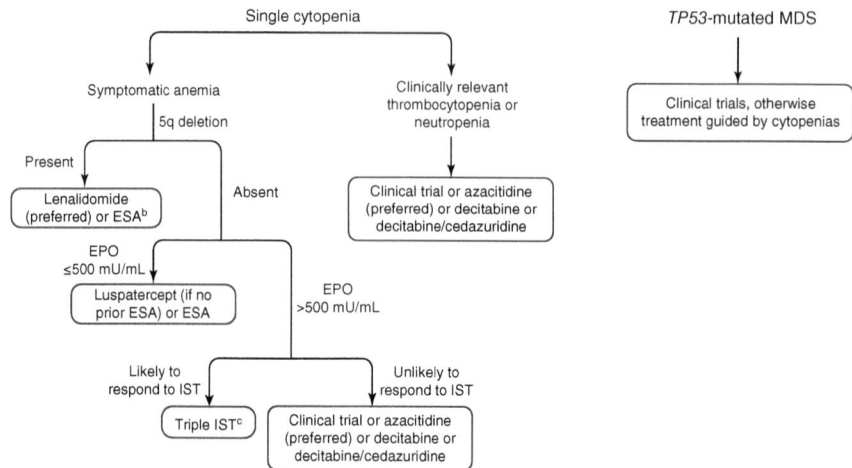

EPO: erythropoietin; ESA: erythropoiesis-stimulating agents; IST: immunosuppressive therapy; MDS: myelodysplastic syndrome
[a]Lower-risk defined as very-low, low or intermediate-risk MDS
[b]ESA defined as recombinant human erythropoietin or darbopoietin alfa
[c]Eltrombopag + hATG + CsA

Fig. 18.3 Management of lower-risk MDS. *EPO* erythropoietin, *ESA* erythropoiesis stimulating agents, *IST* immunosuppressive therapy, *MDS* myelodysplastic syndrome. [a]Lower-risk defined as very low, low or intermediate-risk MDS. [b]ESA defined as recombinant human erythropoietin or darbopoietin alfa. [c]Eltrombopag + hATG + CsA

Treatment

The management of MDS is complex and varies depending on the severity of cyto-penias, risk stratification, defining genetic abnormalities, and the presence or absence of ring sideroblasts. For patients with lower risk MDS (LR-MDS) and iso-lated mild asymptomatic anemia (hemoglobin >10 g/dL), a period of observation may be considered [6]. However, for patients with LR-MDS and symptomatic or severe anemia, a serum erythropoietin (EPO) level should be obtained and a trial of an erythropoiesis-stimulating agent (ESA) should be considered (Fig. 18.3). Of note, serum EPO level > 500 mU/mL and frequent RBC transfusions (>2 per month) predict poor response to ESAs [7]. Patients with 5q deletion LR-MDS should be treated with lenalidomide. LR-MDS patients with *SF3B1* mutation or ring sidero-blasts ≥15% should be treated luspatercept, which has been shown to reduce the severity of anemia and increase the likelihood of transfusion independence [6]. Patients with higher risk MDS (HR-MDS) or treatment-related MDS should be con-sidered for allogeneic HCT if eligible and an HLA-matched donor is available. For patients with transplant-ineligible HR-MDS, hypomethylating agents such as azacitidine, decitabine, or the oral combination of decitabine and cedazuridine should be considered. The discussion of p53-mutated MDS is outside the scope of this chapter, but all such patients should be enrolled in clinical trials if eligible for treatment (Fig. 18.4).

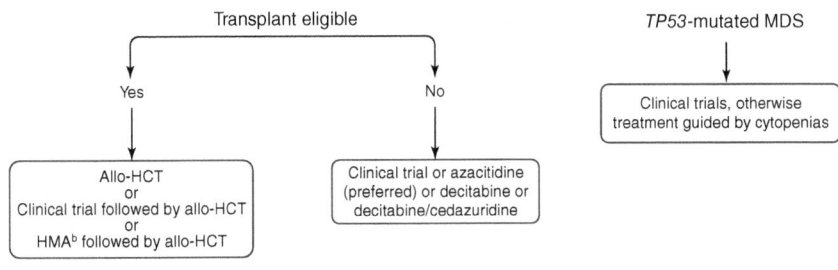

HCT: Hematopoietic stem cell transplant; MDS: Myelodysplastic syndrome
aHigher-risk defined as intermediate, high or very-high-risk MDS
bHMA includes azacitidine or decitabine or oral decitabine and cedazuridine

Fig. 18.4 Management of higher-risk MDS. *HCT* hematopoietic stem cell transplant, *MDS* myelodysplastic syndrome. aHigher-risk defined as intermediate, high or very-high-risk MDS. bHMA includes azacitidine or decitabine or oral decitabine and cedazuridine

Case 2 (Hypocellular MDS)

A 58-year-old female presented to hematology clinic for weakness. CBC was notable for WBC 2.8 × 10⁹/L with ANC 12000, hemoglobin 6.8 g/dL, MCV 103 fL, and platelet count 43 × 10⁹/L. The reticulocyte count was 50,000 × 10⁶/L. Bone marrow biopsy with aspirate showed hypocellular marrow (15%) with trilineage dysplasia. Metaphase cytogenetics demonstrated trisomy 8. A diagnosis of hypoplastic MDS was made. She was treated with horse anti-thymocyte globulin (hATG), cyclosporine (CsA), and eltrombopag with good hematologic response and improvement in bone marrow cellularity.

Aplastic Anemia

Definition

AA is defined as pancytopenia and bone marrow hypoplasia or aplasia. The majority of AA is immune-mediated (80%); however, AA has also been associated with cytotoxic chemotherapy, anti-epileptics (carbamazepine, phenytoin), antithyroid medications (methimazole, propylthiouracil), toxic chemicals (benzene), viral infections (EBV, human immunodeficiency virus, seronegative hepatitis), or inherited bone marrow failure syndromes such as Fanconi anemia, Shwachman-Diamond syndrome, congenital amegakaryocytic thrombocytopenia, or dyskeratosis congenita [8]. AA is also closely associated with acquired clonal hematopoietic disorders such as paroxysmal nocturnal hemoglobinuria (PNH). The severity of AA depends on the degree of cytopenias. Severe aplastic anemia (SAA) is defined as bone marrow cellularity <25% of normal for age and at least 2 of the following: ANC <500, platelet count <20, or reticulocyte count <60,000 [8].

Table 18.3 Aplastic anemia vs. hypoplastic MDS

Feature	Aplastic anemia	Hypoplastic MDS
Single lineage dysplasia	+/−	+/−
Multilineage dysplasia	Absent	Present in ≥10% cells
Excess blasts[a]	Absent	+/−
Bone marrow cellularity	≤25% (adjusted for age)	≤25% (adjusted for age)
Reticulin fibrosis	Absent	Present
MDS defining genetic abn[b]	Absent	Present
Concurrent PNH	Present	Absent
Karyotype	Normal or 6p CN-LOH	7q- or 5q-
Response to IST	+	+

CN-LOH copy number loss of heterozygosity, *IST* immunosuppressive therapy
[a]Defined as >5% in bone marrow
[b]5q-, 7q-, 9q-, 11q-, *SF3B1*, *TP53*

Diagnosis

The diagnosis is established in patients with pancytopenia by obtaining a bone marrow biopsy to identify bone marrow hypoplasia and rule out infiltrative marrow processes and marrow fibrosis. AA is differentiated from hypoplastic MDS based on the presence of severe bone marrow hypoplasia (<10%) in the absence of morphologic dysplasia and MDS-defining chromosomal or genetic abnormalities (Table 18.3).

Treatment

The management of AA is based on disease severity, patient age, functional status, and the availability of an HLA matched donor. For SAA patients ≤40 years of age who are medically fit, allogeneic HCT is recommended over triple immunosuppressive therapy (IST) if a matched related donor (MRD) is available (Fig. 18.5) [8]. If an MRD is not rapidly available, patients should be treated with triple IST, and an alternative HLA-matched donor should be identified for allogeneic HCT [8]. Triple IST refers to the combination of hATG, CsA, and eltrombopag. SAA patients >40 years of age should be treated with triple IST rather than allogeneic HCT due to high rates of transplant-related morbidity and mortality [8]. Although hypoplastic MDS is a distinct disease entity from AA, the mechanism of pathogenesis is believed to be immune-mediated hematopoietic suppression, like AA [9]. Consequently, hypoplastic MDS is also treated with IST, generally the combination of ATG plus cyclosporine. For patients with PNH-associated AA, symptoms generally emerge when the clonal population is >30%. Treatment should only be pursued in the presence of PNH-related clinical symptoms or PNH-associated bone marrow failure.

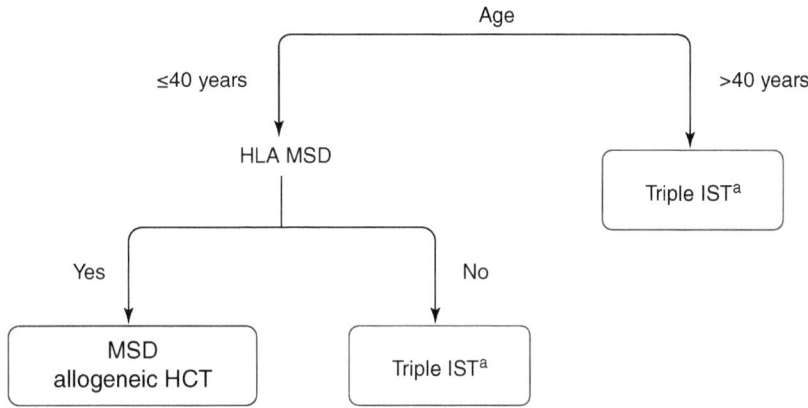

HCT: Hematopoietic stem cell transplant; HLA: Human leukocyte antigen; IST: immunosuppressive therapy
[a]IST defined as eltrombopag + horse anti-thymocyte globulin (hATG) + cyclosporine

Fig. 18.5 Management of severe aplastic anemia

PNH-related clinical findings are complement-mediated and should be treated with terminal complement inhibitors such as eculizumab or ravulizumab [10]. PNH-associated bone marrow failure should be treated similarly to AA with allogeneic HCT if transplant-eligible or IST if transplant-ineligible.

Case 3

A 4-year-old male presented to the emergency room with recurrent abdominal pain and hematochezia. He had recently developed epistaxis and easy bruising, and his medical history was notable for recurrent pneumonia. Physical exam revealed short stature, multiple café-au lait spots. There was no known family history of similar symptoms. CBC showed WBC count 3.4×10^9/L, hemoglobin 10.8 g/dL, MCV 105 fL, and platelet count 65×10^9/L. Peripheral smear was notable for macrocytic anemia, thrombocytopenia, and leukopenia. HbF% was 5%. Comprehensive metabolic panel, vitamin B12 level, folate level, copper level, zinc level, PT, and aPTT were within normal limits. HIV, HBV, HCV, EBV, CMV, and parvovirus serologies were negative. DAT was negative. Lymphocyte telomere length analysis was normal. Chromosomal breakage analysis was performed with diepoxybutane and demonstrated chromosomal hypersensitivity to clastogenic agents. Genetic testing confirmed the presence of homozygous *FANCA* p.Q99X nonsense mutation.

Inherited Causes of Bone Marrow Failure

Fanconi Anemia

Fanconi anemia (FA) is the most frequently observed inherited bone marrow failure syndrome. It arises from germline mutations in *FANC* genes (which are responsible for DNA damage response), and the inheritance pattern is autosomal recessive [11]. FA is characterized by macrocytosis and pancytopenia as well as dysmorphic features including thumb hypoplasia, short stature, and café-au lait spots [11]. This disease should always be considered in patients with unexplained macrocytosis and characteristic congenital abnormalities. The diagnosis is made through chromosome breakage analysis in blood or fibroblasts or germline mutation analysis. Hematopoietic stem cell transplantation (HCT) should always be considered in eligible patients with HLA-matched donors [11]. In patients with pancytopenia who are ineligible for HCT, danazol can be used to stimulate erythropoiesis and decrease transfusion dependence [12].

Shwachman-Diamond Syndrome

Shwachman-diamond syndrome (SDS) is a rare autosomal recessive inherited bone marrow failure syndrome characterized by exocrine pancreatic insufficiency, recurrent infections, and growth retardation in infancy [13]. Patients frequently developed deficiency of fat-soluble vitamins A, D, E, and K secondary to exocrine pancreatic insufficiency. Most cases of SDS (>90%) are associated with mutations in the *SBDS* gene, which is hypothesized to play an important role in neutrophil chemotaxis [14]. In addition to macrocytic anemia and thrombocytopenia, patients commonly present with cyclic neutropenia; therefore, the CBC may need to be repeated over a 3-week timeframe to confirm neutropenia [13]. SDS should be considered in individuals with exocrine pancreatic insufficiency and unexplained neutropenia. The diagnosis is confirmed through genetic sequencing and identification of biallelic *SBDS* pathogenic variants. Treatment is primarily supportive including granulocyte colony-stimulating factor (G-CSF) to decrease the incidence of febrile neutropenia and pancreatic enzyme replacement for exocrine pancreatic insufficiency [13]. The absolute risk of G-CSF accelerating progression to MDS or AML remains unknown. HCT can be considered in SDS patients with severe and/or symptomatic neutropenia refractory to G-CSF [15].

Diamond-Blackfan Anemia

Diamond-Blackfan anemia (DBA) is a rare autosomal dominant inherited bone marrow failure syndrome associated with congenital pure red cell aplasia. DBA is a ribosomal protein (RP) disorder (ribosomopathy) which arises from *RP* gene mutations; *RPS19* gene mutations have been reported in approximately 25% of cases [16]. Patients typically present in infancy with macrocytic anemia and reticulocytopenia in association with congenital abnormalities including craniofacial (hypertelorism), thumb, urogenital (horseshoe kidney), and cardiac abnormalities (atrial or ventricular septal defects) [17]. DBA should be considered in the differential diagnosis of pure red cell aplasia. It should be suspected in infants and children who develop severe anemia with reticulocytopenia; however, there is variable expressivity and many patients are now diagnosed later in life. Increased erythrocyte adenosine deaminase activity and elevated fetal hemoglobin (HbF) are frequently observed due to stress erythropoiesis. The diagnosis is confirmed through germline genetic testing. Treatment varies based on age. Infants ≤1 year of age should be supported with transfusions to maintain hemoglobin 8–10 g/dL [18]. In infants >1 year old, glucocorticoids are typically used to stimulate erythropoiesis [18]. HCT can be considered in patients refractory to steroids [19].

Dyskeratosis Congenita

Telomere biology diseases (previously dyskeratosis congenita, DC) are inherited bone marrow failure syndromes that arise from defects in telomere maintenance. The inheritance pattern of dyskeratosis congenita is variable and can be X-linked recessive, autosomal dominant, or autosomal recessive [11]. Pathogenic mutations in various telomere maintenance genes (including *DKC1, ACD, TERC,* and *TERT*) have been reported in DC [11]. Patients with DC typically present with the clinical triad of dyskeratotic hair/nails, reticular rash, and oral leukoplakia [11]. The diagnosis is made through a combination of the aforementioned clinical criteria and the identification of short telomeres through lymphocyte telomere length analysis. Genetic testing should also be performed to identify suspected causative mutations. Patients are at increased risk of malignancies including head and neck squamous cell carcinoma (HNSCC), stomach/esophageal cancer, liver cancer, acute myeloid leukemia (AML), and pulmonary fibrosis [11]. Treatment includes surveillance for solid tumors including nasolaryngoscopy, esophagoscopy, and HPV vaccination to decrease the risk of anorectal and gynecologic cancers [20]. Pulmonary function tests (PFTs) should be regularly performed to screen for pulmonary fibrosis [20]. HCT should be considered for eligible pediatric patients with BM failure; however, conditioning regimens can increase the risk of secondary non-hematologic malignancies [21]. For HCT ineligible patients, supportive transfusions and danazol may be considered to stimulate erythropoiesis [22].

Congenital Amegakaryocytic Thrombocytopenia

Congenital amegakaryocytic thrombocytopenia (CAMT) is a rare autosomal recessive inherited bone marrow failure syndrome. CAMT arises from homozygous loss of function mutations in the *MPL* gene, which encodes the thrombopoietin (TPO) receptor [23]. Patients typically present with isolated severe thrombocytopenia in infancy resulting in mucocutaneous bleeding and can develop hypocellular bone marrow failure similar to AA later in childhood [23]. The diagnosis is established through genetic testing confirming biallelic *MPL* gene mutations. Treatment is largely supportive with platelet transfusions and antifibrinolytic agents such as tranexamic acid or aminocaproic acid to decrease the incidence of mucosal bleeding [24]. HCT is the only curative treatment option and should be considered in patients with severe thrombocytopenia or progression to bone marrow failure [24].

Severe Congenital Neutropenia

Severe congenital neutropenia (SCN) is a rare inherited bone marrow failure syndrome characterized by recurrent infections. The inheritance pattern of SCN is variable. Although the majority of SCN (50–60%) occurs due to *ELANE* gene mutations (which encodes neutrophil elastase and exhibits AD inheritance), X-linked SCN has been rarely observed in patients with mutations in the Wiskott-Aldrich syndrome (WAS) gene [25]. Interestingly, *ELANE* gene mutations can also cause congenital cyclic neutropenia, but it remains unclear why specific mutations result in congenital cyclic neutropenia vs. SCN. Furthermore, *ELANE*-related SCN is associated with an increased risk of progression to AML whereas the risk of AML is considerably lower in cyclic neutropenia [25]. Patients typically present in infancy with absolute neutrophil count (ANC) <200 cells/uL and recurrent infections including periodontitis [25]. The diagnosis is confirmed through the identification of *ELANE* gene mutations. The mainstay of treatment is G-CSF which reduces the risk of infection. HCT should be considered in SCN patients with high G-CSF requirements or who become refractory to G-CSF [26]. (Table 18.4).

Important Tools

IPSS-M calculator
  https://mds-risk-model.com/

Table 18.4 Overview of diagnosis and management of inherited bone marrow failure syndromes

Disease	Inheritance pattern	Gene(s) affected	Salient clinical features	Diagnostic testing	2° cancers/sequelae	Management
Fanconi Anemia (FA)	AR	FANC (65% FANCA)	Macrocytosis, pancytopenia, hypoplastic thumbs	Chromosome breakage analysis	HNSCC, MDS/AML	HCT, danazol if HCT ineligible
Shwachman-Diamond syndrome (SDS)	AR	SDBS (90%)	Pancreatic insufficiency, infections in infancy	Germline genetic testing	MDS/AML	HCT if AML/MDS, otherwise G-CSF
Diamond Blackfan Anemia (DBA)	AD	RP genes (25% RPS19)	Craniofacial abn, PRCA, ↑eADA, ↑HbF	Germline genetic testing	MDS/AML	Steroids/transfusions, HCT if refractory
Steroids/transfusions, HCT if refractory	Variable (primarily AD)	DKC1, ACD, TERC, TERT, TINF2, etc.	Skin pigmentation, nail dystrophy, oral leukoplakia	Lymphocyte telomere length analysis	Pulmonary fibrosis	HCT
Congenital amegakaryocytic thrombocytopenia (CAMT)	AR	MPL	Isolated thrombocytopenia, mucocutaneous bleeding in infancy	Germline genetic testing	AA, MDS/AML	HCT
Severe congenital neutropenia (SCN)	Variable (primarily AD)	ELANE, WAS	ANC <200, recurrent infection (periodontitis)	Germline genetic testing	MDS, AML, ALL, CMML	G-CSF, HCT if refractory
GATA2 deficiency	AD	GATA2	Monocytopenia, mycobacterial infection	Germline genetic testing	MDS (trisomy 8, monosomy 7)	HCT
Thrombocytopenia-absent radii (TAR) syndrome	AD	RBM8A (1q21.1 deletion)	Neonatal absent bilateral radii, thumbs present	Germline genetic testing	None	Ortho, TTE, avoid cow's milk

AA aplastic anemia, *AD* autosomal dominant, *AML* acute myelogenous leukemia, *ANC* absolute neutrophil count, *AR* autosomal recessive, *eADA* erythrocyte adenosine deaminase, *HCT* hematopoietic stem cell transplant, *HbF* hemoglobin F, *HNSCC* head and neck squamous cell carcinoma, *MDS* myelodysplastic syndrome, *PRCA* pure red cell aplasia, *TTE* transthoracic echocardiogram

References

1. Bodine D, Berliner N. Introduction to the review series on "bone marrow failure". Blood. 2014;124(18):2755. https://doi.org/10.1182/blood-2014-08-587394.
2. Giudice V, Cardamone C, Triggiani M, Selleri C. Bone marrow failure syndromes, overlapping diseases with a common cytokine signature. Int J Mol Sci. 2021;22(2):705. https://doi.org/10.3390/ijms22020705.
3. Cogle CR, Craig BM, Rollison DE, List AF. Incidence of the myelodysplastic syndromes using a novel claims-based algorithm: high number of uncaptured cases by cancer registries. Blood. 2011;117(26):7121–5. https://doi.org/10.1182/blood-2011-02-337964.
4. Khoury JD, Solary E, Abla O, et al. The 5th edition of the World Health Organization classification of haematolymphoid tumours: myeloid and histiocytic/dendritic neoplasms. Leukemia. 2022;36(7):1703–19. https://doi.org/10.1038/s41375-022-01613-1.
5. Ma J, Gu Y, Wei Y, et al. Evaluation of new IPSS-molecular model and comparison of different prognostic systems in patients with myelodysplastic syndrome. Blood Sci. 2023;5(3):187–95. https://doi.org/10.1097/BS9.0000000000000166.
6. NCCN Clinical Practice Guidelines in Oncology: myelodysplastic syndromes. 2022. https://www.nccn.org/professionals/physician_gls/pdf/mds.pdf. Accessed 12 Sept 2022.
7. Park S, Kelaidi C, Meunier M, Casadevall N, Gerds AT, Platzbecker U. The prognostic value of serum erythropoietin in patients with lower-risk myelodysplastic syndromes: a review of the literature and expert opinion. Ann Hematol. 2020;99(1):7–19. https://doi.org/10.1007/s00277-019-03799-4.
8. Young NS. Aplastic anemia. N Engl J Med. 2018;379(17):1643–56. https://doi.org/10.1056/NEJMra1413485.
9. Stahl M, DeVeaux M, de Witte T, et al. The use of immunosuppressive therapy in MDS: clinical outcomes and their predictors in a large international patient cohort. Blood Adv. 2018;2(14):1765–72. https://doi.org/10.1182/bloodadvances.2018019414.
10. Brodsky RA. How I treat paroxysmal nocturnal hemoglobinuria. Blood. 2021;137(10):1304–9. https://doi.org/10.1182/blood.2019003812.
11. Shimamura A, Alter BP. Pathophysiology and management of inherited bone marrow failure syndromes. Blood Rev. 2010;24(3):101–22. https://doi.org/10.1016/j.blre.2010.03.002.
12. Nassani M, Fakih RE, Passweg J, et al. The role of androgen therapy in acquired aplastic anemia and other bone marrow failure syndromes. Front Oncol. 2023;13:1135160. https://doi.org/10.3389/fonc.2023.1135160.
13. StatPearls. 2023.
14. Wessels D, Srikantha T, Yi S, Kuhl S, Aravind L, Soll DR. The Shwachman-Bodian-diamond syndrome gene encodes an RNA-binding protein that localizes to the pseudopod of Dictyostelium amoebae during chemotaxis. J Cell Sci. 2006;119(Pt 2):370–9. https://doi.org/10.1242/jcs.02753.
15. Cesaro S, Pillon M, Sauer M, et al. Long-term outcome after allogeneic hematopoietic stem cell transplantation for Shwachman-diamond syndrome: a retrospective analysis and a review of the literature by the severe aplastic anemia working Party of the European Society for blood and marrow transplantation (SAAWP-EBMT). Bone Marrow Transplant. 2020;55(9):1796–809. https://doi.org/10.1038/s41409-020-0863-z.
16. Engidaye G, Melku M, Enawgaw B. Diamond Blackfan anemia: genetics, pathogenesis, diagnosis and treatment. EJIFCC. 2019;30(1):67–81.
17. van Dooijeweert B, van Ommen CH, Smiers FJ, et al. Pediatric diamond-Blackfan anemia in The Netherlands: an overview of clinical characteristics and underlying molecular defects. Eur J Haematol. 2018;100(2):163–70. https://doi.org/10.1111/ejh.12995.
18. Vlachos A, Ball S, Dahl N, et al. Diagnosing and treating diamond Blackfan anaemia: results of an international clinical consensus conference. Br J Haematol. 2008;142(6):859–76. https://doi.org/10.1111/j.1365-2141.2008.07269.x.

19. Strahm B, Loewecke F, Niemeyer CM, et al. Favorable outcomes of hematopoietic stem cell transplantation in children and adolescents with Diamond-Blackfan anemia. Blood Adv. 2020;4(8):1760–9. https://doi.org/10.1182/bloodadvances.2019001210.
20. Dyskeratosis Congenita and Telomere Biology Disorders: Diagnosis and Management Guidelines, 1st edition. https://teamtelomere.org/wp-content/uploads/2018/07/DC-TBD-Diagnosis-And-Management-Guidelines.pdf.
21. Fioredda F, Iacobelli S, Korthof ET, et al. Outcome of haematopoietic stem cell transplantation in dyskeratosis congenita. Br J Haematol. 2018;183(1):110–8. https://doi.org/10.1111/bjh.15495.
22. Townsley DM, Dumitriu B, Young NS. Danazol treatment for telomere diseases. N Engl J Med. 2016;375(11):1095–6. https://doi.org/10.1056/NEJMc1607752.
23. Germeshausen M, Ballmaier M. CAMT-MPL: congenital amegakaryocytic thrombocytopenia caused by MPL mutations—heterogeneity of a monogenic disorder—a comprehensive analysis of 56 patients. Haematologica. 2021;106(9):2439–48. https://doi.org/10.3324/haematol.2020.257972.
24. King S, Germeshausen M, Strauss G, Welte K, Ballmaier M. Congenital amegakaryocytic thrombocytopenia: a retrospective clinical analysis of 20 patients. Br J Haematol. 2005;131(5):636–44. https://doi.org/10.1111/j.1365-2141.2005.05819.x.
25. Skokowa J, Dale DC, Touw IP, Zeidler C, Welte K. Severe congenital neutropenias. Nat Rev Dis Primers. 2017;3:17032. https://doi.org/10.1038/nrdp.2017.32.
26. Carlsson G, Winiarski J, Ljungman P, et al. Hematopoietic stem cell transplantation in severe congenital neutropenia. Pediatr Blood Cancer. 2011;56(3):444–51. https://doi.org/10.1002/pbc.22836.

Chapter 19
Sickle Cell Disease

Alexis K. Williams and Iberia Romina Sosa

Case

A 21-year-old African American woman presents to the emergency department with severe pain. She has sickle cell disease and is on hydroxyurea. She recently transitioned her care from the sickle cell treatment center at her local children's hospital to an adult program and has had difficulty with the transition. She reports aching, debilitating pain in chest, lower back, and legs that she describes to be 9/10. She is febrile 102F, tachycardic, with a heart rate of 120 bpm, normotensive 110/60 mmHg, respiratory rate of 30, and oxygen saturation of 91%. On chest X-ray, there are new pulmonary infiltrates in bilateral, lower lung lobes.

Clinical Context

Sickle cell disease is a hemoglobinopathy caused by an autosomal recessive mutation in the codon for the sixth amino acid of the β-hemoglobin chain. This mutation results in the substitution of a glutamate for a valine, which results in a conformational change in the affected hemoglobin, hemoglobin S (HbS). Intracellular polymerization of HbS occurs when sickle red blood cells (RBCs) are partially deoxygenated under hypoxic conditions in the microcirculation [1, 2]. A disruption in erythrocyte conformation converts the traditionally biconcave RBC to a

A. K. Williams
School of Medicine, Baylor College of Medicine, Houston, TX, USA
e-mail: Alexis.williams@nyulangone.org

I. R. Sosa (✉)
Department of Hematology/Oncology, Fox Chase Cancer Center, Philadelphia, PA, USA
e-mail: iberia.sosa@fccc.edu

© The Author(s), under exclusive license to Springer Nature Switzerland AG 2024
G. Rivero, I. R. Sosa (eds.), *Consulting Hematology and Oncology Handbook*,
https://doi.org/10.1007/978-3-031-75810-2_19

banana-like "sickle" shape that is classically seen on peripheral blood smear of sickle cell patients (Fig. 19.1). The primary symptomatology of patients with sickle cell anemia (SCA) is due to the sickle shape of the RBC disrupting their deformability through the vasculature and increasing adherence to endothelium. This leads to microvascular occlusion and hemolysis which result in significant organ damage. Patients with SCA are susceptible to autosplenectomy prior to adulthood due to the obstruction caused by the misshapen RBC in the spleen's vasculature resulting in scarring and atrophy of the organ. In general, RBC sickling occurs when greater than 50% of the hemoglobin present in an erythrocyte is HbS. However, concentrations of less than 50% HbS may also lead to clinical consequences if the RBC is exposed to significant hypoxia or dehydration, as may occur in certain anatomical locations such as the renal tubules [3]. Due to the potential for long-term organ damage, SCA is associated with significant morbidity and mortality worldwide. Recent improvements in coordinated care and novel pharmacologic agents have improved outcomes significantly.

Compound sickle cell syndromes include hemoglobinopathies in which the sickle cell mutation is inherited in combination with another hemoglobin mutation. The clinical variability seen in sickle cell disease (SCD) is accounted by the hemoglobin variant that accompanies HbS, including HbC, HbD, HbE, or β-thalassemia (Table 19.1). The inherited combination of HbS and HbC results in a less pronounced conformational change in hemoglobin; hence, these individuals have a milder form of sickle cell disease with less morbidity. HbS can also be heterozygous with β-thalassemia. Thalassemias refer to a spectrum of diseases characterized by a reduced or absent production of hemoglobin. In β-thalassemia, there is an overall decrease or absence in the production of hemoglobin β-chain. Clinical symptoms are determined by the level of HbA produced. Individuals with $HbS\beta^0$ produce less HbA than those with $HbS\beta^+$ and will have a clinical presentation that is virtually indistinguishable from those with HbSS.

Patients with SCA usually require lifelong management of their disease and present with acute exacerbations throughout their lives. On average, patients will

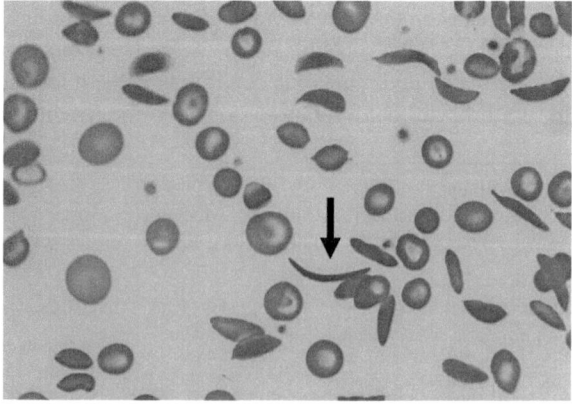

Fig. 19.1 Representation of irreversible sickled cells from a patient with Hb SS (black arrow)

Table 19.1 Comparison of sickle hemoglobinopathies [4]

Genotype	Severity of disease	Hemoglobin composition
HbA (Normal)	N/A	95–98% HbA 2–3% HbA_2 <2% HbF
HbSA	Mild	50–60% HbA <3.5% HbA_2 <2% HbF 25–45% HbS
HbSS	Severe	<3.5% HbA_2 5–15% HbF 85–95% HbS
HbSC	Moderate	<3.5% HbA_2 1–5% HbF 45–40% HbS 45–50% HbC
HbS β^0	Severe	>3.5% HbA_2 2–15% HbF 80–92% HbS
HbS β^+	Mild-moderate	3–30% HbA >3.5% HbA_2 2–10% HbF 65–90% HbS

present to the hospital with vaso-occlusive crises approximately 3 times per year and have an approximate life expectancy to 54 years old [5, 6].

Clinical Manifestations

Patients with SCA have a chronic normocytic anemia caused by intravascular and extravascular hemolysis. This anemia usually has a high reticulocyte count and is polychromatic due to reticulocytes. Symptoms may include fatigue, presyncope, and headache depending on the severity of the anemia.

The most common acute exacerbation of SCA manifests in the form of pain crises. These crises are due to vaso-occlusion of bone and nervous microvasculature and present as nociceptive and neuropathic pain. Pain crises usually cause moderate to severe pain and often require inpatient admission for intravenous pain control [4] and monitoring for complications. Dactylitis, painful swelling of the fingers and toes, is a common complication of SCA in children.

Please refer to section "Special Considerations" at the end of this chapter for a detailed review of clinical manifestations and complications of SCA. Figure 19.2 lists clinical manifestations.

Laboratory Investigation

SCA is commonly a prenatal diagnosis. Hemoglobin electrophoresis of maternal and paternal blood can be used to find pregnancies at risk for SCA. This is routinely done in at-risk populations in the United States. High-performance chromatography or capillary electrophoresis are more sensitive and specific tests that have largely replaced gel electrophoresis for this purpose [1]. In those at risk, chorionic villous sampling for hemoglobin electrophoresis can be done as early as 8–10 weeks.

In infants identified to have SCA, transcranial Doppler is usually done between ages 2 and 16 years to identify risk of stroke [7]. Intervals of transcranial Doppler is determined by the risk of stroke, with patients at higher risk receiving more frequent screening (see "Useful Tools" for information on screening protocols).

In a child or adult presenting with undiagnosed SCA, there are several tests in addition to hemoglobin electrophoresis that may help identify SCA. A simple complete blood count with peripheral blood smear (CBC/PBS) will show a normocytic

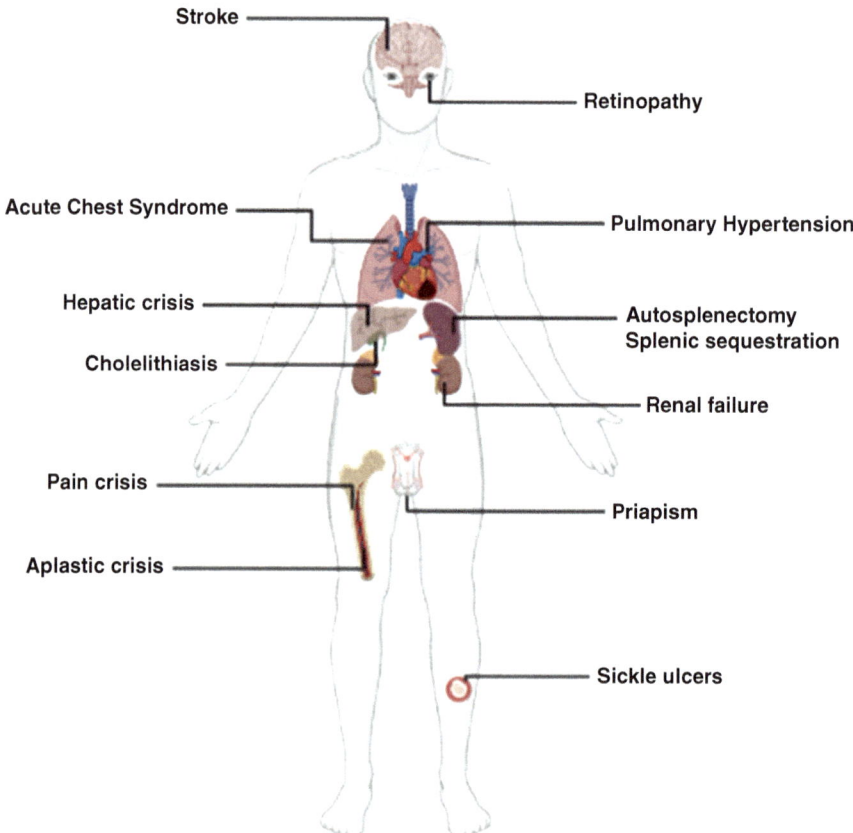

Fig. 19.2 Illustration of the various complications of sickle cell anemia throughout the body

anemia with increased reticulocyte count, polychromasia, decreased numbers of red blood cells, sickle cells, and Howell-Jolly bodies in those patients that have undergone autosplenectomy secondary to SCA. The SICKLEDEX screen uses a concentrated phosphate buffer solution to precipitate HbS while HbA remains in solution [5]. Importantly, the SICKLEDEX screen is not specific for SCA as individuals with sickle cell trait, hemoglobin SC disease, or hemoglobin Sβ-thalassemia will all have a positive SICKLEDEX test.

Management

Management of Acute Pain Crisis

The first step in the management of an acute pain crisis is pain assessment. Pain can be characterized by intensity, duration, location, and tractability or response to medication. Importantly, in pediatric patients who cannot adequately describe their pain, modified assessment tools may be necessary [8]. Scales including the Face, Legs, Activity, Cry, and Consolability (FLACC) scale and the "Faces" scale can help clinicians determine the severity of a child's pain during a crisis. Table 19.2 shows the World Health Organization (WHO) guidelines for pain assessment and treatment.

NSAIDs such as ibuprofen and naproxen are often the first-choice regimen for pain control, especially in patients with mild-to-moderate pain. These medications are especially beneficial for their anti-inflammatory properties. However, NSAIDs have significant gastrointestinal, cardiac, and renal secondary effects that limit their use in patients with SCA [10]. Specifically, NSAIDs may cause acute kidney injury (AKI) and exacerbate chronic kidney disease (CKD) in SCA patients, who are already prone to renal complications [10].

If pain assessment demonstrates the need for opioids, route of administration is another important consideration. Multiple routes of administration, for example, intravenous with oral controlled release, may be best for rapid improvement of pain. In pediatric studies, intranasal dimorphone has also been found to be effective.

Multiple possible adjuvant therapies have been used in sickle cell pain crises, with varying degrees of effectiveness. Intravenous hydration is thought to help patients because a dehydrated state increases sickling thereby leading to vaso-occlusion [8, 11]. In patients with dehydration as a cause of their pain crisis or who

Table 19.2 WHO pain control ladder with suggested therapeutic regimens [9]

Pain level	Suggested therapy
Mild pain	Non-opioid analgesics (NSAIDs) acetaminophen, consider adjuvants
Moderate pain	Weak opioids (hydrocodone, codeine, tramadol), non-opioid analgesics, consider adjuvants
Severe pain	Potent opioids (morphine, methadone, fentanyl, oxycodone, buprenorphine, tapentadol, hydromorphone, oxymorphone), consider non-opioid analgesics, consider adjuvants

have insufficient volume, IV hydration is helpful; however, it may worsen cardiac status in a patient with cardiovascular comorbidities. Other nonpharmacologic therapies that have been used as adjuvants include transcutaneous electric nerve stimulation, acupuncture, and warm or cold compresses [10].

Other options for pharmacologic adjuvant therapy may include the following:

- Low-dose ketamine: As an NMDA antagonist, ketamine may help decrease erythrocyte binding to endothelial walls and therefore reduce vaso-occlusion [8].
- Low-molecular weight heparin: Antithrombotic activity may reduce vaso-occlusion and specifically decrease duration of pain crisis [8].
- Hydroxyurea: May reduce likelihood of pain crises by multiple mechanisms including increased production of fetal hemoglobin (HbF; decreasing erythrocyte-endothelium interaction and thus reducing vaso-occlusion; increasing nitric oxide (NO) and promoting vasodilation; and reducing pro-thrombotic activity in the blood) [5].
- Inhaled nitric oxide: Promotes vasodilation and reduces vaso-occlusion [6].
- Magnesium sulfate: Although the mechanism has not been fully elucidated, magnesium sulfate may have a vasodilatory effect that reduces duration and intensity of pain crises [6].

Regardless of the treatment regimen chosen, multimodal therapy is generally more effective at pain control during a sickle cell crisis.

Transfusion Therapy

Transfusion is an important component of SCA treatment. There are different types of transfusion available to SCA patients depending on the indication (Table 19.3). Transfusions can be done in the acute setting or on an ongoing basis. In patients receiving chronic transfusions, iron chelators such as deferoxamine should be considered to prevent secondary hemosiderosis [2, 11]. In patients who require exchange transfusion, the Exchange Transfusion Calculator can be used to determine the volume of blood required (see "Useful Tools").

Chronic Management of SCA

Hydroxyurea has historically been the most useful drug for control of chronic SCA. The use of hydroxyurea has been revolutionary in prolonging lifespan and decreasing morbidity in SCA patients, decreasing mortality by 40% [12]. Hydroxyurea's primary mechanism of action occurs by increasing the concentration of HbF in erythrocytes. HbF is made of two alpha hemoglobin chains and two gamma globin chains. Since it does not have beta chains, it is not susceptible to sickling. Increasing the concentration of HbF in an erythrocyte to >50% therefore

Table 19.3 Indications for transfusion in SCA

Simple transfusion	Chronic simple transfusion	Exchange transfusion	Partial exchange transfusion
Symptomatic anemia	Cerebrovascular disease	Acute stroke	Hemoglobin S-C disease undergoing major surgical procedure
Aplastic crisis	Pain crises	Acute chest syndrome with severe hypoxia	
Splenic sequestration	Pulmonary disease		
Hepatic sequestration	Cardiac disease	Priapism	
Acute chest syndrome	Complicated pregnancy	Acute multiorgan failure	
Multiorgan failure with severe anemia	Positive intracranial Doppler		

makes the cell less likely to sickle. Unfortunately, hydroxyurea's responses in erythrocytes and across individuals are highly variable, so it must be titrated to achieve optimum response. The starting dose for hydroxyurea is 15 mg/kg/day and can be increased by 5 mg/kg/day every 12 weeks until a maximum dose of 35 mg/kg/day is reached. Since hydroxyurea may cause bone marrow suppression at high doses, titration must be carefully monitored with complete blood count done every 2 weeks to assess for any medication-induced impairment of bone marrow function.

In addition to hydroxyurea, several other agents have been developed for the treatment of SCA and are in various stages of implementation in clinical practice and are listed in Table 19.4. The novel P-selectin inhibitor crizanlizumab is increasingly becoming a routine part of SCA treatment.

While there is currently no pharmacologic cure for SCA, hematopoietic stem cell transplant (HSCT) is currently under investigation as a curative treatment. Allogeneic HSCT from a HLA-matched donor is already being used in children and adolescents, although it requires immunosuppression and has a risk of graft-versus-host disease (GVHD) if the patient is not properly immunomodulated. Furthermore, if the patient does not have an HLA-matched sibling, finding a donor that is HLA-matched can be difficult. Allogeneic transplant has previously been decreasingly successful with increased age, so guidelines currently recommend HSCT only in children. However, recent studies suggest safety and efficacy of allogeneic HSCT with lower intensity ablative regimens [14]. Autologous HSCT with gene editing has been proposed as a solution to the limitations of allogeneic HSCT. For this therapy, SCA patients would have their bone marrow harvested and their stem cells edited to remove or replace the HbS gene before being transplanted with the new stem cells [11]. Autologous HSCT would not require immunosuppression or HLA matching and carries no risk of GVHD; however, the gene editing process is still in the early stages of investigation and may be years away from implementation in clinical practice.

Table 19.4 New agents for treatment of chronic SCA [13]

Agent	Mechanism of action
Crizanlizumab	P-selectin antibody, prevents vaso-occlusion
Rivipansel	E-selectin inhibitor, prevents vaso-occlusion
Panobinostat	Increases HbF
Voxelotor	Stabilizes oxygenated hemoglobin state to prevent sickling
Senicapoc	Blocks K+ channels to prevent cell dehydration
Memantine	NMDA antagonist, erythrocyte adhesion, and cell dehydration
L-glutamine	Reduces vaso-occlusion
Factor Xa inhibitors	Anti-coagulation reduces vaso-occlusion
P2Y12 inhibitors (clopidogrel, prasogurel)	Anti-coagulation reduces vaso-occlusion
N-acetylcysteine	Reduces oxidative stress and decreases inflammation

Prophylaxis

Patients with SCA require certain supportive prophylactic regimens to prevent complications. Most sickle cell patients undergo autosplenectomy in childhood; therefore, SCA patients should be treated as if they are asplenic. Children with SCA receive penicillin prophylaxis until they are 5 years of age [11]. They should also receive vaccinations against encapsulated organisms including *Haemophilus influenzae*, *Neisseria meningitidis*, and *Streptococcus pneumoniae*. Due to hemolysis, patients with SCA have increased cell turnover and therefore increased folate requirements for DNA synthesis. These patients should receive prophylactic folate. Finally, any patient who is hospitalized for sickle cell pain crisis should be provided an incentive spirometer and counseled on use to prevent acute chest syndrome.

Specific Considerations

Stroke

Strokes are a potentially life-threatening complication of SCA with prevalence as high as 4.0% per year in SCA patients. Strokes in SCA patients are not always clinically apparent; many SCA patients will have strokes that are not diagnosed at the time of acute infarction [15]. Strokes in SCA may be ischemic or hemorrhagic, so prompt evaluation for suspicious symptoms is necessary (Fig. 19.3). Most occluded vessels include internal carotid artery (ICA) and the anterior Circle of Willis, including anterior and middle cerebral arteries (ACA, MCA) [17]. Notably, transcranial Doppler has been one of the most effective screening tools for prevention of stroke in SCA patients (Table 19.5) [19].

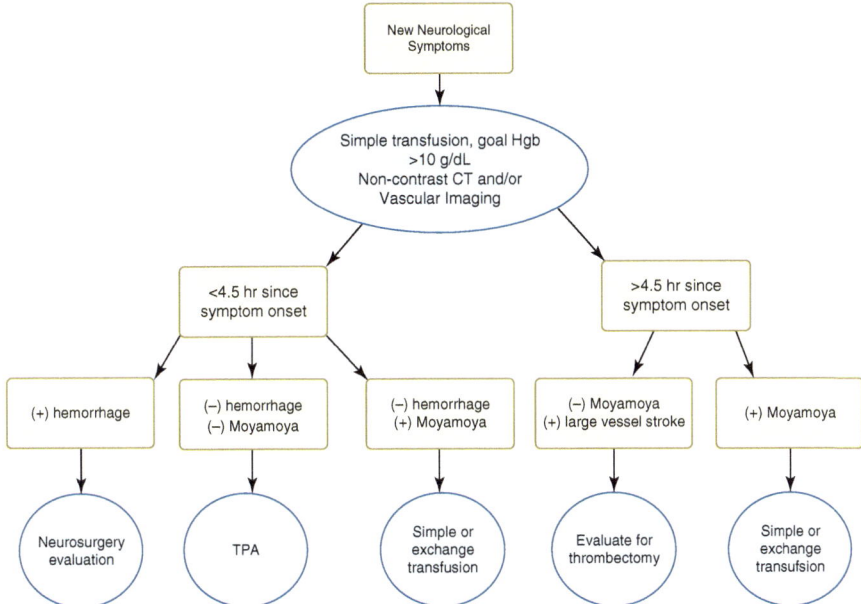

Fig. 19.3 Algorithm for evaluation and treatment of stroke in SCA [16]. Note: Consideration for TPA should be based on established inclusion/exclusion criteria detailed in stroke management and should not delay prompt simple or exchange transfusion

Retinopathy

Blockage of blood vessels in the retina and choroid may lead to changes in vision such as blind spots, flashes or floaters, and loss of side vision. This complication is more common in hemoglobin SC patients. SCA and hemoglobin SC patients should be screened for retinopathy yearly starting at age 10 [16].

Acute Chest Syndrome

Acute chest syndrome (ACS) is defined by a new density on chest radiograph accompanied by fever or respiratory symptoms such as tachypnea, chest pain, cough, wheezing, or decrease in oxygen saturation. Although the trigger for ACS is often unknown, infection and infarction are some common underlying causes [19]. ACS requires urgent medical management; some management strategies are shown in Table 19.6 [4].

Table 19.5 Screening intervals for transcranial Doppler in children with SCA [18]

Flow velocity	Screening protocol
<170 cm/s	Annually
170–185 cm/s	Repeat 3–6 months
185–200 cm/s	Repeat 1–3 months
>200	Repeat 1–2 weeks

Table 19.6 Recommendations for pain control in acute chest syndrome

Pain	Parenteral opioids
Respiratory support	• Oxygen to maintain arterial SpO_2 > 95% • Intubation or ECMO for standard indications [4]
Antibiotics	• Broad spectrum with particular coverage for community-acquired pneumonia (i.e., third-generation cephalosporin) and atypical pneumonia (macrolide)
Transfusion	• Initiate as soon as possible • Simple transfusion for mild to moderate ACS • Exchange transfusion for ACS with severe hypoxia
IV fluids	• As needed to maintain euvolemia and manage pain • Decrease as tolerated to avoid pulmonary edema

Pulmonary Hypertension

Free hemoglobin is a scavenger of NO, so patients with increased hemolysis such as SCA patients may have decreased NO and secondary pulmonary hypertension. The prevalence of pulmonary hypertension in adults with SCA is approximately 6–11%, and pulmonary hypertension can manifest as symptoms of right-heart failure and lead to eventual death [20]. Guidelines from the American Thoracic Society currently do not recommend targeted vasodilator therapy for sickle cell-associated pulmonary hypertension [21].

Hepatic Crisis

Acute sickle hepatopathy occurs in up to 10% of patients due to congestion of hepatic sinusoids. These patients may present with nausea, fever, right upper quadrant pain, and elevated conjugated bilirubin. Supportive treatment is generally sufficient to resolve these crises [22].

Cholelithiasis

Gallstone disease is common in SCA patients; the gallstones in SCA-related cholelithiasis are usually pigmented bile stones secondary to chronic hemolysis. Prevalence of cholelithiasis in SCA may be as high as 70%, with three-quarters of symptomatic patients requiring cholecystectomy [23].

Autosplenectomy

In most patients with SCA, the spleen undergoes episodes of vaso-occlusion and infarction during childhood, leading to atrophy and eventual disappearance of the spleen by adulthood. This disappearance results in increased susceptibility to infection, especially by encapsulated organisms; hence vaccine schedule (Table 19.7) is recommended for this population. Patients with Hgb SC disease and Hgb Sβ⁺ thalassemia may retain their spleens into adulthood and have less vulnerability to infection.

Splenic Sequestration

Splenic sequestration occurs due to widespread trapping of sickled RBCs in the splenic sinusoids. This may result in a significant portion of the body's blood volume being trapped in the spleen, with a drop in hemoglobin of up to 2 g/dL [25]. This complication is generally observed in childhood, as the spleen has usually disappeared in adult patients with SCA.

Renal Disease

The kidney is one of the most vulnerable organs to sickle vaso-occlusion due to the dehydrated, hypoxic, acidotic environment of the renal medulla. Patients with sickle cell trait may present with microscopic hematuria and eventual CKD, while patients with SCA may have more severe manifestations. Up to 18% of deaths in SCA

Table 19.7 Immunization recommendations for children with SCA [24]

Vaccine	Age	Recommended dosing
Hib	<5 years old	3 doses, 8 weeks between each dose
Hib	>5 years old	1 dose
MenB	>10 years old	Bexsero: 2 doses, 4 weeks between each dose OR Trumenba: 3 doses, 4 weeks between first and second dose, 6 months between second and third dose
MenACWY	>2 years old	2 doses, 4 weeks apart
PCV13	2–5 years old	2 doses, 8 weeks apart
PPSV23	2–5 years old	2 doses, 5 years apart, starting minimum 8 weeks after final PCV13 dose
PCV13	6–18 years old	1 dose
PPSV23	6–18 years old	2 doses, 5 years apart, starting minimum 8 weeks after final PCV13 dose

patients are attributable to CKD and eventual development of end-stage renal disease (ESRD) [26].

Aplastic Crisis

Parvovirus B19 is a common infection in children and usually causes erythema infectiosum, or "Fifth disease." Parvovirus B19 infects erythroblasts in the bone marrow and causes a decrease in erythropoiesis. In SCA patients with increased cell turnover, this temporary decrease in erythropoiesis can cause dangerous anemia [27]. Supportive care is the treatment of choice.

Priapism

Priapism is characterized by a prolonged erection that is not associated with sexual stimulation. In SCA patients, vaso-occlusion of the penile vasculature may cause ischemic priapism, in which infarction of penile tissue may occur. Priapism episodes lasting longer than 4 h are associated with irreversible loss of penile tissue. Acute priapism should be treated with aspiration of the corpus cavernosum followed by injection of an alpha-adrenergic agonist. Secondary prevention of priapism in those with repeated episodes occurring in spite of adequate treatment with hydroxyurea includes phosphodiesterase-5 (PDE5) inhibitors (i.e., sildenafil), alpha-adrenergic and beta-adrenergic agonists, and anti-androgenic hormonal therapies [28].

Sickle Ulcers

Skin ulcers are a common manifestation of SCA that most commonly occur in the leg. They are likely due to arteriovenous shunting causing decreased oxygen delivery to the skin. They are most common in the malleolar area and can be extremely painful and slow to heal [29].

Useful Tools

RBC Exchange Transfusion Formula [30]
    RBC replacement volume = RBC volume × ln (HbS% initial/HbS% goal)/donor Hematocrit
    RBC = total blood volume × patient Hematocrit
    HbS = percentage of hemoglobin that is HbS

References

1. Rees DC, Williams TN, Gladwin MT. Sickle-cell disease. Lancet. 2010;376(9757):2018–31.
2. Rodgers GP. Overview of pathophysiology and rationale for treatment of Sickle cell anemia. Semin Hematol. 1997;34(3 Suppl 3):2–7.
3. Scheinman JI. Sickle cell disease and the kidney. Nat Clin Pract Nephrol. 2009;5(2):78–88.
4. Yawn BP, Buchanan GR, Afenyi-Annan AN, Ballas SK, Hassell KL, James AH, Jordan L, Lanzkron SM, Lottenberg R, Savage WJ, et al. Management of Sickle cell disease: summary of the 2014 evidence-based report by expert panel members. JAMA. 2014;312(10):1033–48.
5. Shah N, Bhor M, Xie L, Halloway R, Arcona S, Paulose J, Yuce H. Treatment patterns and economic burden of Sickle-cell disease patients prescribed hydroxyurea: a retrospective claims-based study. Health Qual Life Outcomes. 2019;17(1):155.
6. Lubeck D, Agodoa I, Bhakta N, Danese M, Pappu K, Howard R, Gleeson M, Halperin M, Lanzkron S. Estimated life expectancy and income of patients with Sickle cell disease compared with those without sickle cell disease. JAMA Netw Open. 2019;2(11):e1915374.
7. Adams RJ, McKie VC, Carl EM, Nichols FT, Perry R, Brock K, McKie K, Figueroa R, Litaker M, Weiner S, et al. Long-term stroke risk in children with Sickle cell disease screened with transcranial Doppler. Ann Neurol. 1997;42(5):699–704.
8. Uwaezuoke SN, Ayuk AC, Ndu IK, Eneh CI, Mbanefo NR, Ezenwosu OU. Vaso-occlusive crisis in Sickle cell disease: current paradigm on pain management. J Pain Res. 2018;11:3141–50.
9. Anekar AA, Cascella M. WHO analgesic ladder. In: StatPearls. Treasure Island, FL: StatPearls; 2022.
10. Darbari DS, Sheehan VA, Ballas SK. The vaso-occlusive pain crisis in Sickle cell disease: definition, pathophysiology, and management. Eur J Haematol. 2020;105(3):237–46.
11. Aliyu ZY, Tumblin AR, Kato GJ. Current therapy of Sickle cell disease. Haematologica. 2006;91(1):7–10.
12. Steinberg MH, Barton F, Castro O, Pegelow CH, Ballas SK, Kutlar A, Orringer E, Bellevue R, Olivieri N, Eckman J, et al. Effect of hydroxyurea on mortality and morbidity in adult Sickle cell anemia: risks and benefits up to 9 years of treatment. JAMA. 2003;289(13):1645–51.
13. Cisneros GS, Thein SL. Recent advances in the treatment of Sickle cell disease. Front Physiol. 2020;11:435.
14. Saraf SL, Oh AL, Patel PR, Jalundhwala Y, Sweiss K, Koshy M, Campbell-Lee S, Gowhari M, Hassan J, Peace D, et al. Nonmyeloablative stem cell transplantation with Alemtuzumab/ low-dose irradiation to cure and improve the quality of life of adults with Sickle cell disease. Biol Blood Marrow Transplant. 2016;22(3):441–8.
15. Kassim AA, Galadanci NA, Pruthi S, DeBaun MR. How I treat and manage strokes in Sickle cell disease. Blood. 2015;125(22):3401–10.
16. Downes SM, Hambleton IR, Chuang EL, Lois N, Serjeant GR, Bird AC. Incidence and natural history of proliferative Sickle cell retinopathy: observations from a cohort study. Ophthalmology. 2005;112(11):1869–75.
17. Ohene-Frempong K, Weiner SJ, Sleeper LA, Miller ST, Embury S, Moohr JW, Wethers DL, Pegelow CH, Gill FM. Cerebrovascular accidents in Sickle cell disease: rates and risk factors. Blood. 1998;91(1):288–94.
18. DeBaun MR, Jordan LC, King AA, Schatz J, Vichinsky E, Fox CK, McKinstry RC, Telfer P, Kraut MA, Daraz L, et al. American Society of Hematology 2020 guidelines for sickle cell disease: prevention, diagnosis, and treatment of cerebrovascular disease in children and adults. Blood Adv. 2020;4(8):1554–88.
19. Ballas SK, Lieff S, Benjamin LJ, Dampier CD, Heeney MM, Hoppe C, Johnson CS, Rogers ZR, Smith-Whitley K, Wang WC, et al. Definitions of the phenotypic manifestations of Sickle cell disease. Am J Hematol. 2010;85(1):6–13.
20. Klings ES, Machado RF, Barst RJ, Morris CR, Mubarak KK, Gordeuk VR, Kato GJ, Ataga KI, Gibbs JS, Castro O, et al. An official American Thoracic Society clinical practice guide-

line: diagnosis, risk stratification, and management of pulmonary hypertension of Sickle cell disease. Am J Respir Crit Care Med. 2014;189(6):727–40.
21. Hayes MM, Vedamurthy A, George G, Dweik R, Klings ES, Machado RF, Gladwin MT, Wilson KC, Thomson CC. American Thoracic Society implementation task F: pulmonary hypertension in Sickle cell disease. Ann Am Thorac Soc. 2014;11(9):1488–9.
22. Banerjee S, Owen C, Chopra S. Sickle cell hepatopathy. Hepatology. 2001;33(5):1021–8.
23. Martins RA, Soares RS, Vito FB, Barbosa VF, Silva SS, Moraes-Souza H, Martins PR. Cholelithiasis and its complications in Sickle cell disease in a University Hospital. Rev Bras Hematol Hemoter. 2017;39(1):28–31.
24. Infanti LM, Elder JJ, Franco K, Simms S, Statler VA, Raj A. Immunization adherence in children with Sickle cell disease: a single-institution experience. J Pediatr Pharmacol Ther. 2020;25(1):39–46.
25. Pearson HA, McIntosh S, Ritchey AK, Lobel JS, Rooks Y, Johnston D. Developmental aspects of splenic function in Sickle cell diseases. Blood. 1979;53(3):358–65.
26. Ataga KI, Derebail VK, Archer DR. The glomerulopathy of Sickle cell disease. Am J Hematol. 2014;89(9):907–14.
27. Young NS, Brown KE. Parvovirus B19. N Engl J Med. 2004;350(6):586–97.
28. Ahuja G, Ibecheozor C, Okorie NC, Jain AJ, Coleman PW, Metwalli AR, Tonkin JB. Priapism and Sickle cell disease: special considerations in etiology, management, and prevention. Urology. 2021;156:e40–7.
29. Minniti CP, Eckman J, Sebastiani P, Steinberg MH, Ballas SK. Leg ulcers in Sickle cell disease. Am J Hematol. 2010;85(10):831–3.
30. Schwartz J, Winters JL, Padmanabhan A, Balogun RA, Delaney M, Linenberger ML, Szczepiorkowski ZM, Williams ME, Wu Y, Shaz BH. Guidelines on the use of therapeutic apheresis in clinical practice-evidence-based approach from the writing Committee of the American Society for apheresis: the sixth special issue. J Clin Apher. 2013;28(3):145–284.

Chapter 20
Transfusion Medicine Consultation

Garrett Diltz and Colleen Gilstad

General Principles in Transfusion Medicine

Blood group antigen: Constitute a sugar or protein present on the surface of a red blood cell (RBC). They are serologically defined by antisera thereby permitting agglutination.

Blood group system: A series of one or more RBC antigens that are controlled by a single gene or two or more closely linked genes. The International Society of Blood Transfusion currently recognizes 44 blood group systems containing 354 RBC antigens. This list is updated as more systems and antigens are identified. Table 20.1 shows the characteristics of clinically significant blood groups.

Blood typing: The testing of a blood sample to determine the patient's blood group.

Antibody Screen: A test performed to assess for the presence of antibodies to RBC antigens in an individual's serum.

Crossmatch: Testing the compatibility between a donor and recipient's blood samples.

G. Diltz (✉) · C. Gilstad
Lombardi Comprehensive Cancer Center, Georgetown University School of Medicine, Washington, DC, USA
e-mail: Garrett.p.diltz@medstar.net; Colleen.w.gilstad@medstar.net

© The Author(s), under exclusive license to Springer Nature Switzerland AG 2024
G. Rivero, I. R. Sosa (eds.), *Consulting Hematology and Oncology Handbook*, https://doi.org/10.1007/978-3-031-75810-2_20

Table 20.1 FDA-required blood group antigens on reagent red blood cells

Blood group name	Antigen symbols	Immune vs. naturally occurring	Hemolytic transfusion reaction from antibody
ABO	A, B, AB, A1	Naturally occurring	Yes, acute
Rhesus	D, C, c, E, e	Immune	Yes, delayed
Kell	K, k	Immune	Yes, delayed
Kidd	Jk^a, Jk^b	Immune	Yes, delayed
Duffy	Fy^a, Fy^b	Immune	Yes, delayed
MNS	M, N, S, s	Naturally occurring (anti-M/N), immune (anti-S/s)	Rare (anti-M/N), yes (anti-S/s)
Lewis	Le^a, Le^b	Naturally occurring	Rare
P1PK	P1	Naturally occurring	Rare

ABO Blood Group

Karl Landsteiner discovered the ABO blood group in 1900. Individuals can be clas-sified into type A, type B, type AB, and type O based on the presence of different glycoprotein antigens (A, B, AB, H). These antigens are present on RBCs as well as platelets and other tissues (Fig. 20.1). The absence of an ABO antigen increases the antibody titer in an individual's serum against that antigen. An individual with type A blood has the A antigen and antibodies in their serum against the B antigen (anti-B antibody)). An individual with type B blood contains the B antigen and anti-A antibodies. Individuals with type AB blood contain both the A and B antigens and do not have antibodies against A or B. Individuals with type O blood do not contain A or B antigen and have anti-A, anti-B, and anti-A,B antibodies [1–4].

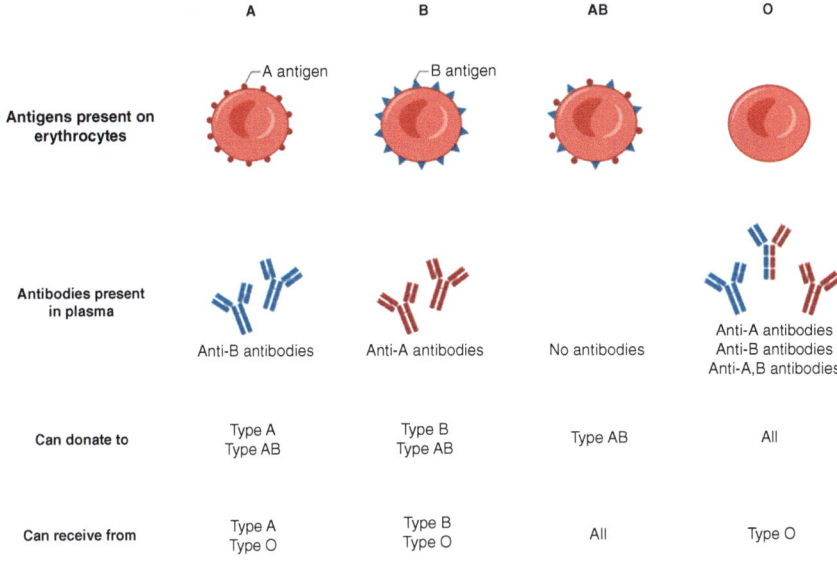

Fig. 20.1 ABO blood types

Rh Blood Group System

The Rh blood group system is the most polymorphic of the human blood groups, currently with 56 antigens identified [3]. It is the second most clinically relevant, after the ABO blood group system. The main antigen in the Rh blood group system is the D antigen. Rh blood typing determines the presence or absence of the D antigen using an anti-D reagent [5]. Anti-D antibodies are not naturally occurring, and most Rh (D) negative patients do not have anti-D antibodies. Antibodies generally arise when there is exposure to blood from another individual (such as prior transfusions or during pregnancy).

Testing Prior to Transfusion

Patients who will receive transfusion products are routinely tested for the ABO and RH(D) antigens, which are essential to ensure safety. Other blood group antigens frequently tested for include MNS, Lewis, Kell, Duffy, and Kidd. These are especially important in patients that are at higher risk for developing alloantibodies. Testing is done with serologic assays based on hemagglutination reactions with RBC antigens against specific antibodies.

Patient RBC   **Test Serum**   **Reaction Result**

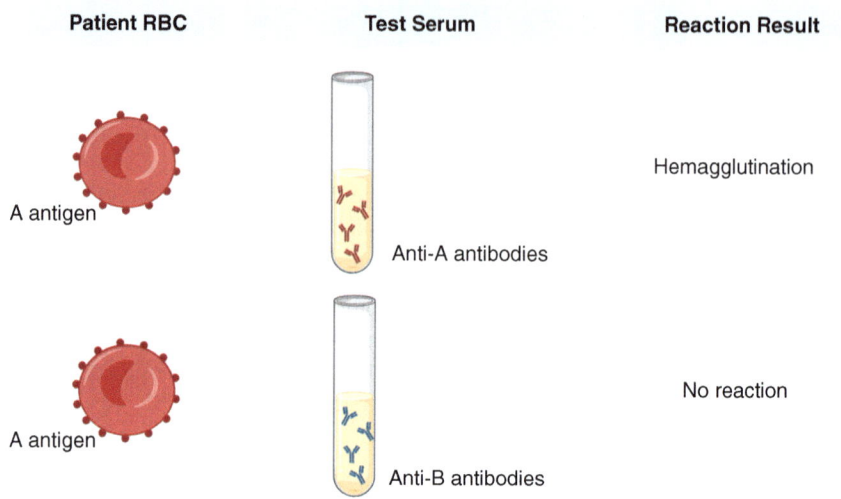

A antigen

Anti-A antibodies

Hemagglutination

A antigen

Anti-B antibodies

No reaction

Fig. 20.2 Forward typing

Forward typing utilizes a patient's RBC mixed with commercially available antibody. *Reverse typing* utilizes patient plasma (which may or may not contain antibodies) with commercially available reagent RBC. If an individual's RBC agglutinates with anti-A serum but not with anti-B serum, this would indicate the patient has type A blood (Fig. 20.2) identified through forward typing. If an individual's RBCs do not react with anti-A or anti-B serum, then this patient's blood is type O. Using reverse typing would allow the same blood type identification by using serum. For example, serum from a patient with type B blood (which will contain anti-A antibodies) will react with type A RBCs but not with type B RBCs (Fig. 20.3).

An *antibody screen* is performed in order to exclude the presence of antibodies to common, clinically significant antigens. In this test, a patient's serum is tested against multiple reagent RBCs with known phenotypes of common, clinically significant antigens.

The combination of blood group typing and an antibody screen is what is colloquially referred to as a "type and screen."

Prior to transfusion, a *crossmatch* is also performed. In this test, a patient's serum is tested against the RBCs from the donor unit to be transfused to verify that there is no agglutination.

In clinical practice, prior to a blood transfusion, a patient will undergo at a minimum forward and reverse typing for ABO antigens, forward typing for Rh(D) antigen, an antibody screen, and crossmatch. Many patients with hematologic disorders can have presence of antibodies against other minor antigens (exacerbated by prior heavy transfusion burdens) that necessitate further nuanced testing [1, 6].

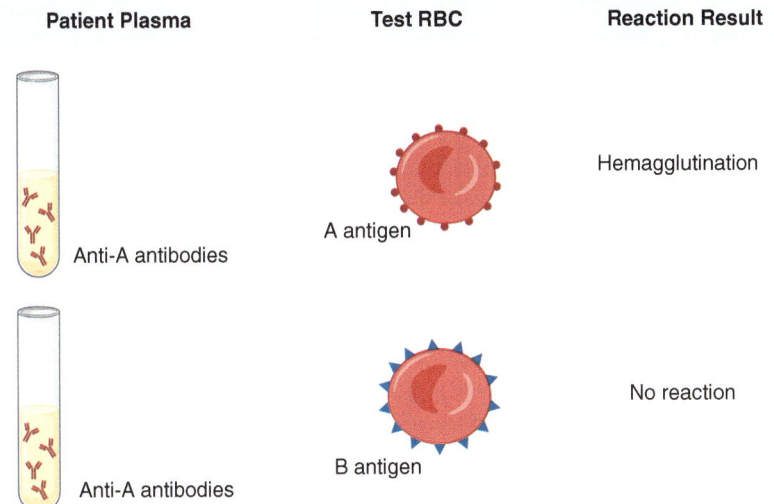

Fig. 20.3 Reverse typing

Transfusion of Blood Components

RBCs (RBCs)

Each unit of RBCs is about 250–300 cc and is thought to raise the hemoglobin level by approximately 1 g/dL or the hematocrit by 3%. RBCs must be refrigerated and can be stored for up to 42 days. Most guidelines recommend transfusion for a hemoglobin <7 g/dL, though one can consider higher thresholds in acute coronary syndromes, acute stroke, symptomatic anemia, acute blood loss, or other special situations as clinically warranted. Emergency red blood cell transfusions use type O, Rh(D) negative blood. Type O, Rh (D) positive blood can also be used in some emergency situations since most Rh (D) negative patients do not have anti-D antibodies as these are not naturally occurring [7, 8].

Platelets

Platelets can be collected using apheresis (one donor) or can be pooled from whole blood products of multiple donors. Advantages of apheresis platelets include exposure to only a single donor and the ability to match donor and recipient characteristics (i.e., HLA type, CMV status, blood type). In both types of platelet collection, there are residual white blood cells (WBCs) and plasma, which can lead to transfusion complications. Platelets are stored at room temperature and generally have a shelf life of only 5 days due to the cumulative increased risk of bacterial infection when stored at room temperature compared to lower temperatures. To decrease the risk of infection, all platelets in the United States undergo bacterial culture or a pathogen reduction method that prevents bacterial and viral DNA and RNA transcription.

General indications for platelet transfusion include thrombocytopenia, dysfunctional platelet disorders, and active platelet-related bleeding. Prophylactic use for prevention of spontaneous bleeding is generally based on platelet counts less than 10 k/uL for otherwise clinically stable patients with bone marrow failure or to prevent bleeding for planned procedures, with transfusion thresholds of 10 k to 50 k/uL, driven by type and invasiveness of procedure [9–13]. Platelets do express ABO antigens and HLA class I antigens on their surface, but not Rh antigens or HLA class II antigens. Platelets are not typically cross-matched, and ABO-matching is not strictly necessary for platelet transfusion. However, if refractoriness to platelet transfusion develops (i.e., post-transfusion increase consecutively <10 k/L), then using ABO-matched or HLA-matched platelets may increase response. This can become especially important for patients with hematologic malignancies that require frequent platelet transfusions, thus increasing risk for platelet refractoriness [14, 15].

Plasma Products

There are several different whole plasma products that are commonly used in practice. Fresh Frozen Plasma (FFP) is a plasma product that is frozen within 8 h of collection. Plasma frozen within 24 h after phlebotomy (PF24) is a plasma that is frozen more than 8 h but less than 24 h after collection. Thawed plasma is a plasma that was frozen (FFP or PF24) and subsequently thawed and kept at room temperature for up to 5 days. Solvent/detergent (S/D) plasma is treated with viral inactivating agents prior to freezing. FFP has a volume of about 200–250 cc and is usable for up to 1 year after the date of collection. Plasma products in general contain all of the coagulation factors and proteins present in the original unit of blood, though the concentrations can differ depending on the method and timing of storage [16, 17]. Other plasma products can also be created by further refining the product, including cryoprecipitate, gamma globulin, albumin, purified coagulation factors, and others. FFP or other plasma products can be used in deficiencies of multiple coagulation factors, such as in severe liver disease, DIC, or massive transfusions. It can also be used in other specific clinical situations if purified products are not available.

Plasma contains antibodies against RBC antigens. Collected blood undergoes an antibody screen (serum is tested against RBC with known antigens), and if positive, plasma products will not be made from that blood. A patient with group A blood can accept plasma from donors who are group A or group AB. A patient with group B blood can accept plasma from donors who are group B or group AB. A patient with group AB blood can only accept plasma from donors who are group AB. A patient with group O blood can accept plasma from donors who are group O, A, B, or AB. Thus, group AB patients are universal plasma donors.

There are several modifications that can be performed to transfusion products to increase safety in certain circumstances.

- *Leukoreduction* removes WBCs by filtration. This can decrease febrile non-hemolytic transfusion reactions, CMV transmission, HLA alloimmunization, and platelet transfusion refractoriness. Leukoreduction can be done either at the time of collection (pre-storage leukoreduction) or prior to transfusion (bedside leukoreduction), though pre-storage leukoreduction is preferred. In many hospital systems and developed countries, there has been implementation of universal leukoreduction [18].
- *Irradiation* subjects RBC or platelet units to 2500 cGy of radiation (targeted to the central aspect of the unit) with the goal of inactivating lymphocytes in the product. Viable donor lymphocytes can attack recipient cells in individuals that are unable to mount an appropriate immune response against them, resulting in transfusion associated graft versus host disease (TA-GvHD) which leads to bone marrow aplasia and other complications that can ultimately be fatal. Leukoreduction is not sufficient to prevent TA-GvHD in vulnerable populations because a small number of viable lymphocytes remain in the blood product. Irradiation increases cost, takes about 30 min, and reduces the shelf life of the irradiated RBC unit (28 days from time of irradiation and not longer than 42 days total in the United States). Platelets can also be irradiated, though the shelf life is not affected. Irradiation is not universally performed and is generally used for intrauterine or neonatal transfusions and for patients with congenital immunodeficiency, hematologic malignancies, stem cell transplants, and directed donations from blood relatives and with other states of immunosuppression due to certain T-cell suppressive medications [19, 20].
- *Washing* is performed on RBCs to eliminate complications that can arise from the residual plasma that remains in the unit. This can be done for patients with prior severe allergic reactions associated with transfusions and patients prone to hyperkalemia. Washing is done immediately prior to transfusion and decreases the shelf life (4 h at 20–24 °C or 24 h at 1–6 °C).

Case Demonstration Part 1

A 32-year-old female has been diagnosed with systemic lupus erythematosus (SLE) for 5 years. Her disease is characterized by hand and elbows arthritis. Additionally, she developed malar rash and progressive deterioration of her renal function with creatinine of 1.56 mg/dL. She follows with rheumatology and is currently on prednisone and mycophenolate. She was admitted for progressive fatigability and abdominal pain. She has had several days of dark, tarry stools. Her CBC showed a WBC of 3.2 k/uL, ANC 0.9 k/uL, hemoglobin 5.8 g/dL, and MCV 83 fL. Her heart rate is 125 beats/min and BP is 98/72. She appears pale and tired. GI bleeding from a gastric ulcer is suspected, and her hospitalist decides to transfuse her with 1 unit of RBC. However, blood bank notifies medical team that several antibodies were detected on antibody screen.

Clinical Context

Identifying and obtaining compatible RBC units can be challenging in patients with serologic complexity. A positive antibody screen or crossmatch can be the result of alloantibodies, autoantibodies, some monoclonal antibodies, or a change in blood type in patients who have undergone an allogeneic stem cell transplant. Alloantibodies can develop from exposure to blood or blood products from other individuals. These can become problematic in patients who require frequent transfusions, such as transfusion-dependent thalassemia or sickle cell anemia. In the event that completely matched blood products are not available in a patient with clear indication for transfusion, immune modulators such as IVIg and steroids have been used preemptively in an attempt to minimize hemolysis [21]. Autoimmune hemolytic anemia can result in autoantibodies that cause positive screening. Prior reviews have demonstrated safe administration of RBC units in patients with autoantibodies, even with serologic complexity. Thus, it is not recommended to withhold an indicated transfusion in this setting even if there is difficulty in finding compatible blood for transfusion [22], though the presence of autoantibodies can make detection of concurrent alloantibodies difficult. Certain therapeutic monoclonal antibodies can also cause panagglutination and affect the antibody screen, specifically anti-CD38 therapies (i.e., daratumumab and isatuximab) and anti-CD47 therapies (i.e., magrolimab). Patients who are planned for these treatments should have baseline type and screening performed prior to starting therapy to use as a comparison when future blood transfusion is indicated [23, 24]. Patients who have undergone allogeneic stem cell transplantation with ABO mismatched donors may have a new ABO type than prior to transplant. For example, a type O recipient who receives blood from a type B donor will have type B RBCs once engraftment occurs.

Laboratory Investigation

When planning to give a transfusion, important laboratory parameters include the following:

- CBC.
- Blood typing.
- Antibody screen.
- Crossmatch.

This patient has symptomatic anemia and an indication for transfusion of at least one unit of RBCs, though she has serologic complexity with multiple antibodies detected. On further questioning, the patient reveals that she received multiple units of blood in the past for excessive bleeding during childbirth, as well as for anemia when she was first diagnosed with SLE. With this history, the patient may have multiple alloantibodies that formed as a result of exposure to antigens from her prior transfusions, or autoantibodies related to her diagnosis of SLE, or both. Oxygen administration can be used to raise plasma oxygen levels in the short term to manage patients with severe anemia to allow for compatible blood to be identified. It will be important to work closely with the blood bank to weigh the risk versus benefit of immediate versus delayed transfusion based on the patient's clinical status and the type of antibody identified. In cases where compatible blood cannot be identified, sometimes "least incompatible" units may be indicated. In this case, the patient's plasma is serologically crossmatched to multiple units, and the one that has the weakest reaction is chosen. If it is not possible to find completely matched units, then prophylaxis with glucocorticoids and IVIg can be given [21].

Case Demonstration Part 2

Several minutes after the transfusion is started, she develops back pain and dizziness. She is pale and diaphoretic appearing. Vitals are obtained and notable for a temperature of 38.6 °C and blood pressure of 86/54.

Clinical Context

This constellation of symptoms is concerning for an acute hemolytic transfusion reaction. Her transfusion should be stopped immediately after she developed symptoms, and initial treatment is supportive with IV fluids and vasopressors. She should have a direct antiglobulin test (DAT), hemolysis markers, DIC markers, and chemistry sent. It is also prudent to perform a gram stain and blood cultures to rule out sepsis from contaminated blood products, as this can present similarly with fever and hemodynamic changes. It is also prudent to rule out non-immune causes of hemolysis, such as ensuring proper storage and administration of the products.

Fortunately, her transfusion was stopped expeditiously, and she stabilizes with fluid resuscitation. Laboratory testing reveals LDH 1200 U/L, haptoglobin undetectable, and total bilirubin 4.5 mg/dL, with indirect fraction 3.8 mg/dL. DAT is sent and results to positive 2+ for IgG and 2+ for C3. This confirms the suspicion of an acute hemolytic transfusion reaction, and an investigation is undertaken to determine the cause, as this most commonly results from clerical or logistical issues that result in ABO incompatibility of blood products.

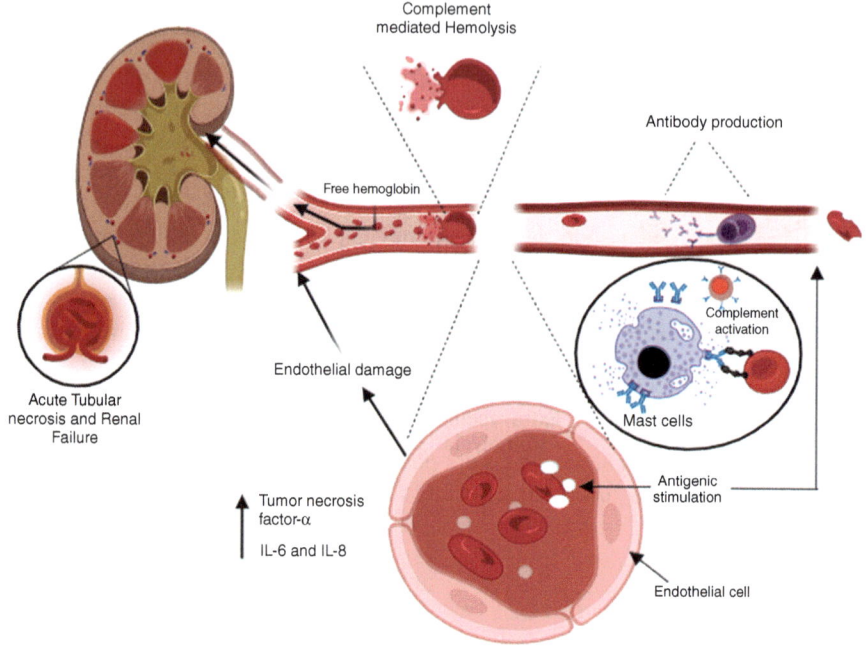

Fig. 20.4 Pathophysiology of acute hemolytic transfusion reactions

Acute hemolytic transfusion reactions occur when ABO incompatible products are administered resulting in significant intravascular hemolysis (e.g., type A blood transfused to a type B recipient) or can also occur due to a reaction to antigens in other blood group systems. This reaction leads antibodies to fix and activate the complement cascade, which can further result in release of pro-inflammatory cytokines and chemokines, resulting in a systemic inflammatory response (Fig. 20.4). Typical clinical manifestations include pain (back/flank), fever, dark urine, oliguria, hypotension and disseminated intravascular coagulation (DIC). The severity of reaction is related to the titer strength of the antibody in the recipient's plasma and the volume of incompatible blood transfused. Management is supportive and includes stopping the transfusion, fluid resuscitation, and vasopressors for blood pressure control. It is important to maintain aggressive hydration in order to maintain urine output and minimize renal damage. In addition, DIC parameters should be monitored regularly with the use of platelets, FFP, and cryoprecipitate for severe bleeding.

A new positive DAT is pathognomonic for immune-mediated hemolysis. This detects IgG or complement (C3) bound to the surface of the RBC. This test can be falsely negative in cases in which the hemolysis is short lived and brisk, resulting in these RBCs being cleared prior to testing.

Hemolysis can also occur with some platelet transfusions. Most platelets in the United States are collected via apheresis and suspended in donor plasma which contains antibodies complementary to blood type. Apheresis platelets are generally used without account of ABO compatibility. Thus, antibodies in ABO incompatible platelets can lead to hemolytic transfusion reactions.

While hemolysis is frequently due to immune causes, non-immune mechanisms can also lead to hemolysis. These include concurrent administration of a hypo-osmolar solution, transfusion of overheated to accidentally frozen blood, and using small bore needles. Importantly, autoimmune hemolytic anemia or drug-induced hemolytic anemia can be exacerbated by transfusion, which can mimic a hemolytic transfusion reaction [25–27].

Laboratory Investigation

Important labs to obtain when suspecting an acute hemolytic transfusion reaction include the following:

- CBC.
- Direct antiglobulin test.
- LDH.
- Total and direct bilirubin.
- Haptoglobin.
- Urinalysis.
- BUN/creatinine.
- D-dimer.
- Fibrinogen.
- Coagulation tests (PT and aPTT).
- Repeat ABO/Rh typing and antibody compatibility.

Case Demonstration Part 3

The patient's symptoms improve with transfusion of appropriate blood products. She undergoes EGD which identifies an ulcer in the gastric antrum, and she is started on a PPI. She is discharged and is seen in follow up with her Rheumatologist 3 weeks later. At this visit, she notes some yellowing of her eyes, and her energy level remains below her baseline. Laboratory testing is sent, which shows hemoglobin 6.7 g/dL. Further testing shows persistently elevated total bilirubin of 5.2 mg/dL, LDH 1050 U/L, and undetectable haptoglobin. A delayed hemolytic transfusion reaction is suspected. Antibody testing is sent and reveals the presence of a new anti-JkA antibody.

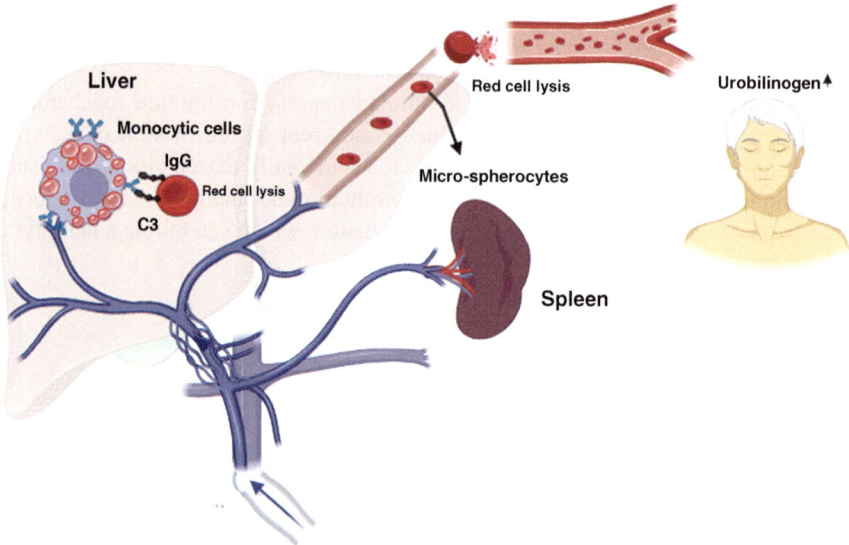

Fig. 20.5 Pathophysiology of delayed hemolytic transfusion reactions

Part 3 Discussion

Delayed hemolytic transfusion reactions occur due to minor antigen incompatibility due to immune responses in patients immunized by prior transfusions, stem cell transplant, or pregnancy. The general time of onset is 24 h to 1 month after the transfusion, and this rarely results in emergent or significant symptoms. Often, laboratory findings are the only signs of the diagnosis or can precede development of symptoms. Potential symptoms include fever, jaundice, and anemia. Testing can show a new antibody on screening or incompatible crossmatch, markers of hemolysis, a positive direct or indirect antiglobulin test, spherocytes or microspherocytes, and reticulocytosis (Fig. 20.5).

Laboratory Investigation

Important labs to obtain when suspecting a delayed hemolytic transfusion reaction include the following:

- CBC.
- Antibody screen.
- Direct and indirect antiglobulin test.
- LDH.
- Total and direct bilirubin.

- Haptoglobin.
- Reticulocyte count.
- Peripheral smear to assess for spherocytes or microspherocytes.

If the only abnormality is detection of a new clinically significant antibody in an otherwise asymptomatic patient without evidence of hemolysis, this is termed *delayed serologic transfusion reaction*. Commonly implicated blood group systems include Rh, Kidd, Duffy, and Kell.

Treatment

Treatment is supportive, though in severe cases immune modulators can be used, such as glucocorticoids, IVIg, or rituximab [25].

Case Demonstration Part 4

The patient is arranged for an RBC transfusion in an infusion center for later that day. A completely cross-matched unit is identified and available. This is administered over 2 h without issue. Her ride is delayed in arriving to take her home, and 1 h later she begins to have difficulty breathing. She alerts the staff, and vitals are notable for a drop in her oxygen saturation to 90% and a respiratory rate of 25 breaths/min. She is afebrile. She is taken to the Emergency Room for further workup and management.

Transfusion Reactions

Blood transfusions cause adverse reactions through a variety of mechanisms in addition to hemolysis, resulting in a variety of clinical manifestations [28, 29]. These can be grouped by their timing of onset in order to best assess patients who develop complications after receiving transfusions (Table 20.2).

Allergic/anaphylactic and acute hemolytic transfusion reactions develop within seconds to minutes of starting the transfusion. Febrile nonhemolytic, transfusion-associated circulatory overload (TACO), transfusion-related acute lung injury, and sepsis can develop within hours. Delayed hemolytic and TA-GvHD develop within days to weeks.

Allergic and anaphylactic reactions occur when recipient antibodies recognize donor antigens/proteins as foreign. This can range from a mild allergic reaction to anaphylaxis. Clinical manifestations can include itching/hives, flushing, bronchospasm, angioedema, nausea/vomiting, and tachycardia/hypotension and in severe

Table 20.2 Blood transfusion complications

Reaction	Frequency	Onset	Clinical findings	Lab findings	Pathophysiology	Management	Implicated products
Acute hemolytic transfusion reaction	1:76,000	Seconds to minutes	Fevers/chills, hypotension, back/flank pain	Hemoglobinuria, positive DAT, DIC	Typically, ABO incompatibility due to clerical error	Stop transfusion, fluid/press or support	RBCs, less commonly platelets or plasma
Allergic/anaphylactic reaction	Allergic: 1–3% with platelets/plasma, 0.1–0.3% with RBC Anaphylactic: 1:20,000 to 1:50,000	Seconds to minutes	Hives/urticarial, resp distress, bronchospasm, angioedema, hypotension	Hypoxia, elevated serum Tryptase	Recipient antibodies recognize donor antigen/protein as foreign	Stop transfusion antihistamines corticosteroids beta agonists and/or epinephrine	RBCs, plasma, platelets
TRALI	<0.01%	Hours	Resp distress, hypotension, fever	Abnormal chest imaging, hypoxia, leukopenia	Donor anti-HLA or anti-neutrophil antibodies target the pulmonary vasculature	Respiratory support, prevention by avoiding high risk donors	RBCs, plasma, platelets
TACO	<1%	Hours	Resp distress, volume overload	Abnormal chest imaging, elevated BNP, hypoxia	Volume overload	Diuresis, stopping or slowing transfusion rate	RBCs, plasma, platelets

Transfusion associated sepsis	1:50,000 with platelets 1:5 million with RBC	Hours	Fevers/chills, hypotension	Bacteremia, leukocytosis, DIC	Pathogens present in donor products	Appropriate sepsis management and antimicrobials, mitigation strategies to minimize infectious risk	Platelets most commonly, though can occur with any product
Febrile non-hemolytic transfusion reaction	1%, lower with leukoreduction	Hours	Fevers/chills, rigors	Normal DAT	Cytokines present in donor products	Supportive care, prevention by using leukoreduced products	All products, but rare with plasma
Delayed hemolytic transfusion reaction	1:800 to 1:11,000	24 h to weeks	Fever, jaundice, anemia	Newly positive DAT or IAT, evidence of hemolysis	Anamnestic response to antigen to which recipient was previously exposed	Supportive care, immune modulators if severe	RBCs

cases death. Management includes stopping the transfusion, antihistamines, corticosteroids, beta agonists, and epinephrine. These reactions can sometimes be mitigated by administering antihistamines and using washed products.

Febrile nonhemolytic transfusion reactions occur due to cytokines present in the transfusion product. Clinical manifestations can include fever, chills, and rigors. Management is supportive, though it is important to exclude other more serious reactions. This can be prevented by using leukoreduced products, as cytokines are thought to be released from donor leukocytes during collection and storage.

Transfusion associated circulatory overload (TACO) results in respiratory distress, volume overload, and pulmonary edema. Pro-BNP may be elevated. It is more common in patients at risk for volume overload, such as babies and the elderly, patients with underlying cardiac or renal disease, and patients receiving multiple transfusions in a short period of time. Management includes diuretics and/or slowing the transfusion rate [30].

Transfusion-related acute lung injury (TRALI) results in pulmonary edema that is not due to volume overload. Clinical manifestations include dyspnea, fever, and hypotension. This is the result of donor anti-HLA or anti-neutrophil antibodies that target to the pulmonary vasculature and cause a subsequent inflammatory response from the recipient, resulting in pulmonary edema. Management is with appropriate respiratory/ventilatory support and prevention [31, 32]. Prevention is best achieved by avoiding use of products from high-risk donors (i.e., multiparous women given increased risk of antibody production), and the incidence has decreased after implementation of a predominantly male plasma donor pool. TRALI is very rare as compared to TACO and, in general, is considered only after exclusion of TACO. If a reaction is suspected to be TRALI, the donor center/blood collection facility must be notified per FDA regulations and to assist with confirming the diagnosis by donor testing.

Transfusion associated sepsis occurs when pathogens grow in a product and are subsequently introduced to the recipient during transfusion. This can result in fevers/chills, rigors, tachycardia, and hypotension. Potential pathogens can include bacteria, parasites, viral hepatitis, and HIV and CMV, among others. Mitigation strategies to minimize infection risk include screening donors for risk factors as well as testing blood products for specific infections. If a septic transfusion reaction is suspected, the blood bank should be notified immediately so that co-collected components can be quarantined to prevent a reaction in another patient.

TA-GvHD is a very rare but serious complication. This results when viable donor lymphocytes can attack recipient cells in individuals that are unable to mount an appropriate immune response against them. This can result in rash, jaundice, abdominal pain, and cytopenias due to bone marrow aplasia. This can be prevented by using irradiated blood products in susceptible patients, such as those with hematologic malignancies and stem cell transplants.

Part 4 Discussion

Given her time of onset and predominant respiratory symptoms, TACO and TRALI are at the top of the differential. She has a chest X-ray, which shows diffuse bilateral pulmonary infiltrates, and pulse oximetry monitoring shows ongoing hypoxia, for which she is started on supplemental oxygen. Laboratory testing is notable for an elevated proBNP of 550 pg/mL and further decline in her renal function with creatinine of 2.60 mg/dL. Her JVP is elevated at 12 cm.

TACO and TRALI can be difficult to distinguish clinically, as both can result in respiratory distress, hypoxia, and pulmonary infiltrates/edema on chest imaging. Obtaining a proBNP and assessment of volume status can be important, as if there is elevated proBNP and/or volume overload, this makes TACO more likely. In this case, her respiratory symptoms are likely due to TACO, and she will need further investigation into her abnormal renal function and predisposition to volume overload.

References

1. Li HY, Guo K. Blood group testing. Front Med (Lausanne). 2022;9:827619. PMID: 35223922; PMCID: PMC8873177. https://doi.org/10.3389/fmed.2022.827619.
2. Mitra R, Mishra N, Rath GP. Blood groups systems. Indian J Anaesth. 2014;58(5):524–8. PMID: 25535412; PMCID: PMC4260296. https://doi.org/10.4103/0019-5049.144645.
3. Red Cell Immunogenetics and Blood Group Terminology: ISBT Working Party [Internet]. ISBT Working Party | The International Society of Blood Transfusion (ISBT). https://www.isbtweb.org/isbt-working-parties/rcibgt.html#:~:text=The%20International%20Society%20of%20Blood%20Transfusion%20(ISBT)%20Working%20Party%20for,cell%20antigens%20(December%202022. Accessed 28 Aug 2023.
4. American Association of Blood Banks. Standards for blood banks and transfusion services. 32nd ed. Arlington, VA: American Association of Blood Banks; 2020.
5. Avent ND, Reid ME. The Rh blood group system: a review. Blood. 2000;95:375–87.
6. Butch SII, Judd WJ, Steiner EA, et al. Electronic verification of donor-recipient compatibility: the computer crossmatch. Transfusion. 1994;34:105.
7. Carson JL, Grossman BJ, Kleinman S, et al. Red blood cell transfusion: a clinical practice guideline from the AABB*. Ann Intern Med. 2012;157:49.
8. Selleng K, Jenichen G, Denker K, Selleng S, Müllejans B, Greinacher A. Emergency transfusion of patients with unknown blood type with blood group O rhesus D positive red blood cell concentrates: a prospective, single-Centre, observational study. Lancet Haematol. 2017;4:e218–24.
9. Kaufman RM, Djulbegovic B, Gernsheimer T, et al. Platelet transfusion: a clinical practice guideline from the AABB. Ann Intern Med. 2015;162:205.
10. Murphy S, Gardner FH. Effect of storage temperature on maintenance of platelet viability—deleterious effect of refrigerated storage. N Engl J Med. 1969;280:1094.
11. McCullough J. Overview of platelet transfusion. Semin Hematol. 2010;47:235.
12. Pham TD, Kadi W, Shu E, et al. How do I implement pathogen-reduced platelets? Transfusion. 2021;61:3295.
13. Yuan S, Otrock ZK. Platelet transfusion: an update on indications and guidelines. Clin Lab Med. 2021;41:621.

14. Cohn CS. Platelet transfusion refractoriness: how do I diagnose and manage? Hematology Am Soc Hematol Educ Program. 2020;2020:527.
15. Schiffer CA, Bohlke K, Delaney M, et al. Platelet transfusion for patients with cancer: American Society of Clinical Oncology clinical practice guideline update. J Clin Oncol. 2018;36:283.
16. Roback JD, Caldwell S, Carson J, et al. Evidence-based practice guidelines for plasma transfusion. Transfusion. 2010;50:1227.
17. Dumont LJ, Cancelas JA, Maes LA, et al. The bioequivalence of frozen plasma prepared from whole blood held overnight at room temperature compared to fresh-frozen plasma prepared within eight hours of collection. Transfusion. 2015;55:476.
18. Mowla SJ, Sapiano MRP, Jones JM, et al. Supplemental findings of the 2019 National Blood Collection and utilization survey. Transfusion. 2021;61(Suppl 2):S11.
19. Davey RJ, McCoy NC, Yu M, et al. The effect of prestorage irradiation on posttransfusion red cell survival. Transfusion. 1992;32:525.
20. Zimmermann R, Wintzheimer S, Weisbach V, et al. Influence of prestorage leukoreduction and subsequent irradiation on in vitro red blood cell (RBC) storage variables of RBCs in additive solution saline-adenine-glucose-mannitol. Transfusion. 2009;49:75.
21. Win N, Needs M, Thornton N, Webster R, Chang C. Transfusion of least-incompatible blood with intravenous immunoglobulin plus steroids cover in two patients with rare antibody. Transfusion. 2018;58:1226–30.
22. Sokol RJ, Hewitt S, Booker DJ, Morris BM. Patients with red cell autoantibodies: selection of blood for transfusion. Clin Lab Haematol. 1988;10:257.
23. Lancman G, Arinsburg S, Jhang J, et al. Blood transfusion management for patients treated with anti-CD38 monoclonal antibodies. Front Immunol. 2018;9:2616.
24. Brierley CK, Staves J, Roberts C, et al. The effects of monoclonal anti-CD47 on RBCs, compatibility testing, and transfusion requirements in refractory acute myeloid leukemia. Transfusion. 2019;59:2248.
25. Panch SR, Montemayor-Garcia C, Klein HG. Hemolytic transfusion reactions. N Engl J Med. 2019;381:150–62.
26. Zantek ND, Koepsell SA, Tharp DR Jr, Cohn CS. The direct antiglobulin test: a critical step in the evaluation of hemolysis. Am J Hematol. 2012;87:707.
27. Soutar R, McSporran W, Tomlinson T, et al. Guideline on the investigation and management of acute transfusion reactions. Br J Haematol. 2023;201:832.
28. Suddock JT, Crookston KP. Transfusion reactions. In: StatPearls [Internet]. Treasure Island, FL: StatPearls; 2023. https://www.ncbi.nlm.nih.gov/books/NBK482202/. Accessed 8 Aug 2023.
29. Goel R, Tobian AAR, Shaz BH. Noninfectious transfusion-associated adverse events and their mitigation strategies. Blood. 2019;133:1831.
30. Zhou L, Giacherio D, Cooling L, Davenport RD. Use of B-natriuretic peptide as a diagnostic marker in the differential diagnosis of transfusion-associated circulatory overload. Transfusion. 2005;45:1056.
31. Eder AF, Dy BA, Perez JM, et al. The residual risk of transfusion-related acute lung injury at the American Red Cross (2008-2011): limitations of a predominantly male-donor plasma mitigation strategy. Transfusion. 2013;53:1442.
32. Skeate RC, Eastlund T. Distinguishing between transfusion related acute lung injury and transfusion associated circulatory overload. Curr Opin Hematol. 2007;14:682.

Chapter 21
Hematologic Consultation During Pregnancy

Giuliana Berardi and Iberia Romina Sosa

Pregnancy Considerations

Anemia During Pregnancy

Case

A 30-year-old G1P0 female presents to the gynecology clinic for a routine first tri-mester visit. She has a history of iron deficiency anemia secondary to her menstrual periods for which she previously saw hematology for parenteral iron infusions. Her baseline hemoglobin (Hgb) is 12 g/dL, and on lab work during clinic visit, her Hgb is 10 g/dL with mean corpuscular volume (MCV) 76. She inquires whether she will need further iron infusions or if taking her daily pregnancy multivitamin and main-taining a balanced diet will be sufficient.

Clinical Context

Anemia in pregnancy is a global problem. According to the World Health Organization, anemia complicates approximately 40% of pregnancies worldwide [1]. Hemoglobin is the oxygen-carrying protein, necessary for the pregnant patient to support oxygen needs for herself and her fetus. Anemia in pregnancy often results

G. Berardi
Fox Chase Cancer Center, Philadelphia, PA, USA
e-mail: Giuliana.Berardi@tuhs.temple.edu

I. R. Sosa (✉)
Department of Hematology/Oncology, Fox Chase Cancer Center, Philadelphia, PA, USA
e-mail: iberia.sosa@fccc.edu

© The Author(s), under exclusive license to Springer Nature
Switzerland AG 2024
G. Rivero, I. R. Sosa (eds.), *Consulting Hematology and Oncology Handbook*,
https://doi.org/10.1007/978-3-031-75810-2_21

297

from inherited or acquired abnormalities in hemoglobin production [2]. The most common acquired defects include physiologic anemia of pregnancy and the deficiency of iron stores but may also include bone marrow failure syndromes and autoimmune hemolytic anemia [2]. Physiologic anemia in pregnancy occurs due to increase in plasma volume when compared to erythrocyte mass [2].

Maternal and fetal outcomes vary according to the mother's hemoglobin and the trimester in which the anemia is identified [2]:

- First trimester (0–12 weeks): Hgb <11 g/dL.
- Second trimester (13–26 weeks): Hgb <10.5 g/dL.
- Third trimester (27–40 weeks): Hgb <11.
- Postpartum: Hgb < 10 g/dL.

The American College of Obstetricians and Gynecologists (ACOG) recommend that all pregnant women undergo screening for anemia in their first trimester regardless of their hematologic history with a serum Hgb or hematocrit (Hct) [2]. A second screening is recommended between 24–28 weeks of pregnancy. A maternal Hgb level indicative of anemia should prompt additional testing for likely etiologies. The evaluation should include laboratory assessment including a complete blood count to evaluate red blood cell (RBC) indices. Mean corpuscular volume is the average volume measurement of RBC and is often decreased in microcytic anemia such as inherited thalassemias or iron deficiency, which is the most common type of anemia in pregnancy [2].

Screening for iron deficiency is not routinely done. The United States Preventive Services Task Force (USPSTF) concluded there was insufficient evidence for routine screening of iron deficiency in the absence of clinical symptoms; however, some experts believe that screening is worthwhile in high-risk populations, such as those previously diagnosed with iron deficiency, diabetes, multiparous females with an interpregnancy interval of <6 months, vegetarians, or women with a low BMI [3, 4].

Notwithstanding physiologic anemia and iron deficiency anemia, other etiologies for anemia in pregnancy are less frequent. Table 21.1 summarizes inherited and acquired causes of anemia that should be considered in the appropriate clinical scenario in a pregnant female.

Clinical Manifestations

The clinical manifestations of anemia in pregnancy often overlap with common symptoms of pregnancy and mirror those of anemic, nonpregnant adults. The most common symptoms include the following [3]:

- Fatigue.
- Dyspnea.
- Pallor.
- Chest pain/arrhythmias.
- Dizziness/lightheadedness.

Table 21.1 Inherited and acquired causes of anemia

Microcytic (MCV < 80 fL)	Normocytic (MCV 80–100 fL)	Macrocytic (MCV > 100 fL)
Iron deficiency ACD[a]/inflammation Sideroblastic Thalassemia Hemolysis	Acute bleeding (not yet compensated) Hemolysis Early iron deficiency ACD/inflammation Anemia of renal disease Hypothyroidism Copper deficiency/zinc poisoning	Megaloblastic (vitamin B12 or folate deficiency) Liver disease Hypothyroidism HIV infection Medications that interfere with nuclear maturation (hydroxyurea, methotrexate) Myelodysplastic syndrome

[a]Anemia of chronic disease (ACD)

Table 21.2 Interpretation of the iron panel

	Iron deficiency	Thalassemia	Anemia of chronic disease
Iron saturation	Decreased	Normal	Normal/decreased
Ferritin	<30 ng/mL	Normal	>30 ng/mL—increased
Total iron binding capacity	Increased	Normal	Decreased
Mean corpuscular volume	Normal/microcytic	Microcytic	Normal/microcytic

- Pica.
- Headaches.

Laboratory Investigations

The laboratory evaluation for anemia will depend on the clinical history and RBC indices. In general, we consider physiologic anemia a diagnosis of exclusion. It is important to investigate for iron deficiency anemia, as it is the most common cause of non-physiologic anemia in pregnancy (Table 21.2) [2, 5].

In addition to a complete blood cell count, based on level of anemia and MCV, the provider should consider ordering a reticulocyte count, ferritin, serum iron, total iron binding capacity, B12, folate, and/or hemoglobinopathy panel. Additional studies may be necessary based on clinical history and RBC indices (Fig. 21.1).

Management

A 55 kg female is estimated to require 1 g of iron from conception to delivery to support the fetus, placenta, and estimated blood loss during labor and delivery [5]. ACOG recommends supplemental oral iron at 27–30 mg daily throughout pregnancy to compensate for the increase iron demands of pregnancy [2]. Despite these recommendations, high quality evidence is lacking to support that this practice improves health outcomes [6]. Standard treatment of iron deficiency is administration of iron at higher levels than found in prenatal vitamins [3].

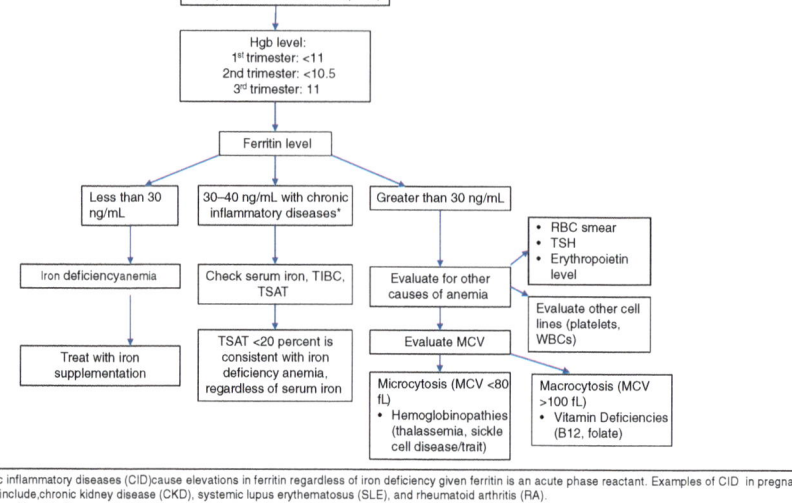

Fig. 21.1 Diagnostic algorithm for anemia in pregnancy

The choice to replace iron orally or intravenously depends on several factors, but both routes can be effective. In general, oral iron is the preferred choice for women treated in their first trimester and those who can tolerate the gastrointestinal side effects [7]. Parenteral infusions are not given during the first trimester but may be used after 13 weeks [7, 8]. It is the preferred mechanism for repletion for women in second and third trimester for whom there is insufficient time to replete iron orally (>30 weeks) and for those who experienced poor tolerance or inadequate response with oral repletion [8]. Different parenteral iron formulations are summarized in Table 17.14, Chap. 17.

Folic acid supplementation is routinely recommended in pregnancy to prevent neural tube defects, and recommended doses (Fig. 21.2) are sufficient to prevent maternal folate deficiency that contributes to megaloblastic anemia [2]. However, a woman may still be at risk for megaloblastic anemia through B12 deficiency if she is a strict vegetarian or has anatomic reasons for poor B12 absorption (Fig. 21.2).

Specific Considerations

- Differentiation of iron deficiency anemia of pregnancy and thalassemia can be difficult and can also coexist. If a pregnant patient still has microcytosis and anemia, despite adequate iron repletion, hemoglobinopathy workup is necessary. Thalassemia should be considered as a diagnosis and a hemoglobin electrophoresis, and possible alpha genotype may be necessary to make the diagnosis.

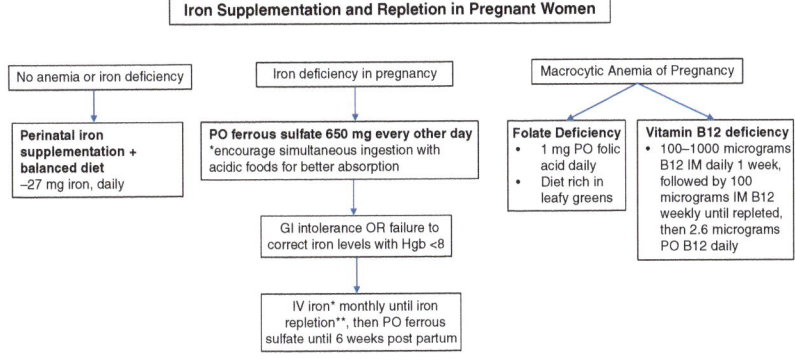

Fig. 21.2 Iron and vitamin repletion

Fig. 21.3 Modified
Ganzoni equation

> **Ganzoni Formula (modified):**
> Total iron deficit (mg) = weight in kg x (Target Hgb –
> Actual Hgb) x 2.4 + Iron
>
> Weight: utilize total weight of pregnant female
> Adjust target Hgb for trimester of pregnancy:
> - 1st trimester: >11 g/dL
> - 2nd trimester: >10.5 g/dL
> - 3rd trimester: >10 g/dL
>
> Iron : 500 mg

- Women with sickle cell disease (SCD) in pregnancy exhibit significant challenges and require a management plan to consider complications of SCD likely to be exacerbated by pregnancy: vaso-occlusive crises, acute chest syndrome, venous thromboembolism, infection, and strokes.
- Macrocytic anemia during pregnancy suggests megaloblastic anemia, particularly vitamin B12 and folate. Following correction of iron deficiency (Fig. 21.3), macrocytic anemia can become unmasked [7].
  - 400 μg/daily of folic acid is required during pregnancy.
  - 2.8 μg/daily of vitamin B12 is required daily for pregnant women.
  - Vitamin B12 deficiency can manifest as hemolytic anemia; thus, attention to hemolysis markers (elevated LDH, indirect bilirubin and/or reticulocyte count and low haptoglobin) and reviewing a RBC smear are imperative.
- Anemia associated with leukopenia or thrombocytopenia during pregnancy may suggest other processes, such as microangiopathic hemolytic anemia, autoimmune hemolytic anemia, or aplastic anemia [1].

- The pathophysiology of aplastic anemia (AA) in pregnancy is generally unknown although there is some speculation it may be triggered by hormonal changes in pregnancy creating an imbalance between erythropoietin and placental lactogen. Pancytopenia is typically accompanied by a hypocellular marrow. Termination of pregnancy is often recommended, and AA will resolve in one third of cases, but relapse is highly likely with subsequent pregnancies.
- Iron deficiency anemia in pregnancy may coexist with hereditary hemorrhagic telangiectasia (HHT). Pregnant women with HHT require IV iron supplementation given the significant iron depletion present, which is unlikely to be adequately replenished with oral supplementation [8, 9].

Thrombocytopenia During Pregnancy

Case

A 27-year-old G1P0 female presents to the hematology clinic after her second trimester evaluation with her OB-GYN. She is 28 weeks pregnant and expecting a baby girl. Her most recent complete blood count (CBC) reveals a platelet count of 101,000/μL and Hgb 11.2 g/dL. Comprehensive metabolic panel is unremarkable. She denies signs or symptoms of bleeding. She has no family history of bleeding or clotting disorders. Her vital signs and physical exam are unremarkable.

Clinical Context

Thrombocytopenia in pregnancy is defined as a platelet count $\leq 150,000$ mm^3 [10]. It is secondary to hemodilution and platelet consumption in placental and splenic tissues, which occurs naturally in pregnancy [10]. However, in most uncomplicated pregnancies, platelet counts usually remain within a normal range of 150,000 to 450,000/μL.

- Gestational thrombocytopenia, a benign self-limited condition, can occur as early as the first trimester but is more likely to manifest as the pregnancy progresses and is most frequently encountered at time of delivery [11].
- 70–80% of thrombocytopenia in pregnancy is gestational thrombocytopenia [10].
- Twin pregnancies are likely to have lower platelet counts compared to singleton pregnancies [10].
- The degree of thrombocytopenia is the most important factor to determine the pathology of thrombocytopenia and differential diagnosis.

Etiologies of Thrombocytopenia in Pregnancy

The differential diagnosis of thrombocytopenia can be broken down based on the *degree* of thrombocytopenia (Fig. 21.4).

Clinical Manifestations

Clinical presentation of different etiologies for thrombocytopenia in pregnancy are reviewed in Table 21.3.

Management

Management of different etiologies for thrombocytopenia in pregnancy are reviewed in Table 21.3.

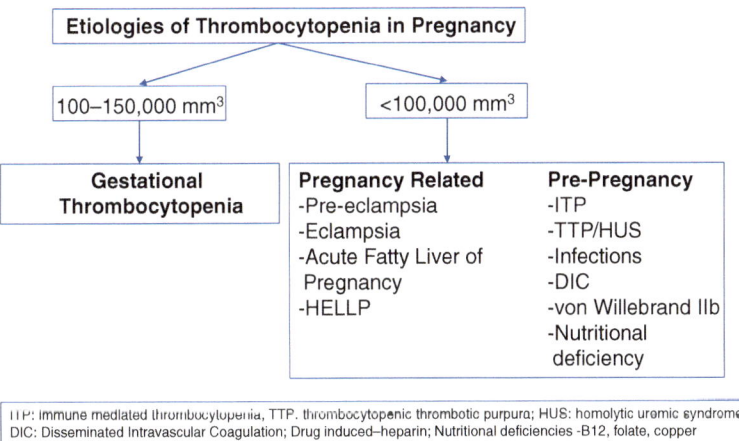

Fig. 21.4 Differential diagnosis of thrombocytopenia in pregnancy

Table 21.3 Clinical Presentation and Management of Thrombocytopenia in pregnancy

Type of thrombocytopenia	Clinical manifestations	Laboratory findings	Complications	Management
Gestational	• Asymptomatic • Common at delivery but can occur anytime	• Normal Hgb • Platelets 100–150,000 cells/μL	None	Monitoring
Preeclampsia	• Occurs in approximately 5% pregnancies • >20 weeks' gestation • New onset hypertension (>160/110) • Women may exhibit severe features such as headaches, visual symptoms, and pulmonary edema	• Platelets <100,000 cells/μL • >0.3 g protein in 24 h urine specimen or >0.3 mg/mg spot urine specimen or • >2+ protein urine dipstick • Cr > 1.1 or doubling of Cr in absence of other renal disease • In severe feature: Serum transaminase 2X ULN	• Disseminated intravascular coagulation (DIC) • Microangiopathic hemolytic anemia • Pre-term birth, oligohydramnios	Delivery
Eclampsia	Preeclampsia + generalized tonic-clonic seizures	As above	As above	Delivery
Acute fatty liver of pregnancy	• >28 weeks gestation • Normotension • Hypotension • Abdominal pain • Nausea • Vomiting • Anorexia	• Severe thrombocytopenia, ~20,000/μL • Hypoglycemia • Transaminitis • Elevated Cr • Hyperbilirubinemia • Leukocytosis • Coagulopathy • Low fibrinogen • Low haptoglobin	• DIC • Acute liver failure • Acute kidney injury • Fetal demise • Recurrence in subsequent pregnancies	• Delivery • Dexamethasone antepartum and postpartum • LCHAD[a] deficiency mutation testing (mother + child)

(continued)

Table 21.3 (continued)

Type of thrombocytopenia	Clinical manifestations	Laboratory findings	Complications	Management
HELLP (hemolysis, elevated liver enzymes, proteinuria)	• Between 28–36 weeks gestation • Hypertension • Proteinuria • Note: Although part of the name, proteinuria or hypertension don't need to occur to meet criteria for this diagnosis • Colicky abdominal pain • Nausea, vomiting, malaise	• Peripheral smear with schistocytes and burr cells • Serum bilirubin >1.2 mg/dL • Low serum haptoglobin • LDH ≥ 2X ULN • Anemia Hgb <8–10 g/dL, unrelated to blood loss • Transaminitis >2X ULN • Thrombocytopenia <100,000 cells/μL	• Bleeding (especially hepatic) • Placental abruption • Acute renal failure • Pre-term birth • Fetal demise	• Delivery • Dexamethasone if <34 weeks gestation • RBC transfusion for Hgb <7 • Plt transfusion if Plts <20,000/μL or plan for C section with platelets less than 40,000/μL
TTP/HUS (thrombotic thrombocytopenic purpura/hemolytic uremic syndrome)	Similar symptoms as nonpregnant adults, such as headache, vomiting, blurred vision, and altered mentation	• Schistocytes on RBC smear • Microangiopathic hemolytic anemia • Normal coagulation factors • Increased creatinine	• Thrombosis—(e.g., transient ischemic attack, pulmonary embolism) • Stillbirth	• PLEX • Regular plasma infusions are recommended for hereditary TTP • Aspirinwhen platelets >50,000 • [a]Delivery does not affect outcome • [a]Eculizumab for HUS • [a]PLEX required for subsequent pregnancies

(continued)

Table 21.3 (continued)

Type of thrombocytopenia	Clinical manifestations	Laboratory findings	Complications	Management
Von Willebrand disease type IIb	• Often diagnosed before pregnancy • Miscarriages prior to pregnancy	• Platelets ~<100,000 cells/μL (mean 20–30,000) • R1306W mutation	Postpartum hemorrhage	• Maintain factor VIII and vWF > 50 IU/dL • Factor VIII replacement • von Willebrand replacement • Tranexamic acid • Platelet transfusion when platelets <20,000
ITP (immune thrombocytopenic purpura)	Most common between 1–12 weeks of gestation Bleeding	• Diagnosis of exclusion • Thrombopoietin level testing *not* recommended	Neonatal thrombocytopenia	• Glucocorticoids • IVIG

[a]*LCHAD* Long-chain 3-hydroxyacyl-CoA dehydrogenase, *ULN* upper limit of normal, *IVIG* intravenous immunoglobulin, *PLEX* plasma exchange

Specific Considerations

- As with nonpregnant patients, it is always important to rule out pseudo-thrombocytopenia with a peripheral blood smear.
- Blood pressure can be informative in the differential diagnosis of thrombocytopenia in pregnancy.

  - Thrombocytopenia with hypertension is suggestive of preeclampsia, eclampsia, acute fatty liver of pregnancy, TTP/HUS, or HELLP.
  - Thrombocytopenia in a normotensive pregnant female suggests gestational thrombocytopenia, ITP, or VWD type IIb.
  - Hypotension may be seen with HELLP and acute fatty liver of pregnancy.

- TTP initially diagnosed in pregnancy may be congenital or acquired TTP. In both cases, you would expect to see a reduced ADAMTS13 activity; however, acquired is immune mediated. The presence of an antibody against ADAMTS13 indicates acquired TTP, whereas lack of an antibody suggests a diagnosis of congenital TTP [11].
- When a diagnosis of ITP is made or already established prior to pregnancy, platelet counts between 20–30,000 cells/microL are considered acceptable during pregnancy [12]. If the patient will require cesarean section or there are plans for neuroaxial anesthesia, platelet counts will need to be raised to 50,000 or 100,000, respectively [12]. The therapy should be initiated at least a week in advance if to allow time for maximal efficacy and time to retest platelet count.
- A woman with ITP who is breastfeeding may provoke a neonatal thrombocytopenia secondary to transfer of maternal IgG anti-glycoprotein antibodies. Cessation of breast feeding usually results in normalization of platelet counts in the neonate [13].
- Aside from physiologic causes of thrombocytopenia in pregnancy, women with von Willebrand Disease type IIb typically have worsening thrombocytopenia given the natural increase of vWF during pregnancy secondary to elevated estrogen levels [14]. Increased vWF causes increased platelet binding and sequestration, resulting in worsening thrombocytopenia. DDAVP should be *avoided* given it increases vWF levels further exacerbating platelet-vWF binding and clearance [10].
- In general, platelet transfusions are indicated when platelet counts are below 50,000 cells/microL prior to administration of epidural anesthesia or caesarean section due to the increased risk of bleeding [10].

VTE in Pregnancy

Case

A 35-year-old obese female, G3P3 presents to the clinic 4 weeks postpartum with increased left lower extremity pain and swelling. She reports that she has been home caring for her 4-week-old infant and has noticed progressive pain and swelling in her left leg. She reports no complications during the pregnancy and delivered a full-term child. She has no history of bleeding or clotting disorders and is not currently on contraception. Her vital signs are within normal limits. Her physical exam is notable for a slightly erythematous left calf that is painful to palpation behind the knee. No rashes or skin breakdown is noted.

Clinical Context

Venous thromboembolism (VTE) in pregnancy encompasses deep vein thrombosis (DVT) and pulmonary embolism (PE). VTE risk is increased in pregnancy secondary to normal physiologic changes that occur during pregnancy resulting in a larger plasma volume with increased venous stasis and pressure placed on veins, particularly pelvic veins due to a large, gravid uterus [15]. Moreover, pregnancy is associated with increased clotting factors (VII, VIII, X, von Willebrand factor), fibrinogen, and plasminogen activator inhibitor type 1 (PAI-1) levels, resulting in a prothrombotic state [16, 17]. These increased levels do not return to normal until after 8 weeks postpartum [17]. Hence, pregnant women are at risk of VTE during both antepartum and postpartum period.

- 1 in 1600 pregnant women will experience a VTE [16] . The risk of VTE during pregnancy is fourfold to fivefold greater in a pregnant woman than the general population and 20 times greater in the postpartum period [18].
- Factors that increase the risk of VTE in pregnancy include history of thrombosis, advanced maternal age (>35 years old), black race, medical comorbidities (e.g., obesity, anemia, autoimmune disorders, coronary artery disease, hypertension, cigarette smoke), and pregnancy complications (e.g., cesarean section, multiple gestations, postpartum hemorrhage/infection, and hyperemesis [18, 19]).
- The most common locations for DVT include left lower extremity and pelvic vein. DVTs account for ~80% of all VTE events in pregnant woman [18]. This is secondary to compression of the left iliac vein by the right iliac artery, which is further exacerbated by a gravid uterus. PE accounts for ~20% of VTE events [18].

Clinical Manifestations

Symptoms of VTE are the same as in a nonpregnant woman. It is important to note that symptoms can often be masked by normal pregnancy [19, 20].

Typical clinical presentation of:

- *DVT:* lower extremity swelling, pain, and erythema.
- *PE:* dyspnea, palpitations, and pleuritic chest pain.

Laboratory Investigations

Laboratory testing, such as basic metabolic panel (BMP), CBC, troponin, and brain natriuretic peptide (BNP), is typically not useful. A D-dimer can be useful if not elevated (DDimer <500 ng/mL rules out a VTE); however, D-Dimer values typically increase during pregnancy and do not return to normal until the postpartum period [19–21]. Variations in D-Dimer levels during trimester of pregnancy have not been well established [19–21], and therefore, this is not a useful strategy to risk stratify pregnant females. Thus, imaging modalities are preferred when there is clinical suspicion for VTE [19, 20].

Management

Common risk scores, such as Wells Score and Revised Geneva Score, have not been found to be useful in assessing risk in pregnant women [21, 22]. LEFt clinical prediction rule (Table 21.4) is predictive in cross-sectional studies, but has not been prospectively validated; thus, it needs to be utilized in combination with imaging (Fig. 21.5) [23].

Anticoagulation is sometimes necessary during pregnancy (Fig. 21.6). Major evidence guidelines recommend the use of low molecular weight heparin (LMWH) as the preferred anticoagulant (Table 21.5) [24]. Like unfractionated heparin (UFH), it does not cross the placenta and it carries a lower risk of osteoporosis and heparin-induced thrombocytopenia. The use of nonpreferred anticoagulants requires special consideration of risk/benefit to mother and fetus.

Specific Considerations

- Pregnant women with an inherited thrombophilia are at the greatest risk for VTE during pregnancy. These women may require prophylactic anticoagulation during antepartum and/or postpartum period despite not having a personal history of VTE. These populations include the following [24, 28]:

  - For women who are homozygous for the factor V Leiden mutation or who have combined thrombophilias, regardless of family history of VTE, expert guidelines *suggest* antepartum antithrombotic prophylaxis to prevent a first VTE.

Table 21.4 LEFt clinical
prediction rule criteria

LEFt clinical prediction rule criteria
Symptoms in left leg (left)
Calf circumference >2 cm (edema)
First trimester presentation (first)

Among patients presenting with 0, 1, or 2–3 variables, DVT
was diagnosed at 0, 16, and 58% of the time, respectively

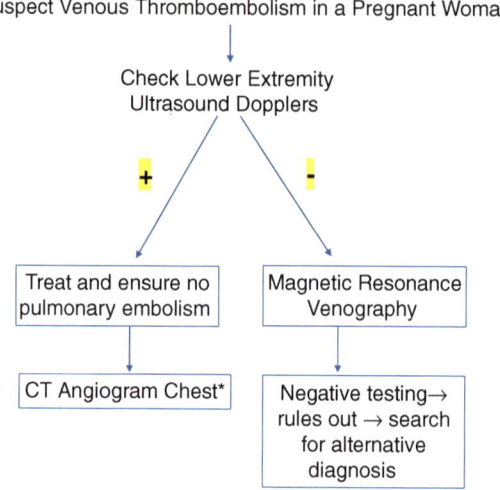

*Risk of untreated pulmonary embolism is greater than risk of radiation exposure to fetus.

Fig. 21.5 Recommended imaging for pregnant female with suspected VTE

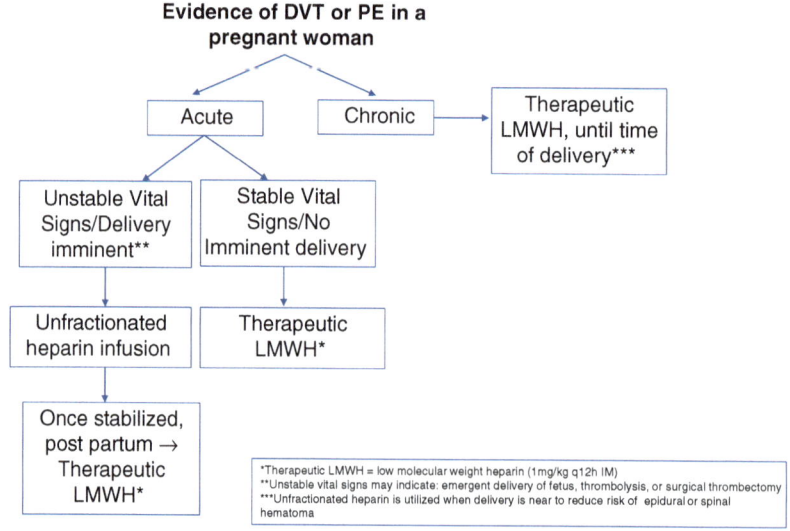

Fig. 21.6 Approach to anticoagulation for pregnant female with VTE

Table 21.5 Anticoagulation in pregnancy

Anticoagulant	Crosses the placenta	Contraindicated	Uses in pregnancy
Unfractionated heparin	–	–	VTE/thrombosis prophylaxis
Low molecular weight heparin	–	–	VTE/thrombosis prophylaxis
Fondaparinux	+/–	–	Treatment of VTE when heparin products unable to be utilized[a]
Warfarin[b]	+	+	None
Direct oral anticoagulants (DOACs)[c]	+	+	None

[a]Fondaparinux can be utilized if a pregnant mother develops heparin-induced thrombocytopenia (HIT) following exposure to heparin products [25, 26]
[b]Warfarin is not recommended in pregnancy because it can cause birth defects and bleeding problems in the baby, owing to its ability to cross the placenta. Exposure during first trimester is especially not recommended. Patients with mechanical heart valves may require continuation of warfarin use because the risk of valve clotting is higher than risk to the baby
[c]Data on DOACSs use in pregnant women is insufficient with some evidence suggesting increased risk of miscarriage; thus, their use is not recommended [27]

- For women with antithrombin III deficiency, it is suggested that if there is a family history of VTE, antepartum prophylaxis should be utilized to reduce risk of first VTE.
- For women with protein C or protein S deficiency, who have a family history of VTE, experts recommend postpartum antithrombotic prophylaxis to prevent a first VTE.

- Antiphospholipid syndrome is associated with high-risk morbidity and mortality in pregnancy. While the most frequent complication is recurrent pregnancy loss, VTE and preterm labor are also highly likely. These patients should be referred to maternal fetal medicine and specialized hematologist.
- Pregnant women with thrombophilia or VTE on therapeutic anticoagulation will need to hold anticoagulation prior to delivery. Bleeding in the epidural space or spinal canal may compress spinal cord and lead to paralysis; hence, anesthesiologists generally wait 6 h after UFH, 12 h after low-dose LMWH, and 24 h after full-dose LMWH, before placement of epidural or spinal anesthetic. Anticoagulation is usually not resumed until 12 h after vaginal delivery, 12 h after spinal or epidural anesthesia, and 24 h after cesarean section given increased risk of bleeding [28].
- Warfarin is generally contraindicated in the antepartum period [29]. However, warfarin can be resumed postpartum and is not contraindicated in breastfeeding mothers given it is not lipophilic [29].

References

1. Stanley AY, Wallace JB, Hernandez AM, Spell JL. Anemia in pregnancy: screening and clinical management strategies. MCN Am J Matern Child Nurs. 2022;47(1):25–32.
2. American College of O, Gynecologists' Committee on Practice B-O. Anemia in pregnancy: ACOG practice bulletin, number 233. Obstet Gynecol. 2021;138(2):e55–64.
3. Auerbach M. Commentary: iron deficiency of pregnancy—a new approach involving intravenous iron. Reprod Health. 2018;15(Suppl 1):96.
4. Siu AL, Force USPST. Screening for iron deficiency anemia and iron supplementation in pregnant women to improve maternal health and birth outcomes: U.S. Preventive Services Task Force recommendation statement. Ann Intern Med. 2015;163(7):529–36.
5. Bothwell TH. Iron requirements in pregnancy and strategies to meet them. Am J Clin Nutr. 2000;72(1 Suppl):257S–64S.
6. Cantor AG, Bougatsos C, Dana T, Blazina I, McDonagh M. Routine iron supplementation and screening for iron deficiency anemia in pregnancy: a systematic review for the U.S. Preventive Services Task Force. Ann Intern Med. 2015;162(8):566–76.
7. Achebe MM, Gafter-Gvili A. How I treat anemia in pregnancy: iron, cobalamin, and folate. Blood. 2017;129(8):940–9.
8. Grzeskowiak LE, Qassim A, Jeffries B, Grivell RM. Approaches for optimising intravenous iron dosing in pregnancy: a retrospective cohort study. Intern Med J. 2017;47(7):747–53.
9. Faughnan ME, Mager JJ, Hetts SW, Palda VA, Lang-Robertson K, Buscarini E, Deslandres E, Kasthuri RS, Lausman A, Poetker D, et al. Second international guidelines for the diagnosis and management of hereditary hemorrhagic telangiectasia. Ann Intern Med. 2020;173(12):989–1001.
10. Ciobanu AM, Colibaba S, Cimpoca B, Peltecu G, Panaitescu AM. Thrombocytopenia in pregnancy. Maedica (Bucur). 2016;11(1):55–60.
11. Reese JA, Peck JD, Deschamps DR, McIntosh JJ, Knudtson EJ, Terrell DR, Vesely SK, George JN. Platelet counts during pregnancy. N Engl J Med. 2018;379(1):32–43.
12. Scully M. Thrombotic thrombocytopenic purpura and atypical hemolytic uremic syndrome microangiopathy in pregnancy. Semin Thromb Hemost. 2016;42(7):774–9.
13. Poston JN, Gernsheimer TB. Management of immune thrombocytopenia in pregnancy. Ann Blood. 2021;6:5–5.
14. Castaman G, James PD. Pregnancy and delivery in women with von Willebrand disease. Eur J Haematol. 2019;103(2):73–9.
15. Goodrich SM, Wood JE. Peripheral venous distensibility and velocity of venous blood flow during pregnancy or during oral contraceptive therapy. Am J Obstet Gynecol. 1964;90:740–4.
16. Marik PE, Plante LA. Venous thromboembolic disease and pregnancy. N Engl J Med. 2008;359(19):2025–33.
17. Bremme KA. Haemostatic changes in pregnancy. Best Pract Res Clin Haematol. 2003;16(2):153–68.
18. James AH, Jamison MG, Brancazio LR, Myers ER. Venous thromboembolism during pregnancy and the postpartum period: incidence, risk factors, and mortality. Am J Obstet Gynecol. 2006;194(5):1311–5.
19. James AH, Tapson VF, Goldhaber SZ. Thrombosis during pregnancy and the postpartum period. Am J Obstet Gynecol. 2005;193(1):216–9.
20. Macklon NS, Greer IA. Venous thromboembolic disease in obstetrics and gynaecology: the Scottish experience. Scott Med J. 1996;41(3):83–6.
21. Touhami O, Marzouk SB, Bennasr L, Touaibia M, Souli I, Felfel MA, Kehila M, Channoufi MB, Magherbi HE. Are the Wells score and the revised Geneva score valuable for the diagnosis of pulmonary embolism in pregnancy? Eur J Obstet Gynecol Reprod Biol. 2018;221:166–71.
22. Lameijer H, Aalberts JJJ, van Veldhuisen DJ, Meijer K, Pieper PG. Efficacy and safety of direct oral anticoagulants during pregnancy; a systematic literature review. Thromb Res. 2018;169:123–7.

23. Chan WS, Lee A, Spencer FA, Crowther M, Rodger M, Ramsay T, Ginsberg JS. Predicting deep venous thrombosis in pregnancy: out in "LEFt" field? Ann Intern Med. 2009;151(2):85–92.
24. Bates SM, Rajasekhar A, Middeldorp S, McLintock C, Rodger MA, James AH, Vazquez SR, Greer IA, Riva JJ, Bhatt M, et al. American Society of Hematology 2018 guidelines for management of venous thromboembolism: venous thromboembolism in the context of pregnancy. Blood Adv. 2018;2(22):3317–59.
25. Dempfle CE. Minor transplacental passage of fondaparinux in vivo. N Engl J Med. 2004;350(18):1914–5.
26. Mazzolai L, Hohlfeld P, Spertini F, Hayoz D, Schapira M, Duchosal MA. Fondaparinux is a safe alternative in case of heparin intolerance during pregnancy. Blood. 2006;108(5):1569–70.
27. McKenna R, Cole ER, Vasan U. Is warfarin sodium contraindicated in the lactating mother? J Pediatr. 1983;103(2):325–7.
28. James AH. Venous thromboembolism in pregnancy. Arterioscler Thromb Vasc Biol. 2009;29(3):326–31.
29. Kline JA, Williams GW, Hernandez-Nino J. D-dimer concentrations in normal pregnancy: new diagnostic thresholds are needed. Clin Chem. 2005;51(5):825–9.

Index